Recent Results in Cancer Research 61

Fortschritte der Krebsforschung
Progrès dans les recherches sur le cancer

D. Metcalf

Hemopoietic Colonies

In Vitro Cloning of Normal and Leukemic Cells

With 54 Figures and 28 Tables

Springer-Verlag
Berlin Heidelberg New York 1977

Donald Metcalf, M.D., F.A.A.
Head, Cancer Research Unit,
Walter and Eliza Hall Institute of Medical Research,
Melbourne, Australia

Sponsored by the Swiss League against Cancer

ISBN 3-540-08232-8 Springer-Verlag Berlin Heidelberg New York
ISBN 0-387-08232-8 Springer-Verlag New York Heidelberg Berlin

Printed in Germany.

Typesetting: William Clowes & Sons Limited, London, Beccles and Colchester/England
Printing and binding: Konrad Triltsch, Graphischer Betrieb, 87 Würzburg, Germany
2125/3140-543210

To Ray Bradley

for his generosity in sharing his first colonies

Preface

The cloning of hemopoietic cells in semisolid medium began some 12 years ago, and when colonies of T= and B=lymphocytes were grown by several groups last year, the last major subclasses of hemopoietic cells had been successfully cultured in vitro.

The time seemed appropriate to write a short general account of this exciting new area of hematology, emphasizing particularly the potential value of these new techniques for direct studies on patients with leukemia and allied diseases.

I had hoped to refer to, or at least record, every paper published in this field, but the literature proved to be larger than I had realized, and furthermore, some areas were so active that chapters had to be rewritten over a period of less than a year.

I regret that what follows is an incomplete account and no doubt, by the time this book becomes available, the material will be even more out of date. However, I have described the basic techniques in some detail and have tried, where possible, to explain how and why the techniques can fail.

It is already possible to see patterns, perhaps even principles, emerging from this work which may well be applicable to other cell populations. These have been emphasized in the text in an attempt to make this review as creative as possible.

Like many biological techniques, semisolid cultures often fail at the worst possible times, and on such occasions life can be very frustrating. However, my colony colleagues around the world are a hardy, persistent lot not easily put down by adversity. The information they have amassed in the last decade is summarized in the pages to follow and, I think, reflects credit on their enterprise and industry.

Melbourne, November 1976

DONALD METCALF

Table of Contents

Chapter 1

Historical Introduction

Why attempt to clone hemopoietic cells in semisolid medium in vitro? As a general explanation, it can be said that the various hemopoietic populations are so inextricably intermixed and their regulatory systems so complex that analysis of hemopoiesis cannot be performed on intact animals. Furthermore, for the analysis of these populations in humans, the ability to manipulate the populations in vivo is essentially nonexistent for practical and ethical reasons.

While these considerations make it clear that hemopoietic populations must ultimately be analysed in vitro, why not use conventional liquid culture systems? Liquid culture systems certainly have many uses in hematology, but such systems are essentially "black boxes"—cell input and output can be monitored, but intermediate events are difficult and often impossible to follow. Furthermore, events cannot be related to individual cells.

The ability to grow clones of hemopoietic cells in semisolid medium permits an analysis of the proliferative and functional activity of individual cells and their progeny. How many progeny can one cell generate and are all cells similar in their capacity to proliferate and differentiate? Do they respond in an identical manner to specific regulatory factors? It will be seen in the account to follow that heterogeneity is in fact the characteristic of even apparently homogeneous hemopoietic cell populations and to recognize and measure this, it is essential that cellular proliferation can be followed on a clonal basis.

As will be discussed in the following chapters, one of the early disappointments in this field was the fact that colonies generated by leukemic cells are usually not distinguishable by shape or appearance from normal colonies. However, this is not universally true, and in some situations normal and leukemic cells produce distinctive colonies readily distinguishable in the same culture dish. In measuring the proliferation of normal versus leukemic cells in such a mixed population, the advantages of a cloning system become obvious.

The techniques for cloning hemopoietic cells in semisolid medium evolved from observations of tumor virologists on the growth in agar of normal and viral-transformed fibroblasts. In this work it was shown that transformed fibroblasts, unlike normal cells, were able to proliferate in the semisolid medium and form colonies of cells (see review by MACPHERSON, 1). Since the colonies were derived from single cells, i.e., the colonies were clones, this phenomenon offered a number of exciting possibilities to the experimental hematologist. With the use of semisolid medium it might be possible to work with cloned populations of leukemic cells and at the same time have a useful method for discriminating leukemic from normal cells. Indeed, it was shown that cells from tissue culture-adapted human lymphocyte cell lines (now known to be transformed by the Epstein-Barr virus) could be cultured in agar medium and could generate colonies of cells which proved of value in analyzing the clonal production of immunoglobulins [2].

Attempts to obtain clonal growth in agar of mouse leukemic cells were made simultaneously and independently by PLUZNIK and SACHS in Rehovot, using Rauscher virus-induced erythroleukemic cells, and by BRADLEY and METCALF in Melbourne, using AKR lymphoid leukemic cells. In both cases these initial attempts failed to obtain colony formation by leukemic cells. In an attempt to achieve success with the growth of the lymphoid leukemic cells, the concepts of PUCK and his co-workers [3] were applied and the value investigated of using feeder layers of various cells, including spleen and bone marrow cells, in the culture system. Colony formation was obtained, but analysis of the system eventually showed that the colonies developing in the agar cultures were composed of neutrophilic granulocytes and/or macrophages and that the colonies were in fact derived from the normal hemopoietic cells included as feeder layers in the cultures [4]. In the cultures of erythroleukemic spleens, those colonies which did develop were similarly identified as normal neutrophilic and macrophage colonies [5] and the role of the spleen cells in supplying a necessary growth factor recognized.

Because the macrophages in these colonies actively phagocytose the metachromatic agar in the surrounding medium, these cells usually contain large amounts of metachromatic granular material. At the time of these early experiments, surface markers were not available for identifying hemopoietic subpopulations, and both groups experienced difficulty in excluding the possibility that the colonies of mononuclear cells were in fact mast cells. Indeed, the initial descriptions of these colonies by the Rehovot group referred to them as colonies of "mast" cells or "mast cell-like" cells [6, 7]. Because of these initial problems, subsequent workers in this field have been reluctant to identify metachromatic cells in colonies as mast cells, and despite the wide variety of culture systems subsequently developed, no descriptions of mast cell colonies have yet been made. It remains uncertain whether any of these techniques have succeeded so far in growing genuine mast cell colonies. However, as will be seen later, a typical culture of normal marrow contains a fascinating variety of colonies, and it is quite possible that mast-cell colonies are present in some of these cultures but have yet to be identified.

With the demonstration that clones of at least two hemopoietic subpopulations could be grown in semisolid agar from normal hemopoietic tissues, many workers became alerted to the possibility that other types of hemopoietic cells might similarly be able to be cloned in agar or comparable semisolid medium. However, from an analysis of the granulocyte-macrophage colony system, it became clear that cell proliferation was dependent on inclusion in the culture medium of a specific growth-stimulating factor (GM-colony-stimulating factor, GM-CSF) to stimulate the proliferation of this pair of related cell populations. Extrapolating from this information, it seemed likely that to obtain successful colony growth of other hemopoietic populations it would be necessary to include in the medium the corresponding regulators for the other cell types.

In an elegant series of experiments, AXELRAD and his colleagues [8, 9] modified the agar culture system, and using the specific erythropoietic regulator erythropoietin, demonstrated that erythropoietic colony formation could be obtained in semisolid plasma gel cultures. Subsequent work with this system has succeeded in growing erythroleukemic cells and indeed in obtaining rapid viral transformation in vitro of cloned erythropoietic cells [10, 11].

As no corresponding regulators were known for other hemopoietic cells, progress in cloning these other types of hemopoietic cells was dependent on chance observations. The agar culture technique for granulocytic and macrophage colonies was adapted by PIKE and ROBINSON [12] to permit the formation of similar colonies by human cells. In this system, underlayers of peripheral blood cells were used to supply the specific regulator, GM-CSF, to the target overlayer cells. Other workers modified the technique further by substituting methylcellulose for agar. In this latter system, it was noted by CHERVENICK and BOGGS [13] that some of the colonies developing were composed not of neutrophilic granulocytes or macrophages but of eosinophils. However, the complexity of peripheral blood underlayers with their mixed populations of cells has so far not permitted further analysis of this particular system.

Based on the principles emerging from the analysis of colony formation by normal mouse granulopoietic and macrophage-forming cells, systems were developed for cloning mouse myeloid leukemic and myelomonocytic leukemic cells in vitro [14, 15, 16]. In work with the latter system, it was noted that these myelomonocytic leukemic cells had the unique ability to stimulate normal marrow cells to form unusual colonies composed of loosely dispersed cells. The significance of this type of colony was not appreciated at the time.

Most of the evidence then available suggested that monocytes and macrophages were an important, perhaps the only, source of GM-CSF. However, studies by McNeill [17] and Parker and Metcalf [18] showed that mitogen-stimulated lymphocytes were also a very rich source of GM-CSF. In the studies of Parker and Metcalf, it was noted that if the lymphocytes had been stimulated by pokeweed mitogen, the conditioned media also had the capacity to stimulate the same loose colonies as were noted previously in cultures stimulated by mouse myelomonocytic leukemic cells. The cells in these loose colonies were eventually identified as eosinophils, and it was shown that the active factor required for their stimulation (EO-CSF) was antigenically different and chemically separable from the GM-CSF stimulating the formation of colonies of neutrophils and macrophages [19]. More potent lymphocyte-conditioned media were subsequently obtained by the addition of 2-mercaptoethanol to the cultures. It was shown by Metcalf and co-workers that highly active conditioned media of this type also were able to stimulate the formation of small colonies of very large cells which were identified as megakaryocytes [20].

During this developmental period, virtually everyone working in the field at some stage had attempted to grow colonies of normal lymphocytes in semisolid medium. These attempts were uniformly unsuccessful, and it was obvious that lymphocytes rapidly died after initiation of the cultures. Although achievement of the clonal growth of lymphocytes remained a "Holy Grail" of experimental hematologists, the problem was shelved temporarily as being too frustrating.

In work on the culture of granulocytic and macrophage colonies using unfractionated mouse peripheral blood, it was accidentally observed that if pleural cavity cells were mixed with the whole blood, colonies of normal fibroblasts developed in the culture medium [21]. Similar colonies could be grown from other hemopoietic populations. Parallel work in liquid cultures resulted in the demonstration that marrow and spleen stromal cells can form similar fibroblast-like colonies [22], and as shall be discussed later, these currently hold great promise as possibly being clones of cells producing specific hemopoietic regulators.

The agar culture system using whole blood supplements was used to study the fibroblast stromal cells in various mouse tumours with an unanticipated result. Some of the transplanted tumours used were mineral oil-induced plasmacytomas, and in cultures enriched by whole blood, it became obvious that plasmacytoma cells were also able to form colonies [23]. Use of supplemental whole blood or red cells in fact permits the clonal growth in agar of most mouse plasmacytoma cells—a cell type which had previously resisted culture attempts in semisolid medium unless first adapted to liquid cultures. At this time, it had recently been shown that addition of 2-mercaptoethanol to liquid cultures of lymphocytes and antibody-forming cells enhanced the proliferation of these cells [24, 25]. Tests on the effects of 2-mercaptoethanol in agar cultures of plasmacytoma cells similarly showed that colony formation by these neoplastic B-lymphocytes was often strikingly enhanced [26].

In retrospect, it is obvious that 2-mercaptoethanol should have been tested immediately in conventional agar cultures of normal mouse lymphoid cells, but the known inability of normal lymphocytes to survive in agar was a mental stumbling block which made such attempts apparently pointless. Eventually 2-mercaptoethanol was used by Metcalf and co-workers in cultures of normal mouse lymphoid cells for other reasons and proved spectacularly successful in permitting the clonal growth of normal B-lymphocyte colonies [27, 28] T-lymphocytes initially proved resistant to culture in single-step agar cultures, but as shall be described later, preliminary culture of lymphocytes in liquid culture with various T-lymphocyte mitogens permits colonies of T-lymphocytes to proliferate in agar [29]. Subsequent improvements in the culture medium now permit the single-step culture of T-lymphocytes (CLAESSON, M., unpublished data).

From this brief historical review, it will be apparent that cloning techniques are now available for all major hemopoietic subpopulations with the exception of hemopoietic stem cells. Efforts are now being made with the aid of these powerful tools to unravel the complexities of the interrelationships between hemopoietic subpopulations and the mechanisms controlling proliferation and differentiation both in normal and neoplastic hemopoietic cells.

At present, the technology for the culture of hemopoietic cells appears to be far in advance of the capacity to grow or clone *functionally active* cells from other tissues. If progress is to be made in understanding the proliferation and differentiation of cells from other tissues, these cells will eventually have to be grown and analyzed in comparable cloning systems. For biologists, it is instructive to consider whether any general principles have emerged from the development of cloning methods for hemopoietic cells which might be used to accelerate the development of comparable technology for other tissue cells. This question will be returned to in Chapter 14, but here it is worth making one further comment. The whole of the period for developing in vitro cloning techniques for hemopoietic cells occupied only 10 years, but progress was erratic, could rarely be planned, and most advances in fact were made accidentally. Nevertheless, the time intervals between the successful culture of each subpopulation progressively shortened (1965, granulocytes and macrophages; 1971, erythropoietic cells; 1972–1974, eosinophils; 1975, megakaryocytes; 1975, B-lymphocytes, T-lymphocytes). Faced with an almost complete lack of information on how to make high efficiency, primary cultures of, for example, functionally active pancreas or kidney cells, this accelerated rate of discovery of hemopoietic cloning methods is a hopeful sign.

The hardware of tissue culture—powdered media, disposable plastic culture vessels, filtration systems, sterilizers, incubators, and laminar flow work stations—have improved greatly in recent years, and it is now possible for most cell biologists to contemplate tissue culture approaches to their problems. It will become clear from the discussion to follow that many principles have emerged from the cloning work on normal and neoplastic hemopoietic cells which probably are generally applicable to other cell systems. The application of these principles can be expected to accelerate progress in understanding these other cell systems.

Analysis has shown that the various hemopoietic cloning systems have unusually high plating efficiencies and that quantitation of hemopoietic cells is both quick and relatively easy using these methods. What has emerged as an unexpected bonus from this work is the fact that these semisolid culture systems are particularly suitable for detecting and analyzing specific regulatory factors. The consequences of these properties of the cloning systems are that the analysis of normal and abnormal hemopoiesis has been revolutionized by the introduction of cloning methods.

It is the purpose of this monograph to describe the various semisolid culture techniques, to review the information produced by those techniques concerning normal and leukemic hemopoiesis, and to assess what problems might be soluble by further applications of in vitro cloning methods.

Chapter 2

An Outline of Hemopoiesis and Current Terminology

It is not within the scope of this monograph to deal with all aspects of hemopoiesis and the reader is referred to the book by METCALF and MOORE [30] for a more extensive discussion of the origin, development, and interrelationships between hemopoietic populations. However, to understand the implications of the results obtained with the in vitro cloning systems, it is necessary at this point to make a brief description of hemopoietic populations and introduce a number of terms to be used in the following chapters. In the interests of simplicity, the description to follow will not be annotated either by detailed evidence or source references.

A. Hemopoiesis

Because mature blood cells (red cells, polymorphs, monocytes, macrophages, eosinophils, platelets, and lymphocytes) have finite life spans, maintenance of stable levels of these cells in the circulation and tissues requires continuous cell production throughout adult life. The necessary cellular proliferation is broadly similar to that which was necessary in embryonic development to form the fully cellular hemopoietic organs from primitive anlagen.

The specific cell populations which proliferate and generate the mature blood cells are best described as consisting of three pyramidal-shaped compartments, or hierarchies, of cells (Fig. 1). The most ancestral cells are multipotential hemopoietic stem cells (stem cell compartment) which are capable not only of extensive self-replication (to form the stem cell compartment itself) but also of generating the various progenitor cells (progenitor cell compartment). Progenitor cells are possibly capable of a limited degree of self-replication but differ from stem cells in that their genomes are derepressed into one or other specific pathway of hemopoiesis, e.g., erythropoiesis or neutrophil-monocyte formation. Proliferation of progenitor cells leads to the formation of cells which for the first time are morphologically identifiable as belonging to specific hemopoietic populations, e.g., proerythroblasts, myeloblasts, etc. (morphologically identifiable compartment). Proliferation of these cells leads to the production of an expanded population of mature cells which appear in the peripheral blood and most of which not only are incapable of further proliferation but have relatively short life spans.

These various hemopoietic populations are located in the same organs except for the more mature lymphoid populations. Thus, in the normal adult, these populations are mainly located in the bone marrow with smaller numbers in the spleen and occasional cells of the first and second compartments being present also in the peripheral blood. In the developing embryo, hemopoietic populations appear first in the yolk sac and after migration into the embryo, are localized first in the liver, then subsequently populate the developing spleen and bone marrow.

The lymphoid populations require additional comment. Although lymphocytes arise from hemopoietic stem cells as do all other hemopoietic cells, two distinct populations of lymphoid

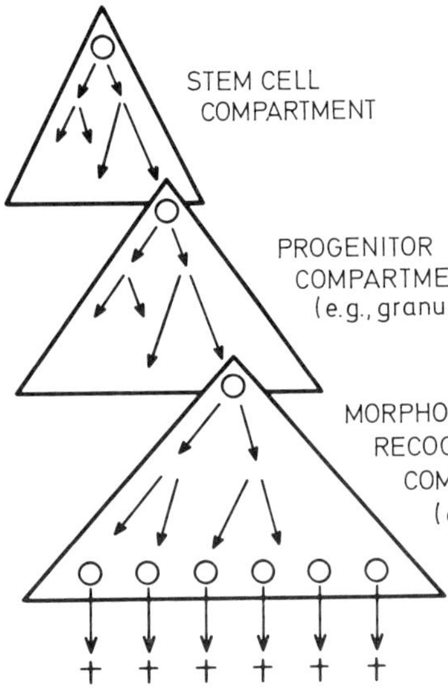

Fig. 1. Schematic representation of the three-tiered structure of hemopoietic populations

cells emerge—one generated mainly in the bone marrow (B-lymphocytes) and the other in the thymus (T-lymphocytes). Cells from the lymphoid progenitor cell compartment onward are located in these organs and also in the specialized lymphoid organs—the lymph nodes, Peyer's patches, tonsils, appendix, and spleen lymphoid follicles.

The important features of this three-tiered structure of hemopoiesis are: (1) the extensive capacity for proliferation and amplification within each compartment, (2) the progressive specialization from one compartment to the next, (3) the inability of cells to move from a mature compartment to a less mature compartment, e.g., of progenitor cells to revert to stem cells, (4) the inability of cells to move from one compartment to a compartment of corresponding maturation in another lineage, e.g., from the granulocyte progenitor cell compartment to the erythropoietic progenitor cell compartment, and (5) the progressive restriction in the final number of progeny able to be generated by cells in succeeding compartments.

As might be anticipated from this description, stem and progenitor cells are relatively infrequent in hemopoietic populations. For example, one cell in 1000 mouse marrow cells is a multipotential stem cell and one cell in 3–400 a granulocytic progenitor cell. Furthermore, members of the various hemopoietic compartments are mixed together in hemopoietic populations. In fact, hemopoietic populations exhibit no stratified architectural pattern (unlike organs such as the skin or testis) which would allow the most ancestral cells to be deduced and identified from their location in the tissue. Finally, stem and progenitor cells are relatively inconspicuous mononuclear cells with no morphological features allowing their certain identification. It follows from these considerations that selective assays are required to detect and enumerate the early members of these various hemopoietic subpopulations.

Hemopoietic stem cells can be identified in the mouse by their ability to generate colonies of cells in the spleen of syngeneic irradiated recipients [31], a property responsible for the other name for these cells—spleen colony-forming cells or units (CFU or CFU-S). No corresponding assays for stem cells exist in other animals or man although their proliferative potential in these species can be deduced indirectly from their capacity to repopulate the hemopoietic tissues of irradiated recipients or recipients depleted of hemopoietic populations for other reasons.

Progenitor cells can be detected and enumerated by their capacity to form colonies in the various in vitro cloning systems to be discussed shortly. These studies have given rise to a somewhat confusing variety of names and abbreviations for progenitor cells, e.g., colony-forming cells (CFC), CFC agar (CFA-A), CFC culture, CFU-C etc.

Morphologically recognizable cells and their progeny can be identified by classical morphological methods which can now be supplemented by sequential studies on pulse-labeled populations. The special names for the various cells within each hemopoietic family (e.g., myeloblasts, myelocytes, metamyelocytes, polymorphs) can be obtained from any standard hematological textbook.

The yolk sac is the only location in which hemopoietic stem cells are generated de novo. Following migration of these cells into the embryo, the supply of stem cells throughout life is maintained by the capacity of these initial cells for extensive self-replication (30). So extensive is this capacity that there are no situations in which stem cell supplies appear to fail, and there are no proven examples in late embryonic or adult life in which new hemopoietic stem cells are generated from other cells. Most stem cells remain quiescent in a non-cycling state throughout life, and there is evidence to suggest that hemopoiesis is maintained by the sequential activation, expansion, and eventual exhaustion of limited numbers of these stem cells.

Within the morphologically-recognizable compartment there is a sequence through which cells pass, e.g., myeloblasts to myelocyte to metamyelocyte to polymorphs, each population being larger in size than the preceding. However, within the stem and progenitor cell compartment, the exact situation is unknown. Cells entering these compartments and proliferating can be assumed to generate increasing numbers of progeny, but the manner in which they leave the compartment is not known. Conceivably, any cell within one of these compartments might be capable on a purely random basis of undergoing selective genetic derepression or activation and entering a succeeding compartment. Alternatively, as is the case in the morphologically recognizable compartment, a specific sequence of events may be associated with or determine exit from the compartment, e.g., the number of preceding divisions the cell has undergone.

Two facts have been established about cells in the stem and progenitor cell compartments: (1) commitment of multipotential stem cells to a specific pathway of differentiation, e.g., the stem cell to progenitor cell sequence is under control of what appear to be "microenvironmental" factors, and (2) proliferation of progenitor cells and their progeny in the succeeding morphologically recognizable compartment is mainly under control of specific humoral factors, e.g., erythropoietin, GM-CSF, etc.

The existence of local or microenvironmental regulatory factors can be deduced from the restricted localization of hemopoietic tissues in the body; from the segregation of hemopoietic populations in the spleen, and from the initial relatively pure populations of hemopoietic cells in spleen colonies generated by CFUs in the spleen. While most agree that commitment of stem cells to one or other type of progenitor cells is a stochastic event, opinions differ on the likely mechanism. Some favor the concept of fixed cellular niches in the hemopoietic tissue with stromal cells or microenvironmental cells forming such niches and functionally differing from cells forming adjacent niches. Random entry of stem cells into an erythropoietic niche would result not only in continuing self-generation on the part of the stem cell but in the transformation of some of the progeny to erythropoietic progenitor cells. The process envisaged might involve cell contact between stem cell and specific receptor sites on the microenvironmental cells. Others envisage that these microenvironmental or "managerial" cells might not be arranged as fixed structures but might be dispersed throughout the tissue and generate short range gradients of specific factors which could trigger entry into an appropriate pathway of differentiation following binding by the stem cells of a significant concentration of the specific factor.

Either process would account for the observed data, the only point of practical importance is that so far it has not been possible to recreate these events in simplified in vitro systems. As a consequence, little is known about the nature of the stem cell to progenitor cell sequence.

With the introduction of in vitro cloning techniques, similar events from the progenitor cell to end cell stage can now be analyzed in isolation in vitro. It is quite apparent that proliferation within the progenitor and morphologically recognizable cell compartments is dependent on adequate concentrations of the appropriate specific regulatory factor. While this makes in vitro analysis relatively simple, it must be cautioned that in vivo events may not necessarily be as simple. It may well be, for example, that microenvironmental factors can also operate on the more mature compartments (just as humoral factors might well influence the stem cell to progenitor cell transition). This reservation should be kept in mind in reading the subsequent chapters. As will be seen, events are complex enough even in vitro but it is possible that even the in vitro systems do not genuinely reflect the full complexity of events occurring in vivo.

B. Terminology

To assist the reader in the following chapters a master list has been compiled in Table 1 of the names and abbreviations of the various hemopoietic cells and regulators. The terms used throughout this book are a combination of those in most common usage and a new systematic terminology for progenitor cells and their regulators. Names used by other workers are included in the synonym list.

C. Glossary

Certain names and terms will be found repeatedly in the text to follow. For the novice, an explanation of some of these terms is now given:

B-Lymphocytes. Subpopulations of lymphocytes mainly involved in humoral immune responses (mediated by immunoglobulin production). Although all synthesize immunoglobulin, plasma cells are a more specialized subset in which immunoglobulin production is extremely active. Derived from progenitor cells in bone marrow (also from the bursa of Fabricius in chickens), but the name is applied regardless of where cells are subsequently located. Note that both T- and B-lymphocytes proliferate extensively in lymph nodes, spleen, and Peyer's patches (that is, in the so-called secondary lymphoid organs). B-lymphocytes are identifiable by membrane immunoglobulin, antibody production, membrane receptors for antigen, the Fc portion of immunoglobulin, and the C3 component of complement.

Table 1 Names and abbreviations of hemopoietic cells and regulators

Cells			Regulatory factor		
Name	Abbreviation	Synonyms	Name	Abbreviation	Synonyms
Stem cell compartment					
Hemopoietic stem cells	HSC	Spleen colony-forming units (CFU-S or CFU)	Microenvironmental regulatory factors		Hemopoietic inductive microenvironment (HIM)
Progenitor cell compartment (committed stem cell compartment)					
Neutrophil and macrophage progenitor cells	GM-CFC	Granulocyte-macrophage colony-forming cells (GM-CFC); in vitro colony-forming (in vitro CFC); colony-forming units, culture (CFU-C); colony-forming units, agar (CFU-A)	Granulocyte-macrophage colony-stimulating factor	GM-CSF	Colony-stimulating activity (CSA), macrophage-granulocyte inducer (MGI)
Macrophage progenitor cells (peritoneal type)	M-CFC	Macrophage colony-forming cells	Granulocyte-macrophage colony-stimulating factor	GM-CSF	
Eosinophil progenitor cells	EO-CFC	Eosinophil colony-forming cells	Eosinophil colony-stimulating factor	EO-CSF	
Megakaryocyte progenitor cells	MEG-CFC	Megakaryocyte colony-forming cells	Megakaryocyte colony-stimulating factor	MEG-CSF	?Thrombopoietin
Erythropoietic progenitor cells	E-CFC	Burst forming units erythroid (BFU-E)	Erythropoietic colony-stimulating factor	E-CSF	Erythropoietin (Epo)
B-lymphocyte progenitor cells	BL-CFC	B-lymphocyte colony-forming cells	?	?	?
T-lymphocyte progenitor cells	TL-CFC	T-lymphocyte colony-forming cells	?	?	?

Chalone. By the original definition, a product of mature cells specifically inhibiting cell proliferation in that cell lineage. Often used loosely for an inhibitor of uncertain origin with usually incompletely characterized inhibitory activity on a particular cell system.

Clone. A cell population derived from the proliferation of one ancestral cell.

Cloning. The process of initiating a population in culture from a single cell. Strictly speaking, the cell should be micromanipulated to a fresh culture or isolated by a ring from other cells. Since most colonies in semisolid medium are clones, the term is often used loosely to describe discrete colony formation of only one cell type by cells contained in a mixed population of cells.

Clusters. Aggregates of cells formed by proliferation in vitro usually containing 3–50 cells.

Colonies. Aggregates of cells formed by proliferation in vitro and usually containing more than 50 cells. For human colonies, a lower limit of 40 cells is commonly used. Some workers use a limit of 20 cells. The criteria used for colonies are important for the interpretation of the data and should be noted with care in reading papers in this field.

Commitment. Usually used in reference to the stem cell to progenitor cell transition. Denotes loss of multipotential state, acquisition of synthetic activities for one special subpopulation and presumably the acquisition of membrane receptors for the specific regulator. Most likely mechanism, selective derepression of the genome.

Colony Stimulating Activity (CSA). A curious term used by some workers to denote the specific chemical factor stimulating neutrophilic and macrophage proliferation in vitro. Use best restricted to impure material with one known biological activity but probably containing a mixture of specific factors.

Conditioned Medium. Medium harvested from cultures of pure or mixed cells and containing many additional substances secreted by, or released from, these cells. Sometimes referred to as "spent" medium although such medium usually still contains adequate levels of nutrients. The growth inhibition sometimes observed with these media is often due to additional toxic or inhibitory factors derived from the cells.

Differentiation. Somewhat broader term than commitment, conveying concept of both commitment and maturation.

End Cells. Cells having reached full cytoplasmic maturation and incapable of further division. Death usually follows shortly after. Note that with lymphoid cells, end cells can avoid subsequent death if restimulated to proliferate by the appropriate antigen. Macrophages may also enjoy this alternative to a limited degree.

Factor. In the present context usually used to refer to a specific chemical substance with a definable property, e.g., the ability to stimulate the proliferation of certain cells, e.g., colony-stimulating factor. The term is an operational one only until chemical extraction procedures have succeeded in purifying the molecule concerned.

Families or Subpopulations. Population subcompartments of one morphological type, e.g., erythropoietic.

Granulocytes. Usually used to denote neutrophilic granulocytes (neutrophils or polymorphs) and less often to denote their immediate morphologically recognizable ancestors. Although eosinophils and mast cells also have granules these cells are usually not covered by the word granulocyte.

Hemopoiesis. Process of formation of blood cells. In this book (and usually) also meant to include the formation of lymphocytes since these are blood cells.

Humoral Factor. A humoral factor is literally something blood-borne, i.e., something detected in the blood, but of course the same factor might also be present in, or produced by, various tissues. The virtue of the expression is to denote that it is a chemical substance which leaves the cell and can act at a distance, traveling to the target cells via the blood. All hormones are humoral factors. Humoral factors may possibly differ from hormones in originating from more than one tissue or cell type. The term is often used loosely to refer to products releasable from cells and theoretically able to act at a distance, e.g., as in conditioned medium but strictly this remains hypothetical until proof is obtained of the presence of the factor in the peripheral blood.

Lymphopoiesis. The specific formation of lymphocytes and usually used to refer to events from the progenitor cell stage onward when cells already have some or all properties of lymphocytes or plasma cells.

Maturation. The progressive sequence of cellular events leading to accentuation of or specialization in one particular activity, e.g., hemoglobin formation or phagocytic activity. Often associated with loss of the capacity for further cell division and used loosely to refer to this state.

Monocyte-Macrophages. Collective term used to cover both monocytes and macrophages. Most tissue macrophages are derived from nonocytes produced in the marrow and spleen which seed in the tissue via the circulation and transform there to macrophages without further proliferation.

Myeloid. Derived from marrow. Often used as synonymous with neutrophilic granulocytes, e.g., as in myeloid leukemia.

Plating Efficiency. Strictly speaking, the percentage of a uniform population of cells able to proliferate in vitro. Often used incorrectly to describe the frequency of proliferating cells in cultures of a mixed cell population.

Poiesis. Formation, e.g., erythropoiesis—formation of red cells.

Poietic. Capable of forming, e.g., erythropoietic—capable of forming erythroid cells.

T-Lymphocytes. Subpopulations of lymphocytes mainly involved in cell-mediated immune responses, responses to viruses and in collaborative interactions with B-lymphocytes. Derived from progenitor cells located in the thymus, but the term applies to these cells wherever they are subsequently located in the body. Identifiable by surface theta antigens, rosette formation with red cells etc.

Underlayers. (Feeder layers) layers of cells incorporated under the cells being cultured, often in thicker agar, to supply growth factors to the cultured cells.

Chapter 3

Techniques for the Clonal Culture of Hemopoietic Cells in Semisolid Medium

Many different methods have now been developed for obtaining colony formation in semisolid agar medium by animal or human hemopoietic cells. Rather than provide an extensive description of all current methods for each separate type of hemopoietic cell, it is proposed to give a general discussion of the principles and to describe one standard method for each cell type. References to other methods will be given where these alternative methods have advantages for special purposes.

A. General Principles

The cloning techniques to be described are designed to obtain *primary* cultures of hemopoietic cells taken directly from animals or patients. When used effectively, they provide information on the number and functional activity of hemopoietic cells in vivo at the time the samples were removed for culture. These solid state cloning systems are not particularly useful for subculture studies, and the long-term behaviour of hemopoietic cells in this type of culture has not been extensively investigated.

The culture systems differ from conventional liquid culture systems in being single-step processes. The cells are suspended in a semisolid culture medium (usually in Petri dishes), and the cultures are incubated without subsequent media changes or supplementation until scoring of cultures is performed—usually 7–14 days later. Since refeeding of cultures or serial transfer of cultured cells are usually not involved, the requirements for performing this type of tissue culture are not as stringent as for other types of culture. As antibiotics are used in the culture medium and replicate cultures invariably performed, loss of occasional cultures from contamination is not critical. Because of this, it is possible to perform this type of culture in a reasonably clean room without special tissue culture facilities, e.g., filtered air or UV lights. Of course, if laminar flow hoods or tissue culture rooms are available, so much the better, but lack of these facilities certainly does not prevent such culture work.

The general requirements for tissue culture-washed glassware, apparatus for filtration of media, and small samples of test material are the same as for other types of tissue culture.

B. Collection of Cells

Marrow cells from mice or other laboratory animals are collected after killing the animal by cervical dislocation or with ether. The skin is cleaned with 70% alcohol, and using boiled instruments, the muscles are carefully stripped from the femur. Holding the tibia at right angles to the femur and pulling along the axis of the femur, the knee joint and lower end of the femur are separated from the femur shaft proper. The upper end of the femur is then severed close to the neck of the femur using scissors. For mice, a No. 21 needle is inserted through the intact cartilagenous sheet at the knee end of the detached femur. The plug of marrow cells is gently extruded into a sterile glass or plastic tube by syringing through the femur shaft 0.5 to 1 ml of Eisen's balanced salt solution or single strength tissue culture medium. The worm-like marrow plug is easily converted to a dispersed cell suspension in 5 ml of the collecting fluid by gently aspirating the suspension up and down 20 times using a sterile 5 or 10 ml pipette. Nucleated cell counts are performed using a hemocytometer and eosin or nigrosin for viable cell counts. *It is essential in all the semisolid techniques to culture a cell suspension of fully dispersed single cells.* If inspection of the cell suspension in the counting chamber reveals undispersed cell clumps, the dispersion procedure must be repeated until no further clumps are seen.

Dispersed suspensions of marrow cells from most species can usually be prepared using oral pipetting, and because of this, trypsinization is rarely necessary. If for some reason dispersion is difficult, preincubation at 37°C with 0.2% trypsin (Difco 1:250) in a salt solution containing 8.0 g NaCl, 0.4 g KCl, 1.0 g glucose, 0.02 g phenol red, 0.35 g $NaH\ CO_3$, 20,000 u penicillin and 100 mg streptomycin per liter for 30–60 min can be employed. The cell suspension is then washed free of trypsin, and gentle oral pipetting may be necessary to complete cell dispersion.

Human marrow samples are best collected in tubes containing 200 u of *preservative-free* heparin to prevent clotting. Samples are diluted by adding 5 ml of Eisen's balanced salt solution or tissue culture fluid, and the cells are dispersed by pipetting. Bone fragments can be separated by allowing these to settle for a few minutes and transferring the supernatant cell suspension to another tube. The marrow cell suspension is centrifuged at 1500 g for 10 min and the buffy coat containing the nucleated cells carefully removed and resuspended in fresh Eisen's solution. This achieves two things simultaneously: (1) it removes most of the contaminating red cells, and (2) it washes the marrow cells free of inhibitory material (ROBINSON, W. A., personal communication).

The nucleated cells in heparinized peripheral blood can be separated from the red cells (1) as a white cell pellet by centrifugation at 1500 g for 15 min, or (2) by layering the blood over a urografin-methylcellulose solution and allowing the red cells to agglutinate and sediment through the urografin-methylcellulose. To prepare the urografin-methylcellulose solution, a 2% solution of methylcellulose is made in distilled water (Methocel MC Premium 25 CPS; Dow Chemical Co. Midland, Michigan). A 20 ml vial of urografin (Shelliger A. G. Berlin) is added to 20.4 ml of distilled water and mixed well. To this urografin solution is added 64.7 ml of methylcellulose solution. The solutions are mixed well and stored in a stoppered container at 4°C.

To remove the red cells from 100 ml of blood, 120 ml of the urografin-methylcellulose solution is placed in a measuring cylinder and the blood gently pipetted into the cylinder as an overlayer. The measuring cylinder is allowed to stand at room temperature, and red cells in contact with the urografin-methylcellulose sediment through the solution. The time required to remove all red cells from a specimen varies from 30 min to 4 h.

The red cell-free supernate is removed using a Pasteur pipette and the cells centrifuged, washed, and resuspended in Eisen's balanced salt solution.

For spleen or lymphoid organ cells, the tissue may be teased apart in Eisen's balanced salt solution using needles, or the organ may be gently forced through a fine stainless steel sieve. Final dispersion of all cell clumps is again achieved by gentle pipetting.

Optimally, cultures are prepared shortly after preparation of the cell suspension so that the lag time for the cells between residence in vivo and incubation at the correct pH in vitro is minimized. Most workers keep their cell suspensions in crushed ice until the cultures are prepared. To minimize the lag time, however, numbering of culture dishes and addition of stimuli or other materials to the dishes should all be done before the cells are harvested.

C. Prefractionation of Cultured Cells

Bone marrow or peripheral blood cells are a heterogeneous group of cells of different families and at different stages of differentiation. In analytical work to determine the nature of the cells generating colonies or clusters, extensive studies have been performed on populations fractionated by one or more of certain separative procedures prior to culture: (1) active adherence separation using a glass bead column [32], (2) buoyant density separation in a continuous bovine serum albumin (BSA) gradient [33], (3) velocity sedimentation separation [34, 35, 36], or (4) electrophoretic separation [37]. In a similar manner, various subpopulations of cells can be selectively enriched by using antibody-mediated lysis of θ-bearing T-lymphocytes, antihemopoietic stem cell sera [38], or antierythroid sera [39]. Alternative methods employ rosette formation with red cells, followed by selection or rejection of the rosetted cells, to enrich for T-lymphocytes or B-lymphocytes [40, 41]. The reader is referred to the papers quoted for detailed descriptions of these techniques.
Prefractionation for quite different reasons is often used in the culture of granulocytic and macrophage colonies. In marrow cell suspensions from most species, there is a sufficiently high concentration of GM-CSF-producing cells to permit some degree of colony formation without supplying an exogenous source of GM-CSF [42]. Where studies on colony formation aim to examine the autonomous or otherwise nature of cell proliferation, it is essential to remove the endogenous GM-CSF-producing cells from the cultured population. A similar problem arises where added materials are being tested for a direct action on colony-forming cells (as distinct from an indirect action via CSF-producing cells).
Different human marrow suspensions differ in their content of colony-stimulating cells and the level of activity of these cells. The magnitude of endogenous stimulation is clearly dependent on the density of the cultured cells, and one simple way to minimize background colony formation is to use fewer cells than 100,000 per ml. The extent of endogenous stimulation of colony formation is also influenced by the type of medium used, the batch of fetal calf serum (FCS), and the length of the incubation period. Variation in these parameters in different experiments or from laboratory to laboratory have led to considerable variability in results, and for some experiments, it is desirable to minimize the number of colony-stimulating cells in cultured cell suspensions.
Three methods exist for selectively removing endogenous colony-stimulating cells based on the fact that most of these cells are relatively dense and adherent:

1. Marrow cell suspensions can be centrifuged through BSA of density 1.060 g/cm^3. Most colony-stimulating cells are denser than 1.060 g/cm^3, and the technique is particularly useful in working with cells from the monkey [43] or from patients with acute (AML) or chronic myeloid leukemia (CML) [44] where most of the proliferating cells are of lighter density than 1.060 g/cm^3. In these special situations, centrifugation through BSA is a simple method for obtaining fractions essentially free of colony-stimulating cells.
2. Most colony-stimulating cells are able to adhere to glass. Marrow suspensions can be allowed to settle in glass Petri dishes at 37°C and the nonadherent cells washed off. Two

cycles of removal of adherent cells over a 2–3 h period effectively remove colony-stimulating cells from most marrow suspensions [45].

3. Most of the cells in the bone marrow with colony-stimulating activity under the usual culture conditions used (i.e., nonactivation of lymphocytes) appear either to phagocytose or adhere to carbonyl iron. If 100 × 10^6 marrow cells are preincubated at 37°C for 1 h with 200 mg carbonyl iron in tissue culture medium containing serum, the colony-stimulating cells phagocytose or adhere to sufficient iron particles to allow them to be effectively removed using a large magnet. If the container holding the cell suspension is placed on the magnet and the cells decanted, the vast majority of colony-stimulating cells remain held firmly to the container wall.

Although most workers until recently have used adherence separation, there is now fairly general agreement that removal of cells using carbonyl iron is the most efficient method for removing colony-stimulating cells.

It must be emphasized that if the primary reason for performing the cultures is simply to enumerate colony-forming cells, there is no particular reason to remove colony-stimulating cells, and it is quite satisfactory to culture unfractionated cells. The endogenously produced GM-CSF (if any) then merely supplements the GM-CSF added to the cultures either in the form of an underlayer or via the addition of conditioned medium.

One final type of fractionation prior to culture of GM-colonies has been used. It has been shown by Broxmeyer and co-workers [46] that polymorphs are inhibitory for GM-colony formation. Analysis of this phenomenon showed that at least one of the mechanisms involved was that the polymorphs suppressed the capacity of endogenous colony-stimulating cells to elaborate GM-CSF in the culture dish. Thus, if high concentrations of cells were used in underlayers and a significant number of these cells were polymorphs, submaximal frequencies of colonies were obtained. However, if an exogenous source of preformed GM-CSF was used, e.g., by adding white cell-conditioned medium, the addition of polymorphs was not inhibitory for colony formation. Thus, in culture systems using underlayers to stimulate colony formation, if the detection of maximum colony numbers is desired, the underlayers and cultured marrow cells should first be freed of polymorphs. The most effective method for removal of polymorphs is centrifugation through BSA (density 1.070 g/cm^3, osmolarity 269 mOsm, for human cells). The polymorphs, being more dense, enter the BSA while the colony-forming cells remain in the supernatant suspension.

For some purposes, e.g., the preparation of a population of colony-forming cells free both of colony-stimulating cells and polymorphs, centrifugation of the cells through BSA is followed by removal of colony-stimulating cells using carbonyl iron.

D. General Preparation of Cultures

The general method for preparing agar cultures is shown in Figure 2. Cultures are prepared in 35 mm plastic Petri dishes (wettable or nonwettable) using a final volume of culture medium of approximately 1 ml. For semisolid agar cultures, a final concentration of 0.3% agar is used. This is achieved by the mixing in a tube or Erlemeyer flask equal volumes of (1) double strength tissue culture fluid and (2) 0.6% agar. Sufficient cells are added to the mixture to produce the final cell concentration required. The concentration of 0.3% agar is critical as higher agar concentrations do not support adequate colony formation and lower concentrations cannot gel satisfactorily. Since in most 1 ml cultures, 0.1–0.2 ml of additional fluid is

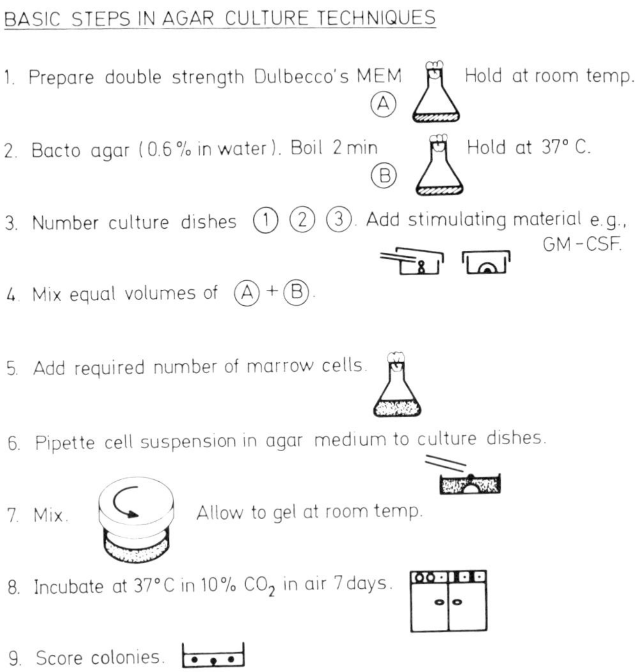

Fig. 2. The basic steps common to all the semisolid culture techniques using agar

added to provide the stimulus for colony formation (see later), it is important to keep to a minimum the volume of medium containing the added cells, e.g., the volume of cells added to 5 ml of agar medium should be less than 0.4 ml.

A satisfactory formula for the double strength medium, which is versatile enough to support the growth of all cells to be discussed, is as follows: Dulbecco's modified Eagle's medium HG instant tissue culture powder, H16 (10.0 g) (Grand Island Biological Company, New York); double glass distilled water, 390 ml; 3 ml of L-asparagine (20μg/ml); 1.5 ml of DEAE dextran (75μg/ml) (Pharmacia, Sweden) (mol wt $= 2 \times 10^6$, intrinsic viscosity $= 0.70$); 0.575 ml of penicillin (200,000 u/ml); 0.375 ml of streptomycin (200 mg/ml); 4.9 g NaH CO_3; 250 ml of unheated FCS.

The medium is millipore filtered and may be stored at 4°C for up to 2 weeks. Before use, the medium is allowed to warm to room temperature or 37°C.

The agar solution is prepared fresh for each culture experiment by boiling 0.6 g of bacto agar (Difco) in 100 ml of double glass distilled water for 2 min, then holding the solution in a water bath at 37°C. Other types of agar, e.g., Noble agar or agarose, can be used but are less satisfactory than bacto agar in supporting colony formation.

The DEAE dextran in the above formula was added to neutralize possible toxic amines in the bacto agar, and the supplementary L-asparagine is used because of the dependency of colony formation by granulocytic and macrophage cells on asparagine [47] and the improved colony growth with some types of CSF, e.g., from human urine (ROBINSON, W. A., unpublished data) if additional asparagine is added.

In a number of early studies trypticase soy broth (Baltimore Biological Laboratories) was included in the formula for the culture medium (3% solution in double glass distilled water with sterilization by millipore filtration). A mixture is made of 4 parts of double strength medium with 1 part of trypticase soy broth and 5 parts of 0.6% agar. Experience has shown (e.g., see METCALF et al., 48) that where culture conditions are poor, possibly because of inadequate FCS, the use of trypticase soy broth can greatly increase granulocytic and macrophage colony numbers and growth rates. However, with good culture media and FCS, the use of trypticase soy broth is certainly not essential and has little influence on colony numbers or growth rates.

Following addition of the cell suspension to the agar medium and *thorough* mixing, the cell suspension in agar medium is pipetted in 1 ml volumes to the culture dishes, using either 5 ml oral pipettes or a Cornwall automatic syringe. It is important to keep the cell suspension well-mixed during pipetting. In a warm culture room, premature gelling of the agar medium is not a problem, and with two people working as a team, up to 500 culture dishes can be prepared in 10–15 min without attempting to maintain the agar medium at 37°C in a water bath. If premature gelling is a problem, the medium should be kept at 37°C during the plating procedure. Premature gelling is difficult to detect by the inexperienced worker as the gelled medium can still be pipetted. However, this medium will never regel in the culture dish and such cultures are useless. A warning sign that premature gelling is commencing is the appearance of rings of solid medium on the walls of the flask holding the culture medium as the level of the medium is reduced.

The cell suspension in agar medium is thoroughly mixed in the Petri dish with any material previously added to the culture dish (see later), then allowed to gel firmly for 10–20 min. Gelling is tested by rocking the dishes gently and looking for movement of any bubbles present on the surface. Gelling should be allowed to occur in a relatively cool room. If the room is too warm, e.g., 30–35°C, gelling may fail to occur or may be so slow that the suspended cells sediment to the bottom of the culture dish as a monolayer.

After gelling, cultures are transferred without delay to a CO_2 incubator operating at 37°C with a fully humidified atmosphere of 10% CO_2 in air.

E. Special Requirements for Colony Formation

The above culture medium will support the proliferation of colonies of neutrophils, macrophages, eosinophils, megakaryocytes, T- and B-lymphocytes, and a variety of leukemic cells, but in each case specific factors must be added before colony formation can occur. These additions are made either to the cell suspension in agar medium before pipetting to the culture dishes or, more usually, the material is added to the empty culture dish. Regardless of the method used, the maximum volume of the additive should not exceed 0.2 ml for a 1 ml culture.

One effective method for supplying specific stimulating factors is the use of an underlayer containing the additive. Some slight delay in colony formation occurs due to the time required for diffusion of active factors from the underlayer into the upper layer containing the cultured cells, but this is usually not critical. Underlayers are best prepared by using the above formula for the medium except that 1% agar is used (instead of 0.6% as the double strength agar) giving the underlayer a firmer consistency of 0.5% agar. Underlayers can be prepared in advance of the preparation of cultures, and if necessary, stored in the CO_2 incubator. Underlayers have two major uses: (1) if high molecular weight inhibitors are present in the stimulating material being used, e.g., in many sera used to stimulate

granulocytic and macrophage colony formation, the density of the underlayer reduces diffusion of these high molecular weight lipoproteins, and (2) where human marrow cells are being stimulated to form granulocytic colonies, the use of peripheral blood cells in underlayers is the standard method for providing stimulating factors.
The various special factors required for the growth of different hemopoietic colonies will now be described in detail.

1. Granulocyte (Neutrophil) and Macrophage Colony Formation (GM-Colony Formation)

GM-colony formation requires continuous stimulation by the specific glycoprotein, colony-stimulating factor, GM-CSF. For mouse cultures, GM-CSF can be supplied to the cultures by adding to each culture dish one of the following:

1. 0.1 ml of a 1:6 dilution of pooled serum from mice injected 3–6 h previously with 5μg endotoxin [49]. This is a stable, reliable, stimulus which can be prepared relatively cheaply and which is capable of stimulating most GM-colony-forming cells.
2. 0.1 ml of serum-free medium conditioned for 48 h by mouse lung tissue [50] This medium is highly potent, stable, and appears to be capable of stimulating all GM-colony-forming cells.
3. 0.1 ml of mouse embryo-conditioned medium [51], another reliable and potent source of CSF.
4. 0.1 ml of dialyzed human urine after batch absorption on calcium phosphate [52]. This is cheap to prepare and stable but is not capable of stimulating all GM-colony-forming cells. Furthermore, colony formation is subject to gross fluctuations with different batches of media and FCS.

For human cells, the standard method for stimulating granulocytic colony formation is the use of an underlayer of 1–2 $\times$ 10^6 nucleated peripheral blood cells from normal human donors or Rhesus monkeys [44]. Considerable variability exists in the effectiveness of such underlayers. This is difficult to control, but variability can be minimized by use of a panel of donors, the activity of whose cells has been pretested and found to be comparable. The polymorphs in peripheral blood underlayers inhibit the production of active material by the colony-stimulating cells [46], and some workers selectively remove such cells by preliminary centrifugation through BSA gradients before culture. Large batches of underlayers can be prepared and stored in a CO_2 incubator for up to 2 weeks before use. Since underlayer activity can be variable and tends to decline on storage, it is wise to use two different batches of underlayers in replicate cultures in every experiment.
Although peripheral blood underlayers have been used routinely by most workers to stimulate colony formation by human marrow cells, such underlayers have a number of serious limitations:

1. The activity of underlayers even from the same donor can fluctuate widely.
2. Underlayers lose activity on storage beyond 1 week.
3. Underlayers seem very prone to fungal contamination, often occurring after storage in the incubator and perhaps due to droplet contamination.
4. Colonies often develop in the underlayers and can be confused with colonies in the target layer, particularly as the so-called "overlayer" containing the target cells often manages to partially get under the underlayer.
5. Because of the use of large numbers of cells in the underlayer, visibility of cells in the overlayer containing the marrow cells is often poor.

For these reasons, efforts have been made to develop a liquid source of GM-CSF, capable of stimulating human marrow cultures, which could be used routinely as a substitute for peripheral blood underlayers. A number of groups have used media conditioned by human peripheral blood or spleen cells (1–50 × 10^6 cells/ml for up to 7 days) [44, 53, 54]. Unfortunately, most media prepared in this way have little or no activity. In some studies, the activity of white cell-conditioned medium was shown to be increased if the white cells were cultured in the presence of phytohemagglutinin [55, 56].

More recently, it has been shown [57] that human placenta is a reliable source of material with colony-stimulating activity for human marrow cultures. Human placentas are stored at 4°C and used within 12 h of delivery. The outer membranes are removed and the placental tissues cut into 5 mm^3 pieces. After being rinsed 3 times in Eisen's balanced salt solution, six pieces are placed in each flat-sided plastic tissue culture bottle containing 20 ml of RPMI-1640 (Gibco, Grand Island, New York) containing 5% FCS. The bottles are incubated flat for 7 days at 37°C in a fully humidified atmosphere of 10% CO_2 in air. The conditioned medium is harvested by filtering through a double layer of cotton gauze to remove pieces of placenta, centrifuged at 10,000 g for 20 min to remove cellular debris and precipitated material, then stored at −15°C until used.

Untreated placental-conditioned medium appears to contain inhibitory material as evidenced by the higher numbers of colonies obtained when 0.1 ml of 1:2 or 1:4 dilution of conditioned medium is used. The level of inhibitory material in the conditioned medium appears to increase as incubation is continued beyond 7 days. A preparation with increased colony-stimulating activity can be prepared by preliminary calcium phosphate gel absorption of crude placental-conditioned medium followed by Sephadex column chromatography. Such preparations, after concentration, are capable of delivering a supramaximal stimulus for colony formation in the absence of high dose inhibition.

These preparations of placental-conditioned media have been shown to stimulate eosinophil colony formation in addition to the formation of neutrophilic, granulocytic, and monocytic colonies.

With all species except the mouse, the cultured marrow cells themselves are capable of generating some GM-CSF and thereby exhibiting some endogenous stimulation of colony formation. Although cultures without exogenous stimulation have been used in some studies, their use for most studies on granulocytic and macrophage populations is quite unsatisfactory and should be avoided for two major reasons: (1) because CSF levels are relatively low, colony development and growth rates are grossly suboptimal, and (2) relatively large numbers of cells need to be cultured, rendering colony counting inaccurate even if small colonies do develop.

2. *Sources of GM-CSF for Species Other Than Mouse or Man*

The general culture technique for GM-colony formation has been adapted by various workers to permit the culture of cells from a variety of species. These variations will not be discussed in detail since they introduce no new principles. The most commonly used methods for stimulating colony formation are the use of underlayers of white cells, medium conditioned by white cells, or serum containing normal or elevated levels of GM-CSF. In general, cultures are best stimulated by GM-CSF derived from the same species. Some useful references for the culture of cells from different species are: chicken [58], rat [59], dog [60], and monkey [43].

It is clear that little difficulty exists in culturing cells from most animal species. However, some caution needs to be exercised in accepting technical details and data from studies in species other than the mouse or man. These studies have not been extensive, and perusal of some of the papers published reveals many of the errors in technique discussed in this chapter. As a consequence, the data obtained may not be optimal and, to some degree, may be misleading.

3. Eosinophil Colony Formation

For human marrow cultures, satisfactory eosinophil colony formation can be stimulated either by underlayers of peripheral blood cells or by placental-conditioned medium. No special additives are required.

For mouse cultures, eosinophil colony formation requires stimulation by a specific type of CSF known to be different from GM-CSF [19]. The eosinophil CSF can be produced in liquid cultures of mouse spleen or lymph node cells following the addition of pokeweed mitogen and/or 2-mercaptoethanol (2–5 $\times$ 10^6 cells/ml are incubated for 7 days in media containing 5% heat inactivated human plasma with 0.05 ml/ml medium of freshly dissolved pokeweed mitogen (Gibco, Grand Island, New York) (diluted a further 1:15 with water) and/or a final concentration of 2-mercaptoethanol of 5 $\times$ 10^{-5} M). The lymphocyte-conditioned media are harvested after 7 days of incubation and can be used in volumes of 0.2 or 0.1 ml. Such conditioned media also contain GM-CSF and, in addition, the factor stimulating megakaryocytic colony formation so these cultures develop a complex mixture of colonies. Not all batches of human plasma support the production of these factors, and batches must be pretested.

4. Megakaryocyte Colony Formation

As mentioned above, megakaryocyte colony formation by mouse bone marrow cells can be stimulated by the addition of 0.2 ml of highly active preparations of the same type of lymphocyte-conditioned media used to stimulate eosinophil colony formation [19, 20]. No other special additives are required.

5. B-Lymphocyte Colonies

B-lymphocyte colony formation by mouse lymph node or spleen cells can be obtained by adding to the standard agar culture medium sufficient 2-mercaptoethanol to produce a final molar concentration of 5 $\times$ 10^{-5} [28]. Colony formation is improved if the double strength medium is modified slightly so that the medium contains a final serum concentration of 5–15% unheated FCS depending on the batch of serum—distilled water being used to replace the remaining FCS in the standard formula listed earlier.

Unlike the preceding types of colony formation. B-lymphocyte colony formation shows a marked nonlinearity with respect to the number of cells cultured. In cultures containing 200,000–1 $\times$ 10^6 cells, good colony formation occurs using the above system, but with cell concentrations below 100,000/ml, relatively few colonies develop, and these reach only a small size before dying prematurely. Since the frequency of B-lymphocyte colony-forming cells is at least one per 100 cells, this phenomenon causes practical difficulties when experiments require the production of small numbers of discrete, well-separated, colonies.

Nonlinearity in the B-lymphocyte colony-forming system can be overcome by the addition of 0.1 ml of fresh 10% washed sheep red cells to each culture dish [28]. Colony formation is then linear and even with 1000 or fewer cells per dish, colonies achieve a good size. The practical problem posed by the use of sheep red cells is that the plates are opaque and colonies are difficult to identify. Cultures must be cleared by the addition of 0.5 ml of 3% acetic acid before colony counting. An alternative method for obtaining linearity is the addition of 20μg endotoxin to each culture dish [61]. Not all commercially available endotoxin preparations are effective, but with an active preparation, good linearity and colony growth can be achieved with optically clear culture dishes. Endotoxin potentiation also depends on the batch of FCS being used, and this requires pretesting of various batches (see later).

6. T-Lymphocyte Colonies

A system for obtaining human T-lymphocyte colonies in agar was described by ROZENSZAJN et al. [29]. This involved overnight incubation of peripheral blood cells in liquid with phytohemagglutinin, followed by culture of the cells in agar on underlayers containing PHA. In this system, approximately 20 colonies developed per 10^5 cultured cells. The culture method has been modified and improved by CLAESSON in this laboratory (CLAESSON, M., unpublished data) so that approximately 10^3 colonies develop per 10^5 cultured cells. This latter system will now be described.

Peripheral blood is collected in sterile flasks using 10 u of preservative-free heparin per ml of blood. Since polymorphs are inhibitory in this culture system, these are removed by separation over Ficoll-paque. The blood is diluted 1:2 in normal saline and 9 ml of diluted blood layered over 2.5 ml of Ficoll-paque (Pharmacia, Uppsala, Sweden) (density 1.077 g/cm^3). The tube is centrifuged at 200 g for 30 min and cells at the interface removed. The cell suspension is washed twice and resuspended in Eisen's balanced salt solution containing 10% FCS.

T-lymphocyte colonies can be grown either as a one-step procedure (culturing the separated mononuclear cells immediately in agar) or as a two-step procedure (an initial liquid incubation step followed by culture in agar). The agar culture procedure is the same in the one-step and two-step procedures.

For the liquid incubation step, 1×10^6 white cells are incubated in 1 ml of Eagle's minimal essential medium containing 10% FCS and 2μl phytohemagglutinin (Burroughs Wellcome, Reagent grade, London) at 37°C in 5% CO_2 in air for 18 h. The cells are then washed twice and resuspended. Cell aggregates are dispersed by mechanical agitation using a vortex mixer and viable cell counts are then performed.

Ten to fifty thousand freshly separated mononuclear cells (one-step procedure) or 2500–25,000 PHA presensitized cells (two-step procedure) in a volume of 0.2 ml are added to 5 ml of agar medium (equal parts of double strength Dulbecco's modified Eagle's medium and 0.9% agar). The final concentration of FCS is similar to that used in cultures of B-lymphocytes (5–15%). Phytohemagglutinin is added to give a final concentration of 2μl/ml, and to potentiate colony formation, 0.1 ml of 10% triple-washed sheep red cells is added per ml of agar medium. Volumes of 1 ml of agar medium containing the cell suspension are plated in 35 mm Petri dishes and allowed to gel. Cultures are incubated at 37°C in 10% CO_2 in air for 5–7 days and colonies scored after lysing the sheep red cells either by adding 0.5 ml of 3% acetic acid or 0.5 ml of 0.17M ammonium chloride, if viable colony cells are to be harvested.

The use of a final agar concentration of 0.45% rather than 0.3% should be noted. With the use of 0.3% agar, many lymphocyte colonies develop as rafts of cells on the surface of the agar and these are impossible to count accurately. The use of a more rigid agar matrix appears to restrain lymphocyte mobility, and the colonies develop in 0.45% agar with essentially similar three-dimensional morphology to other types of hemopoietic colonies developing in 0.3% agar.

F. Technique for Growth of Erythropoietic Colonies

Techniques have been described for the culture of mouse or human erythropoietic colonies either in plasma gel cultures or in cultures containing methylcellulose. As these techniques are quite different from the general agar culture method, the plasma gel method will be described in detail.

The most useful description of the improved plasma gel culture method is that of McLeod et al. [9]. Cultures can be prepared in 1.1 ml volumes in 35 mm plastic Petri dishes or in 0.1 ml volumes in disposable microtiter plates (6 mm diameter) (Cooke Engineering Company, Alexandria, Virginia).

The composition of the ingredients used are:

1. Supplemented Eagle's minimal essential medium with Hank's balanced salt solution prepared as follows: 10 ml of minimal essential medium with Hank's balanced salt solution (10 × concentrated), 1 ml of minimal essential medium nonessential amino acids (100 ×), 1 ml minimal essential medium sodium pyruvate solution (100 mM = 100 ×), 1 ml L-glutamine (200 mM = 100 ×), 1.25 ml of 5% $NaHCO_3$ solution (autoclaved at 15 lbs. for 10 min), and made up to a final volume of 100 ml with water (deonized, distilled, sterilized by autoclave); penicillin and streptomycin are added at a concentration of 100 u per ml and 50 μg per ml respectively. This supplemented medium, which is not filtered after being made up, is stored at 4°C and kept no longer than 3 weeks.
2. Bovine plasma (citrated) stored at −20°C.
3. Beef embryo extract, reconstituted to original volume with supplemented medium stored at −20°C and diluted 1:5 in medium NCTC-109 before use.
4. FCS preheated to 60°C for 30 min and stored at −20°C.
5. Erythropoietin (anemic sheep plasma) (Step III Connaught Medical Research Laboratories, Willowdale, Canada) diluted to 10 U/ml in supplemented medium, stored at −20°C and diluted before use 1:4 in NCTC-109 for use at a final concentration of 0.25 U/0.1 ml.
6. L-asparagine (Nutritional Biochemicals, Cleveland, Ohio) 2 mg/ml in supplemented medium, stored at −20°C and diluted before use 1:10 in NCTC-109 so that 0.1 ml contains 0.02 mg L-asparagine.
7. NCTC-109 medium (Microbiological Associates, Bethesda, Maryland) containing penicillin 100 U/ml and streptomycin 50 μg/ml.
8. BSA (Fraction V) (Sigma Chemical Co. St. Louis, Missouri), a 10% stock solution prepared using double detoxification with the resin AG-501-X8(D) (Biorad Laboratories, Richmond, California) as described by McLeod et al. [9] and stored at −20°C. Before use, 0.5 ml of 7% sodium bicarbonate is added to each 20 ml of the BSA. Phenol red solution 0.5 ml (4 g/100 ml in phosphate buffered saline) is added per 100 ml of 10% BSA.

The culture medium is prepared in a plastic tube, mixing the following, or multiples of the following, and holding the mixture in an ice bath:

1. 0.1 ml beef embryo extract
2. 0.2 ml of FCS
3. 0.1 ml BSA (10%)
4. 0.1 ml L-asparagine (0.02 mg)
5. 0.1 ml erythropoieten (0.25 U)
6. 0.1 ml marrow or fetal liver cells in supplemented Eagle's minimal essential medium—Hank's.
7. 0.2 ml NCTC-109

The mixture is checked to ensure that no cell clumps are present, then 0.1 ml of bovine citrated plasma at room temperature is added per 0.9 ml of mixture, then 1 ml of the mixture added to each Petri dish or 0.1 ml to each microtiter well. Cultures are allowed to gel at room temperature and incubated in a fully humidified atmosphere of 5% CO_2 in air.

Each new batch of bovine plasma, beef embryo extract, FCS, and BSA is pretested for its ability to support the production of erythropoietic colonies and can be reused if stored.

While the erythropoietic colonies grow equally well in the large Petri dishes or the microtiter vessels, the use of microtiter wells facilitates the subsequent removal of the plasma clots for fixation and staining and increases the ease and precision of scoring colonies. The use of microwells also reduces the volumes of culture medium and erythropoietin used and the time spent in scanning cultures for the small erythrocytic colonies.

The addition of erythropoietin is essential for the formation of normal erythropoietic colonies. Commercially available Step III material is satisfactory for stimulating such colony formation. However, this preparation is known to contain inhibitory material which prevents the use of very high concentrations of erythropoietin to stimulate colony formation. High dose inhibition of colony formation can be avoided if the erythropoietin-containing material is subjected to further purification [62].

A major disadvantage of the plasma clot system is the impossibility of harvesting colony cells from the culture medium following gelling. This difficulty can be overcome by the use of methylcellulose as the gel medium. The technique employing methylcellulose has been described in detail by ISCOVE et al. [63].

G. Procedures for Potentiating Colony Formation

For each of the above special culture systems, there are certain materials which can be added to the cultures to increase the number and/or growth rate of the colonies developing. For special purposes, it may be desirable to obtain maximum possible colony growth, e.g., prior to harvesting and analyzing the cells from individual colonies. In these situations use of the materials to be listed can be helpful.

The most important of these additives is of course the serum used in the cultures, and this will be referred to later in this chapter and in Chapter 4.

Before listing the various additives for each culture system, one general comment must be made. Additives can only *improve* colony growth, they cannot by themselves *stimulate* colony formation. Thus, an additive cannot stimulate granulocytic colony formation in the absence of GM-CSF or erythroid colony formation in the absence of erythropoietin.

There seems to be a certain confusion in the minds of some workers regarding this distinction, and reports have been published of "serum stimulation" of colony formation where it is clear that the authors thought the serum itself was responsible and not the specific regulator present in that serum. Serum is of course necessary to support colony formation, and a "good" serum will support better colony formation than a "poor" serum. However, if no regulator is added, and the serum is first fractionated to remove the small amounts of regulator present in the serum, no colony formation can occur. The situation becomes complex with granulocytic and macrophage colony formation since, in most species, cells are present in the marrow which can produce GM-CSF, the specific regulator required for granulocytic and macrophage colony formation. This GM-CSF production depends on cells remaining alive in vitro and is therefore serum-dependent.

Space does not permit a detailed discussion of the possible mechanisms involved in the potentiating effects of the various additives to be listed. In no case is the mechanism known, but certain possibilities exist: (1) the additive may protect the specific factor from degradation or inactivation, (2) the additive may cause the production or activation of increased amounts of the specific factor, or (3) the additive may improve the viability of the colony-forming and colony cells or increase their responsiveness to the specific factor.

1. Granulocytic and Macrophage Colonies

The formation of granulocytic and macrophage colonies by mouse (but not necessarily other species) bone marrow cells can be potentiated by the addition of:

(1.) Sera from various species except FCS [48, 64]. The potentiating factor is macromolecular, but its nature and origin are unknown. Levels of the potentiating factor are increased in mouse serum by preinjection of endotoxin but not by irradiation. Potentiation is observed with all sources of GM-CSF and a useful dose for mouse or human serum is 0.1 ml of 1:4 dilution serum. Since most sera contain lipoproteins that inhibit colony formation, the use of undiluted serum often inhibits, rather than potentiates, colony formation.

(2.) Intact red cells or lysates prepared from them. Rat, sheep or human red cells strongly potentiate colony formation by mouse marrow cells and a useful dose per ml of culture is 5×10^8 cells [65].

(3.) In a number of laboratories, the addition of 2-mercaptoethanol (final concentration 5×10^{-5}M) has been found to double the number of colonies developing, but the effect has not been seen in all laboratories and may depend on the use of certain (? suboptimal) batches of FCS.

(4.) As discussed earlier, the addition of trypticase soy broth can strongly potentiate colony formation if poor batches of FCS are being used.

(5.) In the presence of moderate or low GM-CSF concentrations, the addition of living or freeze-thawed lymphoid (spleen, thymus, lymph nodes) or marrow cells can have a moderate potentiating effect on colony numbers and growth rates [66]. Potentiation of colony growth is also observed if colonies are crowded in a culture dish regardless of the number of original cells cultured, suggesting that the colony cells themselves are capable of autopotentiation.

2. Megakaryocyte Colony Formation

Megakaryocyte colony formation by mouse bone marrow cells can be strongly potentiated by substituting human serum (preheated to 56°C for 30 min) for the FCS in the culture medium listed previously. Colony numbers and size can be increased four to fivefold by this procedure. Only about one in three human sera has this striking potentiating effect, and selection of a suitable serum requires pretesting. The same active sera also potentiate granulocytic and macrophage colony formation, but this potentiating activity does not correlate with the capacity of human sera to stimulate B-lymphocyte colony formation.

3. Erythroid Colony Formation

Addition of β-mercaptoethanol or α-thioglycerol to give concentrations of 10^{-4}M has been reported to increase by fivefold the number of erythroid colonies developing in cultures of mouse bone marrow cells [62]. Responsiveness to erythropoietin is also increased by these additives.

The use of 1% BSA in the culture medium for erythroid colony formation is an example of an additive that is almost essential for good colony growth and is particularly necessary to obtain linearity of colony formation with numbers of cells cultured when working with low seeding densities.

4. B-Lymphocyte Colony Formation

As mentioned above, addition of red cells or endotoxin is essential for good B-lymphocyte colony formation when low numbers of cells are cultured. Fresh red cells should be used, and both human and sheep red cells are effective in cultures of mouse B-lymphocytes. Mouse red cells are also effective, but since mouse peripheral blood itself contains many B-lymphocyte colony-forming cells, addition of mouse red cells can lead to a spurious increase in the number of B-lymphocyte colonies developing due to the presence of B-lymphocyte colony-forming cells in the washed red cell preparations [28].

H. Phytohemagglutinin-Primed AML Cultures

In conventional underlayer-stimulated agar cultures of cells from patients with AML, the leukemic cells from most patients are unable to form colonies and characteristically form small clusters of cells. The morphological appearance of these clusters is not different from that of normal granulocytic or macrophage clusters, and the cultures therefore do not provide a method for discriminating normal from leukemic cells.

A radically different culture system has been described by DICKE et al. [67] in which leukemic, but not normal, human granulocytic cells are able to proliferate. The system depends on an overnight preincubation of the marrow or peripheral blood cells with phytohemagglutinin before the cells are cultured in agar.

Marrow cells are collected in 2 ml Hank's solution containing 300 u of preservation-free heparin and 20 mM Hepes buffer, pH 7.2. The cells are dispersed by oral pipetting and a buffy coat prepared by centrifugation at 1000 g for 10 min. The cells in the buffy coat are resuspended in 7 ml of Hank's solution and layered on 3 ml of Ficoll-paque (Pharmacia, Uppsala) (density 1.07 g/cm^3). This tube is centrifuged at 600 g (at level of the interface) for 30 min and cells at the interface harvested using a Pasteur pipette and suspended in 15 ml of Hank's solution. These cells are washed twice by centrifugation, the last time using α-medium [68].

After preparation and washing of the cells, 8×10^6 cells are added to 4 ml of α-medium containing 10% FCS and 10% horse serum. This suspension is divided between two Falcon tissue culture tubes (16 × 125 mm), each containing 2 ml. PHA (Wellcome, London) 8 μg per ml is added to one tube and the other used as a control. The tubes are incubated for 15–20 h at 37°C in an atmosphere of 5% CO_2.
After preincubation, the cells are centrifuged at 1000 g for 10 min and resuspended in 2 ml of Hank's solution. The cells are washed three times in all, the last wash being with α-medium containing 10% FCS and 10% horse serum. The cell suspension is adjusted to 1 ml and nucleated cell counts performed (recovery of viable cells usually approximates 50%). A fixed volume of 0.175 ml is added to 7 ml of agar medium (equal volumes of double strength α-medium and 0.6% agar) and 1 ml volumes plated in three cultures over underlayers of peripheral blood cells and three cultures over blank underlayers (underlayers contain α-medium in 0.5% agar with a final concentration of 10% FCS and 10% horse serum).
Immediately after plating, one-tenth of each culture dish is examined for aggregation and cell clumps. Usually the size of cell clumps is three to ten cells and the number of such aggregates varies from 0–200 per dish. Plates in which cells are markedly agglutinated are discarded. The cultures are incubated for 7 days in a CO_2 incubator, and after this period, colony and cluster counts are performed, scoring as colonies aggregates of 50 or more cells.
In this method leukemic cells are able to form colonies in the absence of stimulation by an underlayer of peripheral blood cells, but normal granulocytic colony formation remains dependent on stimulation by GM-CSF supplied by the conventional peripheral blood underlayers. It will be noted that this two-stage method was modeled on the two-stage PHA stimulation culture technique for T-lymphocyte colony development developed by ROZENSZAJN et al. [29]. However, colony formation by T-lymphocytes is dependent on the inclusion of PHA in the second-stage agar culture, whereas in the present system for obtaining colony formation by AML cells, phytohemagglutinin is omitted from the second stage of the culture system.

I. Agar Cultures in Diffusion Chambers

It has been shown that mouse or human marrow cells can be prepared in semisolid agar cultures in diffusion chambers and that these can be successfully incubated by insertion into the peritoneal cavity of irradiated mice [69, 70]. The technique is cumbersome in comparison with conventional Petri dish cultures, and so far the granulocytic and macrophage colonies developing have not differed from those grown in Petri dishes. Furthermore, because unknown factors diffuse into the chambers from the host, the exact nature of these factors cannot be defined unlike the situation with Petri dish cultures.
However, the system does have the capacity to directly demonstrate the in vivo existence of diffusible factors affecting hemopoietic cells and in suitable circumstances the technique will probably prove to be a useful ancillary method, supplementing information from Petri dish cultures.

J. Incubation of Cultures

For several reasons, cultures are best not removed from the incubator until final scoring: 1. Cultured cells are very susceptible to pH changes. The low buffering capacity of the culture system and the loose fitting culture dish lid permit rapid pH changes. 2. The humidified atmosphere of the incubator allows water to condense on many culture dish lids. If the cultures are moved, some of this water can run under the dish lid and sometimes contaminate the cultures. 3. The gels are delicate and any jerking or banging of the culture trays can fracture the gels and reduce or prevent colony formation. Where cultures have to be checked at intervals during the incubation period, trays must be handled very gently and the cultures should not be left out of the incubator for more than a few minutes.

One of the critical factors common to all the above types of colony-forming systems is the necessity to use an adequate CO_2 incubator. From trials on many types of incubators, National incubator (National Appliance Company, Portland, Oregon) (or incubators with the same basic design system) has proved superior. The correct mixture of 10% CO_2 in air is achieved by adjusting the mixing valves and using the pH indicator in the culture medium (phenol red) to achieve the correct pH of 7.2–7.4 (a yellowish, salmon-pink, color). The small volume (1 ml), large surface area, and loose fitting nature of the Petri dish lid gives semisolid cultures only a minimal buffering capacity. If the incubator door is opened repeatedly during the working day, the pH of the cultures will become alkaline and remain so for many hours. Under such conditions colony formation is extremely poor. To correct this, it is essential to have a bypass valve capable of flushing the incubator with pure CO_2 for 30–45 s each time the door is opened. The gas flow rates that are optimal for these cultures are below those indicated on the lowest markings on the flow meters. Use of higher gas flow rate is uneconomical and often dries out the cultures.

Water-jacketed incubators seem to maintain a more even temperature than other incubators, but it should be remembered that there is a continuous water loss from such jackets. When water levels fall, drying and poor colony formation occur first on the top shelves of the incubator and at the edges of other trays. This is a warning sign that overheating is occurring because of low water jacket levels. Incubators with fan attachments should not be used as the air movement leads to plate contamination because of the humid atmosphere and the loose-fitting Petri dish lids.

Under *no* circumstances should antibacterial or antifungal agents be placed in the water bath of the incubator. These become dispersed in the atmosphere of the incubator and are extremely toxic. Contamination of the water bath in the incubator is inevitable but rarely causes contamination of culture dishes. Water bath contamination does eventually lead to a slow deterioration in the quality of the cultures, and when colony formation becomes progressively poorer (about every 2–3 months), the incubator needs to be stripped down and thoroughly cleaned with detergent and water, then allowed to dry with the door open for 24 h before reuse.

Alternative incubating systems can of course be devised in laboratories lacking a CO_2 incubator. For example, perspex boxes can be built which are gassed after loading, then sealed and placed in a standard bacteriological incubator or a warm room. A tray of water needs to be included during loading of such boxes. The system is cumbersome and prevents ready access to cultures, but it is capable of supporting satisfactory colony growth. Alternative systems are also possible using sealed containers in which CO_2 is generated from bicarbonate powder.

K. Problems

1. Unsatisfactory Serum

The most common practical problem encountered with these techniques is the variability of commercially available serum. All workers in this field have experienced episodes where poor or no colony growth was traced ultimately to particular batches of FCS or horse serum. There is no satisfactory method for predicting the suitability of a batch of serum, and serum batches can only be checked by pretesting in the type of cultures being used. It is important to note that assays for serum suitability using other types of cultures do *not* necessarily select suitable batches for agar culture. Ideally, samples of a serum batch are pretested before purchase of the batch. Serum appears to retain its capacity to support colony formation better if stored at 4°C than at −15°C, and it is unwise to store sera for periods longer than 6 months.

Various possibilities have been raised to account for the toxicity or unsatisfactory growth supporting properties of certain serum batches. Some workers consider that complement is a prime factor and recommended heat inactivation at 56°C for 30 min. Heat inactivation is not used routinely in the author's laboratory, and while on occasion it has improved the quality of some serum batches, this has not been a consistent finding. On storage, some sera develop thick layers of light density lipoprotein. Removal of this material after centrifugation often improves the capacity of a serum to support colony formation. These lipoproteins often make millipore filtration difficult or impossible, and since sera are usually supplied in sterile containers by the manufacturer, in many laboratories the serum is not subjected to a second filtration during preparation of the double strength medium. This also avoids another possibility—that toxic material is released from the millipore filters. It is suggested that some sera are better than others in activating this toxic material.

2. Drying of Cultures

A problem common to all gel cultures performed using Petri dishes which have large surface areas and loose-fitting lids is the tendency for the cultures to dry out on continued incubation, particularly if the cultures are maintained beyond 7 days. As drying occurs, the agar concentration rises and concentrations above 0.45% are inhibitory for most colony formation. As a consequence, partially dried out cultures usually exhibit either suboptimal colony growth or, if drying is severe, no colony formation.

Drying of cultures can be detected by (1) obvious thinning of the agar layers with rings of dried agar on the dish walls, (2) an uneven hilly surface on the agar culture, (3) a rubbery texture which prevents colonies being picked off, using a pipette. If there is doubt about an incubator's capacity to maintain fully hydrated conditions, test cultures should be weighed before and after incubation. A weight loss of more than 10% in the cultured material is excessive and indicates that the cultures are drying abnormally.

Excess drying of cultures is usually preventable by minimizing gas flow rates in the incubator and by maintaining a fully humidified atmosphere within the incubator. This is achieved by keeping the water bath in the bottom of the incubator full of distilled water and by having the incoming gas enter the incubator through the water bath, preferably using a finely dispersed gas flow achieved by fitting a scintered glass gas dispersion fitting on the end of the tubing. An alternative method is to puncture the tubing with multiple pin holes. Under conditions of full humidification, water should be condensed on the doors and walls of the incubator and on many of the culture dish lids.

For incubators of poor design or if there is no water bath in the bottom of the incubator, the humidity can be raised by inserting stainless steel trays of water in the bottom of the incubator and by taping a sheet of filter paper to the back wall of the incubator arranging the sheet so that the lower edge is in the water bath at the bottom of the incubator.
A commonly used method to minimize drying is to place two 35 mm Petri dishes containing cultures in a 60 mm Petri dish together with an open third 35 mm Petri dish containing distilled water. The system is simple and effective but tedious when large numbers of cultures are being produced, and a better solution is to attempt to obtain adequate humidity throughout the whole incubator.

3. Failure of Cultures to Gel

One problem which is common when first attempting these techniques is failure to obtain proper gelling before the cultures are incubated.
Failure to obtain gel formation is very obvious as the culture dishes contain a mixture of small fragments of agar floating in liquid medium. Under such conditions, colony formation rarely occurs. If gelling has occurred abnormally slowly, the colony-forming cells have had time to fall to the bottom of the dish and while colony formation can occur, the colonies are not spherical but two-dimensional plaques on the bottom of the culture dish.
Cultures usually fail to gel for one of three reasons: 1. The medium has cooled too quickly and has already gelled in the flask. This gelling has been unnoticed and the gelled medium pipetted into the culture dishes, permanently disrupting the gel. 2. The culture room or hood is too hot. In this situation, gelling can be obtained by removing the tray to a cool room, or if temperatures are very hot, *briefly* placing the tray in a cold room or refrigerator. 3. Too large a volume of liquid stimuli or additives has been included in the basic agar medium.
In general, if cultures do not gel within a few minutes, they are unlikely to within 20 min and should be removed to some cooler area. Never put away a tray of incompletely gelled plates as these will never completely gel in the incubator.
After preparation, cultures should not be left out of the CO_2 incubator for more than 20–30 min. If by accident, cultures are forgotten and not placed in an incubator for 1–2 h, it is better to repeat the experiment as subsequent colony formation will be subnormal.

L. Scoring of Cultures

For scoring the above types of cultures, by far the most convenient method is to use an Olympus dissection microscope with a stereo zoom lens system (Olympus Optical Co., Tokyo, Model SZ III). Light is transmitted through the cultures from a source in the base plate. The curved mirror is adjusted so that colonies appear white on a black or dark background. For granulocytic, macrophage, eosinophilic, and lymphocyte colonies a magnification of $\times$ 30 or $\times$ 35 is suitable, but for megakaryocyte colony counting a magnification of $\times$40 is necessary. For accurate colony counts, it is convenient to place the culture dish on the base of a larger (50 mm) culture dish, the bottom of which has been scored with a diamond pencil in a grid pattern. Care needs to be taken when counting colonies at the edges of these cultures since the gels exhibit a distinct meniscus at the periphery and the agar layer is thickest at the edge of the dish.

For scoring of erythropoietic colonies, the very small size of the erythroid colony cells necessitates the use of an inverted microscope.

In all the hemopoietic cloning systems, a characteristic feature of the cultures is the variation in size and shape of colonies. In addition, in most of the culture systems, larger numbers of small aggregates of cells develop (clusters). By convention, discrete aggregates of 50 or more cells are scored as colonies. Aggregates of 3–50 cells are scored as clusters.

Although this necessitates a succession of subjective judgments during the scoring of cultures, with a minimum of experience, individuals quickly acquire the ability to make the discrimination between colonies and clusters.

Exceptions to the above general rule are: (1) human granulocytic colonies where aggregates of 40 or more cells are scored as colonies and aggregates of 3–40 cells as clusters, and (2) megakaryocytic colonies where because of their small size, aggregates of three or more cells are scored as colonies.

M. Harvesting and Cytological Examination of Colony Cells

Harvesting of colony cells from agar for cytological examination or functional studies can present some problems. For this reason, methylcellulose was introduced as a substitute for agar since colonies can be removed from the medium and the colony cells readily washed free of surrounding methylcellulose.

For work with colonies grown in agar, it has been shown that predigestion with agarose is a useful procedure for freeing colonies [71]. However, most batches of agarose appear incapable of liquifying the average agar culture and in many laboratories the results have been disappointing.

In practice, the difficulties in harvesting colonies turn out to be more imagined than real, and relatively little difficulty is experienced in harvesting colonies or in preparing useful cell suspensions from harvested agar colonies.

1. Orcein Staining of Picked Off Colonies

For the routine typing of mouse granulocyte-macrophage colonies, the identification of megakaryocytic colonies or the enumeration of total cells or mitotic cells in a colony, a very simple procedure gives reliable results. A small Pasteur pipette is used to pick off individual colonies under direct vision. The Pasteur pipette ideally is no more than 8–10 cm in total length with a firm rubber bulb and a fine tip 1–2 cm in length with an internal diameter of 0.2–1.0 mm. The bulb of the pipette is held loosely between thumb and forefinger and the stem of the pipette between the third and fourth fingers with the edge of the hand resting firmly on the base plate of the dissection microscope. The culture dish is held firmly with the left hand and the pipette introduced at an angle of 45°. The colony is *not* sucked up the pipette, instead a very slight suction is used merely to hold the colony against the end of the pipette, the colony being scooped out of the agar with a movement of the pipette towards the stationary left hand. The colony with a small volume of surrounding agar (approximately 1 mm^3) is not allowed to move far up the pipette and is promptly placed on a marked microscope slide. It is convenient to make three rows of five squares 2–3 mm squares) on the reverse side of the microscope slide using a wax pencil.

With practice, even single cells can be removed with this general technique but using a finer pipette. Until expertise is achieved, it is wise to check under the dissection microscope that the colony was in fact removed completely from the agar and that the agar droplet deposited on the slide contains the entire colony.
The Pasteur pipette can be washed in hot water and reused repeatedly. Colonies are allowed to dry and may be stored in a dust-free container for several days before scoring. Storage beyond 1–2 weeks is unsatisfactory as the agar yellows and colonies become difficult to stain.
When dry, a coverslip is placed over the colonies and drops of freshly filtered 0.6% orcein in 60% acetic acid run under the coverslip. The acetic acid dissolves the agar and allows uniform staining of the colonies usually within 1 h unless excessive volumes of agar were removed. If two to three drops of glycerine are added per 100 ml of stain, drying under the coverslip is slowed, and it is unnecessary to seal the edges of the coverslip. The colonies can then be examined wet at × 100, × 400 or × 1000 magnifications, according to needs.
Such stained preparations can be kept for a short interval at 4°C but usually overstain with time. It is unwise therefore to stain colonies if there is insufficient time to count these within 2–3 h of preparation.
For routine estimation of the proportion of granulocytic, mixed or macrophage colonies in cultures of mouse bone marrow cells [72], it is necessary to sample a minimum of 45 sequential colonies.

2. *Cytocentrifuge Preparations of Colony Cells*

In general, colonies removed from agar and smeared in the manner of blood films are quite unsatisfactory as too many colony cells are damaged, or very frequently the agar fails to permit proper spreading of colony cells. A technique for pre-fixing and squashing individual colonies was described by TESTA and LORD [73] and can give good results. The advantage of methylcellulose cultures is that smearing and staining of individual colonies is a much simpler procedure.
Most often the morphology of colony cells is best demonstrated by preparing suspensions of pooled colony cells and preparing cytocentrifuge preparations. Pooled colonies can be collected in tissue culture medium or buffered saline preferably containing 10–20% serum. The colonies are collected in a small pointed plastic centrifuge tube of 0.5 ml volume. A suspension of the pooled colony cells freed from surrounding agar is made by gently aspirating the colonies through a finely drawn Pasteur pipette. This cell suspension can be placed directly in a cytocentrifuge cup and the cell preparation subsequently fixed in methanol and stained with May-Grunwald-Giemsa.
Studies by DAO (DAO, C., personal communication) showed that individual colonies could be aspirated from agar cultures through a fine Pasteur pipette into a small volume of distilled water. The resulting cell suspension could be placed as three or four droplets on a microscope slide. If these droplets are *immediately* cytocentrifuged, the spreading and drying of these small droplets is sufficiently rapid to prevent lysis of the cells and achieves a quite satisfactory spreading of the cells. The slides can then be fixed and stained as before. This is one of the few methods which permits total colony cell counts on well spread cells.

3. *Preparation of Cell Suspensions from Pooled Colonies*

Pooled colonies can be harvested from cultures and colony cells resuspended by pipetting through a fine Pasteur pipette. Such colonies are best collected in a small plastic tube (0.5 ml capacity) with a pointed tip. If the cells are then centrifuged at 700 g for 5 min and washed 2–3 times using balanced salt solution, sufficient agar is removed to permit a wide variety of membrane marker studies, e.g., rosette formation or antigen binding [74].

N. Staining of Eosinophil Colonies

In cultures of mouse marrow cells, the largest of the eosinophil colonies can be recognized and counted in unstained cultures because of the characteristic, loosely dispersed arrangement of the colony cells [19]. However, in cultures of human marrow cells, eosinophil colonies are usually compact and not distinguishable from other compact colonies in the cultures. Even in the mouse, compact eosinophil colonies and clusters do develop which cannot be distinguished from other colonies and clusters with a similar general shape.

To accurately count the number of these eosinophil colonies in a culture, it is necessary either to establish the proportion of eosinophil colonies from a random sample of the colonies and then calculate the total number from the total colony count or to differentially stain the entire culture dish and perform a direct eosinophil colony count.

Methylcellulose cultures have been used for the first method [13] since individual colonies may be picked out of the culture medium using a Pasteur pipette, smeared on microscope slides, and stained. The colonies are typed, and the frequency of eosinophil colonies calculated from the total colony count. The method is technically feasible but is tedious, usually samples only a small proportion of available colonies, and cannot document the number or size of clusters developing in the cultures.

A more informative method for analyzing eosinophil proliferation in a culture dish is to culture the marrow cells in agar and stain the entire culture dish (DRESCH, C., personal communication). The method works best if only a single layer culture is used, as the double thickness of an agar underlayer together with the cells in the underlayer can obscure visibility and make scoring difficult. It is preferable therefore to stimulate human colony formation using 0.1 ml of placental conditioned medium.

The cultures are stained unfixed using Dominici stain: 0.5 g eosin yellowish (G. T. Gurr, London) and 0.5 g orange (G. T. Gurr, London) in 100 ml distilled water. This solution is diluted 20 times with water and sufficient phloxine added to give a final concentration of 0.0012%. This stock solution can be kept in a dark bottle at room temperature. Immediately before use, the solution is diluted fivefold in water and 4 ml of the diluted stain is added to the culture dish. After addition of the stain, the agar of the culture is gently detached from the edge of the culture dish using a metal spatula. The cultures are allowed to stain at room temperature for 1.5–2 h, then the excess stain removed using a Pasteur pipette. The cultures are then fixed by the addition of 4 ml of absolute methanol for 10–15 min. This methanol is then removed and the cultures counterstained for 15 min by the addition of 4 ml of a 0.2% solution of methyl green in water. The intact agar culture is then gently tipped onto the surface of a 60 mm Petri dish filled with water. The agar culture floats on the surface of the water and is picked up on a 3 × 2 inch glass microscope slide using the same general technique as in picking up stripping film during the preparation of autoradiographs. Excess water is blotted from the edge of the agar culture and the culture is allowed to dry overnight at room temperature.

The stained preparations are covered completely with microscope oil and scored using a conventional microscope either at × 100 or × 1000 magnifications. The red granules of

eosinophils are more visible if a yellow Wratten KI filter is used. Groups of more than 40 cells are scored as colonies and groups of 3–40 cells as clusters.
While the scoring of eosinophil colonies and clusters is easy in cultures of human cells, granule formation is less evident in some mouse eosinophil colonies, particularly in the large, loosely dispersed colonies.
Other methods for differentially staining colony eosinophils have been described by SHOHAM et al. [75].

O. Staining of Erythroid Colonies

Although the very small size and pink color of many of the cells in erythroid colonies makes it possible often to identify erythroid colonies in unstained cultures, it is usually essential to verify the fact that the cells contain hemoglobin by using a benzidine stain. Full details for the technique of staining erythroid colonies and the subsequent scoring of these colonies are given in the paper by MCLEOD et al. [9].

P. Examination of Agar Colonies by Electronmicroscopy

Individual colonies can be removed using a Pasteur pipette and processed for electronmicroscopy by fixing initially in 5–10 ml of a solution of 2% paraformaldehyde and 2.5% gluteraldehyde in 0.08 M sodium cacodylate buffer for 1 h at room temperature. The fixed colonies are then centrifuged, the fixative removed, and the pellet resuspended in 50% horse serum. The resuspended colonies are centrifuged gently in 4 × 0.5 cm Spinco cellulose nitrate centrifuge tubes to form a loose pellet in which individual colony cells remain well separated from each other. The pellet is then overlaid with 2.5% gluteraldehyde which serves to cross-link the horse serum surrounding the cells.
The bottom of the centrifuge tube containing the pellet is cut off, washed overnight in 0.1 M cacodylate buffer, and post-fixed for 2 h in 2% osmium tetroxide. Following a wash in water, the pellet is stained for 2 h in 2% aqueous uranyl acetate and then dehydrated in a graded series of acetone. The acetone dissolves the cellulose nitrate cap covering the pellet which is then embedded in Spurr's low viscosity resin [76]. After 48 h polymerization at 60°C, thin sections are cut with glass knives, stained with uranyl acetate in 70% ethanol followed by lead citrate, and examined in a Philips 300 electron microscope.
An alternative is to fix and embed the entire agar culture. This method has been described in detail by VAN NOORD et al. [77].

Q. Transfer of Developing Colonies

A very useful technique for determining whether hemopoietic colony growth is dependent on, or influenced by, a particular factor is to transfer individual developing colonies to culture

dishes containing agar medium, no other cells and with or without the factor under study.
Recipient single layer agar cultures are prepared in advance and five small circles marked on the bottom of each Petri dish using a wax pencil. Donor cultures are prepared, ideally using as few cells as possible, so that discrete developing colonies are well separated from other cells or colonies, e.g., by using 10,000 mouse marrow cells for GM-colonies.
Technically, it is simpler to transfer small colonies of five to ten cells usually from day 2 or 3 cultures. Individual colonies are picked out of the agar using a small sterile Pasteur pipette, removing as little of the surrounding agar as possible (a suitable agar volume around the picked off colony is 1–2 mm^3). The colony is then deposited on or slightly under the surface of the recipient agar culture dish over one of the marked areas. The recipient culture dish is returned to the incubator without delay and incubation continued for 2–5 more days. At this time, the transferred colonies are reharvested, stained with orcein, and colony cells counted and typed.
The principle involved in this technique is that the volume of the transferred droplet is only 1/1000th that of the recipient culture. Any diffusible factor in the agar droplet surrounding the transferred colony in the original culture will diffuse into the agar of the recipient culture which itself lacks the factor. If that factor is necessary for colony survival and/or growth, the ultimate concentration of the factor is now too low and the transferred colony ceases growing and/or dies.
Although the technique is simple, it is capable of giving highly reproducible and dramatic answers concerning the action of various specific factors [78, 79, 19, 61].
A variant of this technique is the transfer of single colony or colony-forming cells. In this technique, it is not sufficient simply to deposit the cell on the surface of the recipient dish. The transfer pipette must be stabbed into the agar culture and the transferred cell deposited at the end of this track [80]. Some difficulty can be experienced in preventing the cell floating up the pipette track and being lost on the surface of the agar. This can be prevented by using 2 ml of agar medium in the culture dish, the greater depth of agar allowing the cell to be firmly planted in the agar.

R. Liquid-on-Agar Cultures

Although the advantages of working with colonies (clones) of hemopoietic cells will be referred to repeatedly throughout this book, it must be emphasized that for most of the hemopoietic colonies (except B-lymphocytes) the supporting matrix of the gel is inert and supplies nothing special to the growing cells.
Provided adequate concentrations of the special stimulating factors are supplied, the same hemopoietic cells can proliferate in an essentially identical fashion in liquid cultures. Indeed, if these are left undisturbed, globular aggregates of proliferating cells develop which in many cases are genuine colonies.
For certain purposes, e.g., where many "colony-type" cells must be harvested for biochemical studies, marrow cultures can be set up in liquid culture. Many plastic culture dishes appear to be slightly cytotoxic, and better cell growth is obtained if an underlayer of medium in 0.5% agar is used. The cell suspension in single strength medium is then added as a 1 ml overlayer. Since the effectiveness of the stimulus is dependent on its concentration, either a double dose should be added to the 1 ml of liquid overlayer, or preferably the stimulus should be added to both the underlayer and liquid overlayer.

After incubation, the cultures are rocked gently to suspend sedimented cells and the cell suspension harvested using a Pasteur pipette.

S. Comments

This discussion has attempted to describe the basic techniques used in the culture of hemopoietic cells in semisolid medium. Once learned, the techniques are relatively simple and reliable. While the preparation of cultures can safely be left to an intelligent, well-trained technician, it is my very strong opinion that the scoring of culture dishes must be done by the investigator and must *not* be left to a technician.

It is of great practical assistance in setting up cultures for the first time if someone else in the same city or region already is using the techniques successfully. If so, media and reagents can be exchanged to test their adequacy and the performance of the incubator. When the techniques are established, it is useful to again exchange standard stimulating preparations so that colony counts obtained in one laboratory can be cross-standardized with another.

In all new fields there is a period during which the waters are muddied by the precipitous publication of data based on poor technology, often applied improperly to various problems. If the reader takes note of the comments made in this chapter, it will be possible to identify many of these misleading publications and to avoid making similar errors.

Chapter 4

General Features of Hemopoietic Colony Formation

Hemopoietic colonies that develop in semisolid cultures appear to be generated by specific hemopoietic progenitor cells. In this context, progenitor cells are defined as cells that are intermediate in differentiation between the multipotential stem cells and the morphologically identifiable members of a particular hemopoietic family. It is possible that these progenitor, or colony-forming, cells may share a number of morphological features in common, e.g., size, nuclear-cytoplasmic ratio, and shape of the nucleus, despite the fact that each is specifically derepressed into one particular pathway of differentiation and each is capable of responding to only one specific set of regulatory molecules. Lymphoid colony-forming cells are a possible exception to this generalization. Both B -and T-lymphocyte colony-forming cells appear to be so numerous as to be likely to be more mature cells, and the evidence on their physical properties is in agreement with this conclusion.

As a further generalization, it can be stated that the cellular proliferation necessary for the formation of each type of colony requires continuous stimulation by an appropriate specific stimulating factor.

In the discussion to follow, features shown in common by the various hemopoietic populations during colony formation will be described since these give some insight into the basic biological processes operating.

A. Colony Formation

Immediately after the preparation of a culture dish, the cells being cultured are distributed uniformly in the three-dimensional matrix of the semisolid culture medium. In carefully prepared cultures where the cell concentration is less than 100,000/ml, microscopic inspection reveals no cell aggregates and extremely few pairs or triplets of undispersed or reaggregated cells. Studies in which the location of individual cells was plotted, then followed sequentially for the next few days of incubation, revealed essentially no movement of cells in the matrix of the culture medium [72]. The conclusion is that reaggregation of cultured cells to form pseudocolonies does not occur in properly prepared cultures containing fewer than 100,000 cells/ml. In cultures containing much higher cell numbers, e.g., 1×10^6/ml, it is very difficult to obtain uniform dispersion of cells, and some aggregation of cells can occur prior to gelling of the medium. Interpretation of such cultures can be difficult if the original cells survive during the incubation period.

In most agar culture systems using normal hemopoietic cells, in the first 1–2 days of incubation, there is widespread death and disintegration of most of the cells originally placed in the culture dish. In general, this is due to the death of relatively mature end cells in the various hemopoietic families, no doubt accelerated by the somewhat abnormal culture conditions. It also seems that in cultures lacking the specific growth stimulator for a particular subpopulation, death of even the mature cells of that subpopulation occurs more rapidly although this has not been formally documented.

Whatever the reasons for the early death of many cultured cells, the phenomenon causes a dramatic clearing of the culture dish which now contains only a few surviving cells. These cells enlarge, then commence proliferation to form colonies or smaller aggregates.

The early cell death and the enlargement of colony-forming cells make it particularly easy to follow the early events in colony formation even using the relatively low magnification of a dissection microscope. Optical conditions are ideal for time-lapse cinematographic studies although none have been reported so far, due possibly to the stringent requirements of the cultures for pH stability and high humidity.

Cells proliferating to form colonies can be located at any depth in the agar. It is usual to find colonies concentrated at the periphery of the culture dish due (1) to the circular mixing movement most workers use during preparation of the cultures, and (2) to the prominent meniscus in the culture dish which causes the cultures to be distinctly thicker at the edges than in the central region.

In at least two culture systems, the granulocyte-macrophage and erythroid-forming systems, there is a striking degree of symmetry and synchrony in the initial few divisions of the colony-forming cell (81; AXELRAD, A. A., personal communication). As shall be discussed shortly, the onset of differentiation in some of the colony cells soon leads to loss of this initial symmetry in most colonies.

In most types of culture, the first few divisions of the colony-forming cell and its progeny lead to the formation of a tight aggregate of cells. However, the initial shape of this aggregate is not necessarily spherical. Indeed, it is more common for the cells to be arranged in a linear, Y-shaped, or cigar-shaped array.

After the first 3 or 4 days of colony growth, the cells in most normal hemopoietic colonies begin to disperse. Some normal colonies can continue to grow as tightly packed aggregates, but this is a relatively uncommon growth pattern. However, in cultures of some types of neoplastic hemopoietic cells, e.g., plasmacytomas, the formation of tight colonies is more common.

The different patterns formed by dispersing colony cells give rise to an almost infinite variety of colony shapes, and this variability is one of the fascinations of working with cultures of this type. In most cases, colonies remain roughly spherical in shape and may either retain a tight central region or the whole colony may become a uniformly dispersed cloud of cells. Less commonly, dispersion of cells occurs early, then ceases, giving rise to the spectacular multiple colonies made of irregularly shaped groups of tight cell aggregates. As shall be discussed in some detail later, progressive dispersion of colony cells can cause colonies to no longer be apparent to the eye against a background of dispersed single cells. This can become a real problem in scoring cultures of human marrow cells.

If an enlarging colony comes into contact with the upper or lower surface of the gel, the colony often develops as a flat, two-dimensional circular aggregate, and if the colony contains macrophages, these cells can become firmly adherent to the bottom of the culture dish and become stellate in shape.

Mitotic activity tends to be highest early in colony formation and to progressively decline with time due (1) to maturation of an increasing proportion of colony cells to postmitotic cells, and (2) to progressive deterioration of the culture medium. In most of the culture systems using normal hemopoietic cells, mitotic activity and colony growth cease after 7–14 days of incubation, and death of colony cells follows shortly after.

B. Asynchronous Onset of Proliferation

Not all hemopoietic cells potentially capable of proliferating in a particular type of culture commence proliferation simultaneously. In fact, it is quite characteristic that there is a linear increase with time in the number of such cells that have commenced proliferation. Thus, with granulocyte and macrophage colony formation by mouse marrow cells, there is a lag period of 16 h followed by a progressive increase with time in the number of colony-forming cells that commence proliferation during the next 3–5 days [82, 83] (Fig. 3). Similarly in B-lymphocyte colony formation by mouse cells, a lag of 24 h occurs followed again by a progressive rise with time in the number of proliferating cells [28].

The mechanisms responsible for this phenomenon have not been characterized. In the case of granulocytic and macrophage colony formation by mouse cells, most of the colony-forming cells are in active cell cycle when the cells are removed from the body for culture, and selective killing of the cells in the S phase of the cell cycle does not alter the basic asynchrony of the initiation process [84]. A cell cycle-based delay of some cells entering mitosis is therefore unable to account for the asynchrony in initiation of proliferation. Furthermore, the resting period involved for some cells is up to 4–5 days which is much longer than the probable total cell cycle time for such cells *in vivo* (approximately 12–15 h).

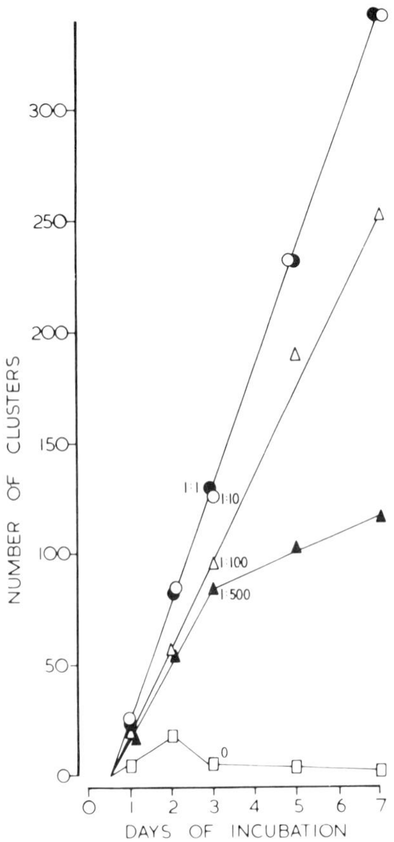

Fig. 3. The asynchronous initiation of proliferation of GM-colonies and clusters in cultures of mouse bone marrow cells. Note the progressive increase with time in the number of cells that have commenced proliferation and the fact that increasing concentrations of GM-CSF shorten this lag period. (From METCALF, [83]. Reproduced with permission from J. Cellular Physiology)

In all tissue culture systems there is a lag period between removal of cells from the body and commencement of proliferation in vitro which may represent a time interval during which the cells adjust to the abnormal in vitro environment. However, it is not explicable at present why this adaption process should exhibit such asynchrony, since in other culture systems, e.g., in liquid cultures of lymphocytes stimulated by phytohemagglutinin, no such asynchrony in the initiation of proliferation is observed. The average length of the lag period can be shortened to some extent by increasing the concentration of the specific regulator, e.g., GM-CSF for initiation of granulocytic and macrophage colony formation [83] (Fig. 3), but the onset of cell proliferation remains asynchronous.

The situation with neoplastic hemopoietic cells has not been studied as extensively, but there also appears to be a superficially similar asynchrony in initiation of proliferation by leukemic cells. However, in line with the greater uniformity in size of colonies formed by some leukemic populations, the duration of the period of asynchronous initiation of proliferation seems to be shorter than for normal cells.

C. Homogeneity and the Clonal Nature of Colonies

It is the most striking feature of all the semisolid culture systems for hemopoietic cells that colonies are composed of pure populations of cells of only one lineage. For example, in cultures supporting both erythroid and granulocytic colony formation, colonies are composed either wholly of erythropoietic cells or wholly granulopoietic cells but never a mixture, even though the two types of colonies may be adjacent to one another in the culture dish. There is one notable exception to this rule: most neutrophilic granulocytic colonies eventually contain two populations of cells — granulocytes and macrophages.

When more than one stimulating factor is present in a culture of marrow cells, the fact that individual adjacent colonies are composed wholly of cells of a single type suggests strongly: (1) that colonies are clones, each derived from a single cell, and (2) that the progeny of colony-forming cells are genetically predetermined to remain in the same pathway of differentiation. As shall be discussed in following chapters, the progeny of individual colony-forming cells can exhibit a remarkable degree of homogeneity and colony populations provide overwhelming evidence of the influence of somatic genotypic influences in hemopoiesis.

Several lines of evidence indicate that colonies are clones derived from *single* colony-forming cells:

1. For neutrophilic and macrophage colonies, micromanipulated single colony-forming cells from monkey marrow have been shown to give rise to colonies, some of which can be a mixture of both granulocytes and macrophages [43].
2. Time-lapse photography of erythroid colonies developing from mouse fetal liver cells has documented that each colony arises from a single cell (Axelrad, A. A., personal communication).
3. For B-lymphocyte colonies, analysis of the cells in individual colonies for membrane immunoglobulin and their capacity to bind to specific haptens has indicated that colonies are clones whose members have a uniform pattern of membrane immunoglobulin and a uniform capacity to bind specific haptens [28].
4. Cells isolated physically in the culture dish, e.g., by plastic rings, have been shown to be able to generate granulocytic and macrophage colonies [6].

Table 2. Origin of colonies and clusters from single light density cells from patients with CML

Patient	% Myeloblasts in light density fraction	Number of light density cells per culture dish	Total number of clusters and colonies per culture dish
O'K	75%	199	185 ± 27
		397	405 ± 50
CO	85%	390	324 ± 70
		780	456 ± 120

Both patients had CML. Peripheral blood cells were fractionated by centrifugation through BSA of density 1.062 g/cm^3. Supernatant light density cells were cultured in the presence of 0.1 ml human placental-conditioned medium or on underlayers of monkey peripheral blood white cells.

5. Regression coefficients for the titration curves of colony numbers versus the number of cells cultured have provided strong indirect evidence that colonies arise from individual cells [4, 6].
6. Because of the high plating efficiency of hemopoietic cells in agar, in certain situations the number of discrete colonies or clusters developing equals the number of cells cultured, again indicating that individual colonies must have arisen from single cells. An example of this situation is seen in cultures of light density fractions from the blood of patients with CML where every cell can be capable of forming a colony or cluster (METCALF, D. and KOLBER, S., unpublished data, Table 2).

D. Cloning Efficiency of Hemopoietic Colony-Forming Cells

As has just been mentioned, the cloning efficiency of hemopoietic colony-forming cells appears to be very high in the few systems which have so far been analyzed. It should be realized that colony formation by hemopoietic cells is a *primary* culture system, and experience with primary cultures of other types of cells has suggested that a cloning efficiency efficiency of 1% might be a quite reasonable expectation.

Many authors use the term "cloning or plating efficiency" incorrectly and usually with reference simply to the *frequency* of a cell per 100 or 1000 starting cells. However, the term refers specifically to the efficiency with which cells of a known, *uniform* type are able to grow in vitro.

The hemopoietic tissues contain such a mixture of unrelated cells that cloning efficiencies of particular colony-forming cells cannot possibly be estimated from cultures of unfractionated cells. Only when fractionation procedures have produced a purified, homogenous, starting population of colony-forming cells can the question of "cloning efficiency" be raised. Of course, if the cloning efficiency of such an apparently homogeneous population turns out to be very low, it might be that the population still contains a mixture of cells (albeit of the same morphology) embracing several subpopulations, only one of which is able to grow in vitro. For this reason, estimates of plating efficiency usually tend to be underestimates.

In several situations with hemopoietic cells, a minimum estimate can be made of plating efficiency of colony-forming cells, and the estimates indicate a very high plating efficiency, possibly approaching 100%:

1. In cultures of light density cells from monkey bone marrow where there was known size and cell cycle heterogeneity, one cell in three was able to form a colony or cluster. With micromanipulated single cells, the results indicated a plating efficiency of 70–110% [43].
2. Cultures of light density fractions from patients with CML indicated in some cases a plating efficiency of approximately 100% for colony and cluster formation (see Table 2).
3. In unfractioned spleen and lymph node cultures, approximately one cell in 30 can form a colony and once cell in six a cluster. This plating efficiency of at least 15% can be doubled since the colony-forming cells are known to have properties of B-lymphocytes and less than half the spleen or lymph node populations are B-lymphocytes [28].

Estimates of plating efficiency are important to establish since in each colony-forming system, colony-forming cells are only a minority or a small minority of the cells cultured. If, for example, one cell in 1000 marrow cells forms a colony, it is important to know exactly what this means. Was only one colony-forming cell present or were more present but inhibited by other cells in the culture dish? Such questions become particularly important where widely divergent frequencies of colony and cluster-forming cells are encountered in cultures of marrow cells from patients with various diseases.

Leukemic populations, even transplantable leukemias, are by no means uniform in their capacity to proliferate in agar cultures. In some situations, for example, with patients with CML, the plating efficiency is almost uniformly high. However, with other leukemias, few cells are able to form colonies or clusters. It has yet to be established whether this indicates a genuinely low frequency of colony or cluster-forming cells in these latter leukemias or simply a low plating efficiency due to unsatisfactory culture conditions or the action of inhibitory cells.

E. Variation in Size and Shape of Colonies and Clusters

It is a characteristic feature of all normal hemopoietic colonies that there is a gross variation in the size and shape of colonies, even between colonies of one morphological type, and in fact colonies can vary in size from 50 to 5000 cells (Fig. 4). While some of this heterogeneity can be ascribed to the asynchronous onset of proliferation of colony-forming cells, size

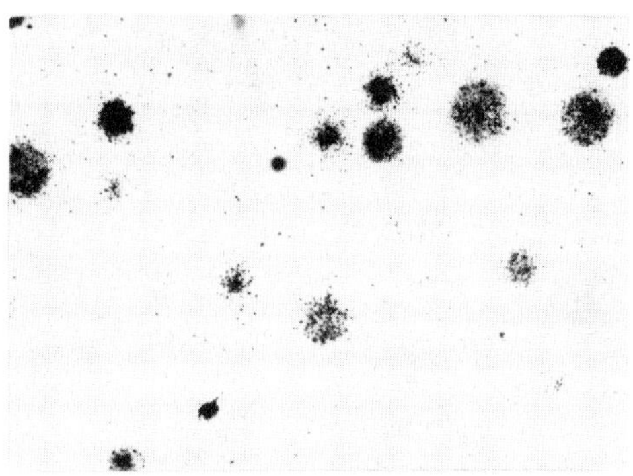

Fig. 4. Portion of an unstained culture of mouse bone marrow showing granulocytic and/or macrophage (GM) colonies of varying size and shape. (From METCALF and BRADLEY [221]. Reproduced with permission of Appleton-Century-Crofts)

heterogeneity persists even on extended incubation of the cultures. Cessation of growth of homopoietic colonies is associated with maturation to nondividing end cells and in some cases to death of colony cells. Conversely, progressive growth of colonies indicates the occurrence of cell divisions in which a significant proportion of the progeny remains capable of division. As shall be discussed later, cell division in colonies is dependent on the concentration of specific regulators and the degree of responsiveness of colony-forming cells to such regulators.

Consideration of these various factors indicates that individual colony-forming cells, even within one hemopoietic subpopulation, must vary (1) in their capacity to proliferate, i.e., in the number of cell divisions of which they are capable, and (2) in their level of responsiveness to a given concentration of stimulating factor. Confirmation of the intrinsic heterogeneity of colony-forming cells with respect to capacity for proliferation and responsiveness to stimulation has come from the demonstration that cells can be segregated by physical methods into subpopulations with distinctive characteristics [36]. Since the variability between colony-forming cells is detectable by observation of the colonies finally generated by these cells, it follows that the progeny of the colony-forming cells must, to some degree, continue to exhibit the particular traits of the parent colony-forming cell. However, no analyses have yet been reported on the variability or otherwise of cells within a developing colony with respect to proliferative capacity or responsiveness.

The growth pattern in vitro of cells from tissue culture-adapted transplantable hemopoietic tumors is quite different from that of normal hemopoietic cells. Cells from animals with transplanted plasmacytomas, lymphoid leukemias, or myeloid leukemias that are able to proliferate in agar generate colonies of much more uniform size and morphology than those generated by normal cells (see Fig. 5). Since most such tumors are probably clonal populations derived from single cells, this difference in growth pattern possibly provides

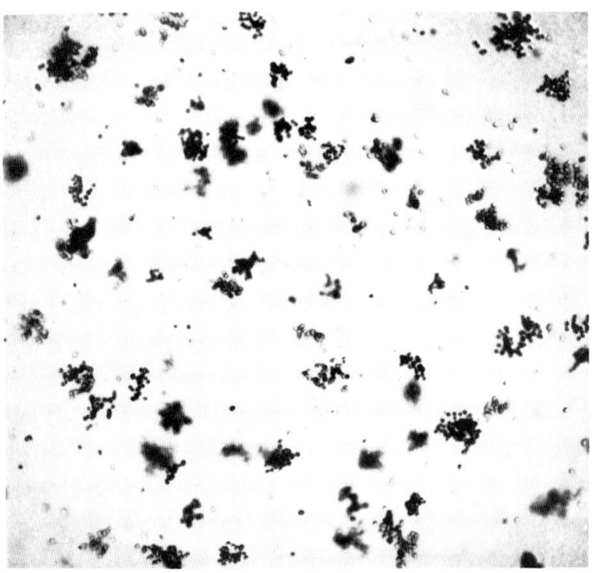

Fig. 5. A culture of mouse lymphoid leukemic cells showing the development of a large number of colonies of relatively uniform size and appearance

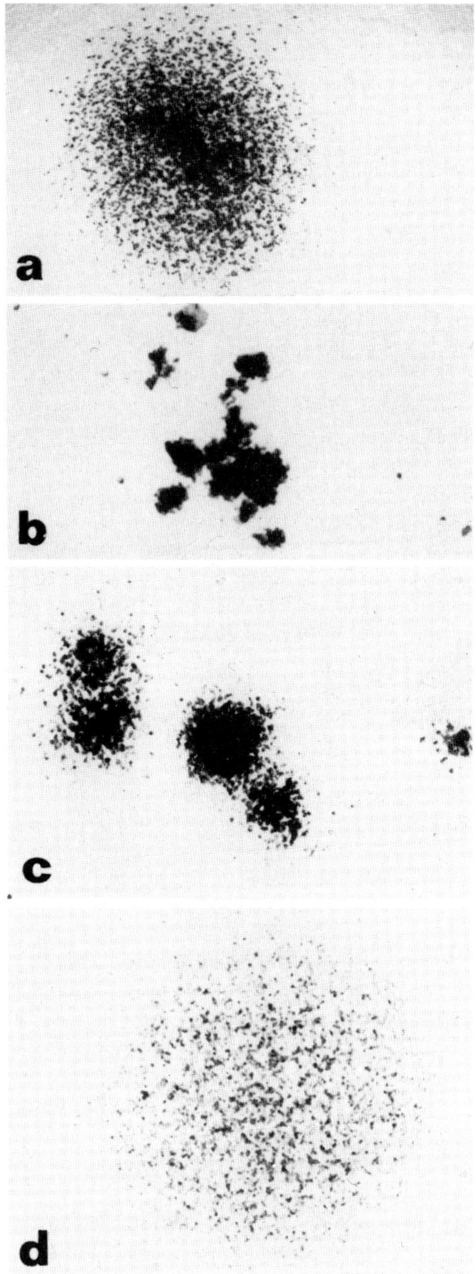

Fig. 6a–d. Varying shape of 7-day colonies formed by mouse bone marrow cells. (a) a granulocytic colony, and (b) a multiple granulocytic colony, both stimulated by mouse lung-conditioned medium, (c) four macrophage colonies stimulated by human urine, (d) an eosinophil colony stimulated by mouse lymphocyte-conditioned medium. (From METCALF [133]. Reproduced with permission of Cold Spring Harbor Laboratory)

supporting evidence for the conclusion that the variability in normal colonies is the phenotypic expression of somatic genetic differences between normal hemopoietic cells. On the other hand, the uniformity of growth patterns seen in cultures of established tumor lines may simply reflect selection pressures occurring during the initiation and maintenance of such transplantable tumor lines both in vivo and in vitro. In this context, it is noteworthy that leukemic cells, taken directly from patients with CML (a monoclonal disease) generate colonies which have the same variability in size and shape as those generated by normal human marrow cells.

In addition to size variation, some types of normal hemopoietic colonies exhibit a marked variation in shape. Thus, with granulocytic colonies grown from normal mouse marrow, colonies may be multicentric aggregates of cells, single spherical type aggregates, single aggregates with a tight center and a loose outer mantle of cells, or loosely dispersed aggregates of uniformly dispersed cells (Fig. 6). The basis for this extraordinary variability in shape is explained in part by an examination of the differentiation of the cells comprising the colonies. For example, when granulocytic colony cells differentiate to polymorphs, the mature cells appear to have a greater mobility than more immature cells and are capable of considerable migration in the surrounding agar. Widely dispersed granulocytic colonies are usually found to be composed of polymorphs and metamyelocytes. Conversely, colonies composed wholly of early stage granulocytic cells are usually compact in shape. It is not clearly established whether differentiation precedes dispersion of colony cells or whether random centrifugal movement of colony cells precipitates differentiation, but the former possibility seems more likely.

The formation of multicentric tight granulocytic colonies is caused by an early separation of individual cells in the developing colonies, but it is unknown why this process of separation fails to continue during subsequent divisions, leading to a single loose aggregate of cells rather than to several dispersed aggregates of tightly packed cells. Such multiple colonies are seen in cultures of mouse bone marrow cells stimulated by very high GM-CSF concentrations [36].

F. Cluster Formation

A minimum of 50 cells is usually designated as the lower size limit for normal hemopoietic colonies. In most of the culture systems, it is characteristic that, in addition to colonies, more numerous aggregates of smaller size develop in the cultures. These aggregates are termed "clusters," and, as is the case with colonies, cluster size is again heterogeneous [82].

Two general explanations are possible to account for the development of clusters: (1) colony and cluster-forming cells may be a homogeneous single population and the difference in the population size of the progeny generated may be due simply to the operation of stochastic processes leading to end-cell differentiation and cessation of further growth, or (2) cluster-forming cells may differ from colony-forming cells although belonging to the same family of hemopoietic cells. The latter interpretation would suggest that although the two populations are definably different (on the basis of proliferative capacity), they are in fact related populations.

In most systems, clusters outnumber colonies by 5–10:1 and the ratio of cluster-forming cells to colony-forming cells in a tissue tends to parallel the general proliferative activity of the colony-forming cells. In at least one tissue, the mouse bone marrow, GM-cluster-forming cells

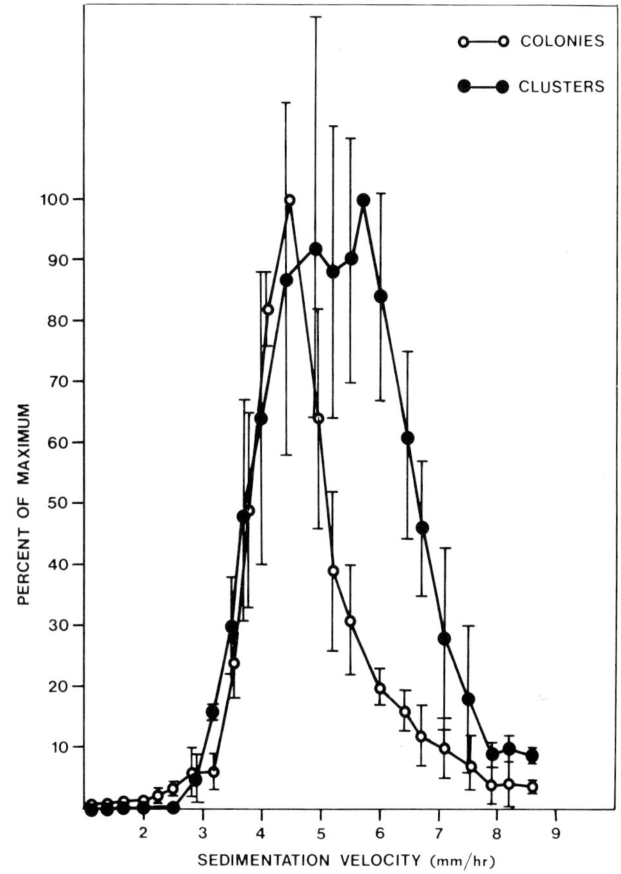

Fig. 7. Velocity sedimentation separation of C57BL mouse bone marrow cells showing that the cells forming GM-clusters sediment more rapidity than the cells forming GM-colonies. Mean data from five experiments, vertical bars are standard deviations. (From METCALF and MACDONALD [36]. Reproduced with permission from J. Cellular Physiology)

have been shown to be larger cells than colony-forming cells, and the two can be partially segregated by velocity sedimentation separation [36] (Fig. 7). However, in other properties, e.g., buoyant density or cell cycle status, the two populations resemble one another.

At least in the granulocyte-macrophage system, the most reasonable interpretation of the nature of cluster-forming cells appears to be that most are the immediate progeny of colony-forming cells. It should be emphasized, however, that this interpretation may not necessarily be true in other situations. In one special instance, that of AML in humans, the leukemic cells are usually capable only of cluster formation [85]. This contrasts with the situation in CML where the leukemic cells are able to form both colonies and clusters. It cannot be assumed from these observations that AML cells are derived from more mature cells than CML cells. AML cells are clearly abnormal and their capacity for only limited proliferation in agar does not, by itself, permit any conclusions regarding the state of differentiation of the leukemic cells in comparison either with CML or normal granulopoietic populations.

G. Differentiation in Colonies

One of the most striking features of normal hemopoietic colonies in vitro is the progressive differentiation of colony cells as the colonies age. This differentiation is apparent from the progressive loss of the capacity to proliferate, the change in morphology of the colony cells, and the acquisition of specialized functional activities and cell surface markers. Indices of differentiation so far recorded in hemopoietic colonies are listed in Table 3.

Although colony cells usually differentiate to the stage where they can readily be identified on simple morphological grounds, it must be emphasized that differentiation is rarely as complete in agar cultures as in vivo. Thus, the nuclear morphology of polymorphs may be normal, but their cytoplasmic content of neutrophilic granules is subnormal [85]; eosinophil granules fail to develop the crystalline structures indicating full maturation [75]; the cytoplasm of megakaryocytes often does not develop clearly demarcated budding platelets [20, 88]; maturing B-lymphocytes do not lose their cytoplasmic basophilia, and maturing plasma cells do not develop the highly organized lamellar system of rough endoplasmic reticulum characteristic of end-stage plasma cells in vivo [28].

The reasons why colony maturation stops short of completion in vitro are not known, but because of the many cell types involved, it is tempting to speculate that a single common mechanism may be involved. While this might be the absence of some hormone, factor, or metabolite in vitro, a simpler explanation is that death may occur prematurely in most cells attempting to differentiate in vitro, thus preventing completion of the process.

The development of morphological and functional signs of maturation is usually paralleled by a progressive loss of the capacity to proliferate. This correlation is of course familiar in vivo but might not necessarily have held true in vitro. However, observations suggest that cessation of proliferation is as closely linked in colony cells with the acquisition of specialized morphology and function, as is true of corresponding hemopoietic populations in vivo.

Table 3. Indices of differentiation in hemopoietic colony cells in vitro

Type of colony	Morphological changes	Special functions	Cell surface markers
Granulocytic-macrophage	Polymorphs—granules [31] Macrophages — excentric nucleus and vacuolated cytoplasm [72]	Peroxidase positive granules [31, 86] Phagocytosis adherence [72, 87]	Fc receptors [74] C3 receptors [74]
Erythropoietic	Normoblasts and enucleated cells [8]	Hemoglobin synthesis [8]	—
Eosinophilic	Eosinophil granules [19, 75]		Fc receptors [74]
Megakaryocytic	Giant size, multilobulate nucleus [20]	Shedding of platelets [88] Acetylcholinesterase [20]	—
B-lymphocytes	Maturing plasma cells and lymphocytes [28]	Immunoglobulin and antibody synthesis [28]	Fc receptors [28] I^a Membrane IgM, IgG_{2a} [28]
T-lymphocytes	Maturing lymphocytes		Sheep red cell rosettes [29] (Thy-1) antigen [89]

The clear evidence that differentiation occurs in normal hemopoietic colonies in vitro makes it possible to ask certain questions of leukemic cells proliferating in similar cultures. Does the division of leukemic cells ultimately cease in vitro? Is this linked with morphological or functional evidence of differentiation? Is the differentiation normal or abnormal, and what factors induced differentiation? These questions will be discussed in detail in the relevant chapters, but as a generalization, it can be said that the cells in leukemic colonies can exhibit some degree of differentiation. Depending on the leukemic population, this differentiation can also be linked with a restriction in the capacity to proliferate, and both can be manipulated experimentally.

It must of course be emphasized that the capacity of some leukemic cells to differentiate in vitro is not particularly novel since the same leukemic populations can usually differentiate in vivo to nondividing end cells. However, the fact that the processes can be manipulated experimentally during colony formation makes the semisolid culture systems very useful methods for analyzing the mechanisms controlling such leukemic cell differentiation.

It was initially hoped that the situation with hemopoietic colonies might be similar to that existing with fibroblasts, where transformed or neoplastic colonies are readily distinguishable from normal colonies because of loss of contact inhibition and the consequent heaping up of colony cells. One of the minor disappointments of the development of hemopoietic cloning systems for normal and leukemic cells has been the realization that by gross morphology, leukemic colonies are usually not distinguishable from normal colonies. Certain exceptions to this generalization will be discussed in subsequent chapters.

H. Asynchrony of Differentiation

Although progressive differentiation usually occurs in the cell populations in most colonies, this process develops asynchronously. Except in colonies sampled very early or very late in the culture period, most colonies contain a mixture of cells at varying stages of differentiation. Furthermore, colonies composed of undifferentiated cells may develop adjacent to colonies of fully differentiated end cells.

The implications from these facts are similar to those which can be drawn from the heterogeneity of individual adjacent colonies. Since the cells in any one colony are bathed in the same nutrients or regulatory factors, the events permitting or forcing individual cells to differentiate must either be entirely stochastic or determined by the genetic preprograming of individual cells. Unlike the situation in some tissues, e.g., skin or testis, there is no obvious stratification of differentiating cells in colonies such as concentric layers of more differentiated cells. Similarly, differentiated cells do not occur as distinct aggregates within a colony.

However, there are two situations in which some regional segregation of differentiated colonies is observed: (1) in many granulocytic colonies, a tight central region of relatively undifferentiated cells is surrounded by a loose outer mantle of metamyelocytes and polymorphs, and (2) in mixed granulocytic and macrophage colonies, it is common to observe that the tight central region is composed only of granulocytes, while the loose outer mantle contains most of the macrophages. As described earlier, both of these situations may arise simply from the great mobility in agar of polymorphs or macrophages. Thus, the observed regional segregation may be the result of differentiation and not the result of a gradient of some differentiating factor emanating from the center of the colony. However, the possible existence of microgradients generated within colonies has not been definitely excluded.

I. Role of Specific Stimulating Factors in Colony Formation

1. Survival of Colony-Forming Cells

While some cells such as human polymorphs or macrophages from most species appear capable of prolonged survival in agar cultures, in general, hemopoietic cells survive for only short periods in such cultures unless the specific factor required to stimulate their proliferation is present in the culture in adequate concentrations.

This rule applies particularly to the hemopoietic progenitor cells initially generating colonies in vitro. Observations have shown, for example, that most GM-colony-forming cells either die or permanently lose their capacity to proliferate if cultured for more than 24 h in cultures lacking GM-CSF [83] (Fig. 8). Similarly, transfer of developing colonies to cultures lacking GM-CSF is followed almost immediately by cessation of proliferation and usually by premature death of the colony cells [78, 79].

This has suggested to some that these so-called "stimulating factors" are in fact nothing more than "survival" factors that are necessary to allow survival in vitro. In this hypothesis, progenitor cells and their progeny are envisaged as being capable of autonomous proliferation without the provision of anything other than nutrient building blocks and energy sources.

Because of the dose-response relationships observed between the concentration of stimulating factors and the degree of proliferation, this survival hypothesis is improbable, but it is difficult to design experiments to positively exclude such a possibility.

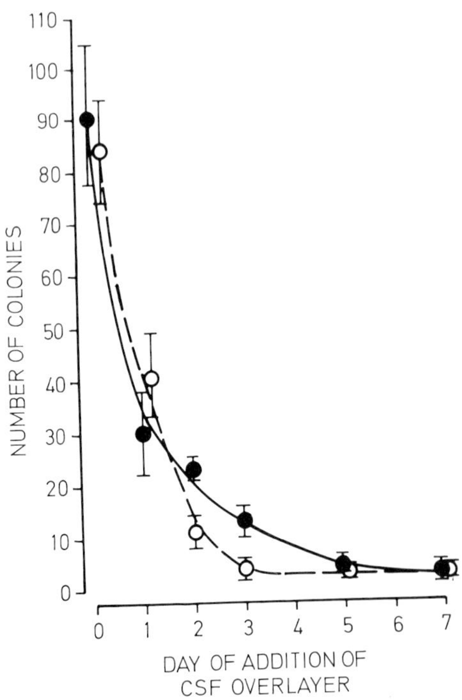

Fig. 8. Decreasing numbers of GM-colonies developing when mouse marrow cells are incubated in agar 0–7 days before addition of an overlayer containing GM-CSF. Two separate experiments. Mean data and standard deviations of six cultures at each time point. (From METCALF [83]. Reproduced with permission from J. Cellular Physiology)

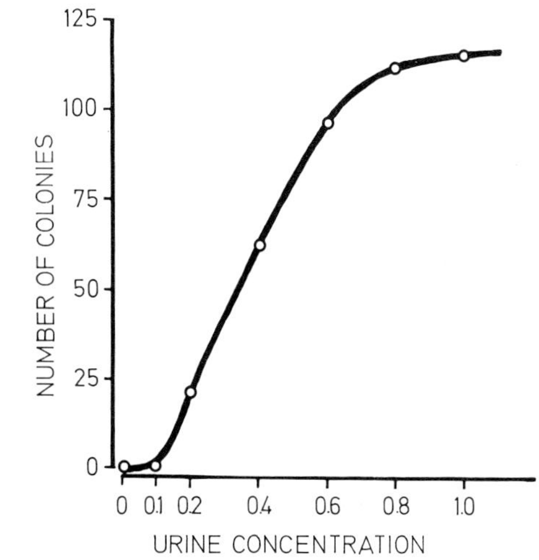

Fig. 9. Sigmoid dose response relationship in cultures of mouse bone marrow between the concentration of human urine GM-CSF and the number of GM-colonies developing. (From METCALF and MOORE [30]. Reproduced with permission of North-Holland, Amsterdam)

The situation is not unique for cultures of hemopoietic cells. For example, cultured neurones also will not survive in vitro in the absence of nerve growth factor (NGF) (90). Possibly the best evidence for the nature of stimulating factors comes from observations in vivo on correlations between factor levels and the level of proliferative activity of the specific target cells and particularly on the effects of injected stimulating factors. Thus, NGF or erythropoietin, when injected in vivo, produce the same type of growth stimulation as observed in vitro. If it is then argued that cells cannot survive in vivo without a specific stimulating (survival) factor, the question becomes merely semantic and could then be extended to whole organs or the organism itself.

2. *Proliferation of Colony-Forming Cells*

Colony formation by normal hemopoietic cells is completely dependent on the presence of adequate concentrations of the specific stimulating factor in the culture medium.

Hemopoietic colony formation therefore simultaneously permits two types of application: (1) it provides a method of enumerating hemopoietic progenitor cells, and (2) it detects and provides a method for assaying specific growth-stimulating (colony-stimulating) factors operating on hemopoietic populations.

In the following chapters dealing with specific types of colonies, apparent examples of factor-independent colony formation by normal cells will be discussed. At this stage, the situation can be summarized by stating that none of these is a genuine example of factor-independent proliferation, and all hemopoietic colony formation appears to be dependent on specific factors, operating in a highly selective manner on the appropriate target cell population.

As might be anticipated, there are dose-response relationships between the concentration of a particular factor and the number and size of the colonies developing. In Figure 9 is shown a dose-response curve for the relationship between the concentration of GM-CSF in the culture and the number of granulocytic and macrophage colonies developing. This sigmoid curve is characteristic of the relationship between specific stimulating factor and colony formation for all types of hemopoietic cells. In its central region there is a linear relationship between concentration and colony numbers which permits assays to be performed on the concentrations of the factor by counting the number of colonies developing. At low factor concentrations, the relationship departs from linearity, and abnormally low numbers of colonies develop. As will be discussed later, this is in part due to the heterogeneity of colony-forming cells with respect to their responsiveness to stimulation by various concentrations of the factor. As the factor concentration is decreased, progressively fewer of the less responsive cells will be stimulated. In part, however, the abrupt loss of colony-stimulating activity at low factor concentrations is due to the use of an arbitrary minimum size for colonies. The proliferation of aggregates of subcolony size is still factor-dependent but is not scorable because of the size limit restriction.

As factor concentrations are increased to the point where all available progenitor cells have been stimulated to proliferate, the number of resulting colonies reaches a plateau level. In early studies on both granulopoietic and erythropoietic colony formation in vitro, it was observed that colony numbers fell progressively as factor concentrations were increased beyond those stimulating plateau colony numbers ("high dose inhibition"). For a time, this raised the possibility that colony-forming cells might exhibit a biphasic responsiveness to specific stimulating factors and actually be inhibited by very high factor concentrations. However, subsequent work has excluded this possibility by showing that the inhibition observed was an artifact due to the use of impure preparations of stimulating factors which contained inhibitory or toxic contaminating material.

One early possible explanation of the observed relationship between the amount of stimulating factor added and the number of colonies developing was that colony formation was dependent on the total *amount* of stimulating factor in the culture dish rather than the *concentration*. Experiments have shown, however, that colony formation is related to the concentration, not the total amount, of factor present in the culture. Indeed, assays for residual factor in cultures containing fully developed colonies have shown that relatively little of the factor is actually consumed or broken down during colony development [83].

In all cases so far analyzed (GM, eosinophil, and B-lymphocyte colony formation), the stimulating factor must be present *continuously* from the time of initiation of the cultures. Withdrawal of the stimulating factor from the developing colony immediately causes cessation of proliferation, and death of colony cells follows. The implication is that the stimulus is not simply a trigger initiating, or completing, the first cell cycle of the colony-forming cell. The exact molecular basis for a continuous proliferative stimulus of this type has never been investigated. Only low molar concentrations of the factors are involved (around 10^{-11}M), and these factors are macromolecular glycoproteins.

Both erythropoietin and GM-CSF have a very rapid action on target cells, stimulating RNA synthesis within minutes [91, 92]. Noncycling cells can be stimulated by GM-CSF to enter the S phase of the cell cycle within 3 h [93], but an action on protein synthesis is relatively delayed. None of these observations provides an adequate explanation of the continuous requirement for the factor but suggest that if the factor is removed, these vital functions of the target cells might cease or decline equally rapidly leading to cessation of proliferation. Until reliable radiolabeled preparations of each purified factor are available, it is not possible to determine whether the factor binds to the target cell, whether it enters the cell and whether it is degraded or utilized by the target cell during the stimulation process.

In addition to the clear relationship between the concentration of stimulating factor and colony numbers, there is an equally obvious relationship between size of such colonies and factor concentration [95] (Fig. 10). Since colonies arise from single cells and colony size is

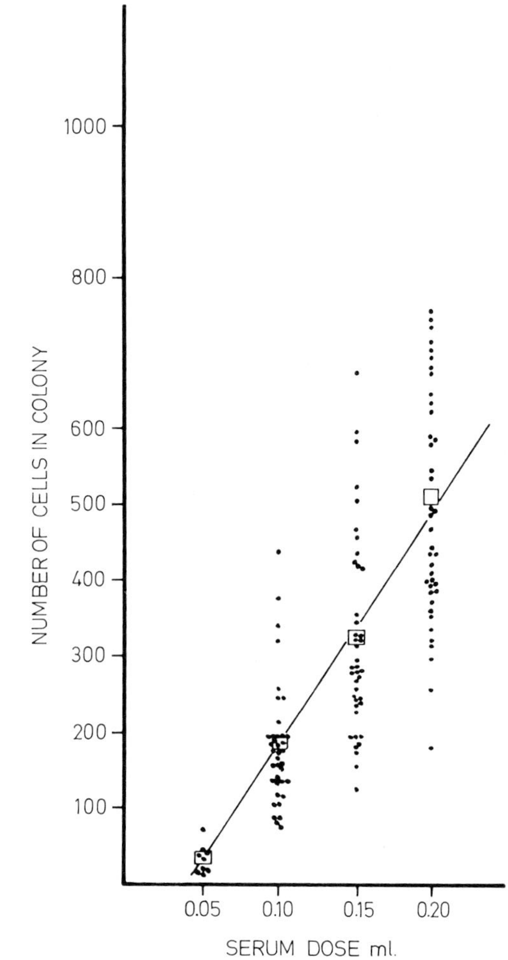

Fig. 10. Effect of increasing concentration of mouse serum GM-CSF on size of GM-colonies at 7 days of incubation in cultures of mouse bone marrow cells. (From ROBINSON et al [95]. Reproduced with permission from J. Cellular Physiology)

assessed at a fixed time point, e.g., 7 days after initiation of the cultures, several possibilities might account for this observed relationship: (1) stimulating factors may shorten cell cycle times in dividing colony cells, (2) stimulating factors may influence the differentiation of colony cells and at high concentrations permit or force cells to remain relatively undifferentiated and capable of further divisions, or (3) stimulating factors may permit better survival of colony cells and thus allow colony size to increase at a more rapid rate than if the increase in colony cell numbers was being eroded continuously by death of colony cells.
Observations on GM-colony formation by mouse bone marrow cells have shown that all of these possibilities occur although (2) may be the most important single process in the development of a very large colony at high GM-CSF concentrations. Mean cell cycle times were observed to be shortened from 17 h to 12 h by increasing GM-CSF concentrations [81]. However, colonies grown in the presence of high GM-CSF concentrations always contained a high proportion of myeloblasts and myelocytes, and conversely with very low CSF concentrations, granulocytic colonies at 7 days were usually composed only of metamyelo-

cytes and polymorphs. In general, the largest colonies tend to have the highest proportion of cells still capable of division. By causing colony cells to remain relatively undifferentiated, high concentrations of the stimulating factor tend to permit an almost geometric expansion of colony numbers. Any tendency in this direction will ultimately have a much greater impact on colony growth rates than a simple shortening of cell cycle times by a few hours. Finally, as mentioned earlier, GM-colony-forming cells cannot survive in vitro in the absence of GM-CSF, from which it can be extrapolated that in the presence of very low GM-CSF concentrations, early cell death may be more evident than with higher GM-CSF concentrations. It must be emphasized, however, that the relationship between colony growth rates and GM-CSF concentrations is clearly evident within 2 or 3 days of initiation of cultures. At this time, no cell death has occurred in any colonies, so cell death can be only a minor determinant of the differing colony growth rates as seen in the usual culture dish.

J. Duration of Proliferation in Colonies

In most of the culture systems using semisolid medium, colony growth ceases between 7 and 14 days of incubation. Cessation of colony growth is usually associated with evidence that colony cells have matured to nondividing forms. However, some caution needs to be exercised in concluding that the degree of proliferation exhibited before end-cell differentiation is an accurate reflection of the full capacity of these cells for proliferation in vivo.

As described earlier, these culture systems do not employ changes of fresh medium, and it is quite possible that a significant depletion of essential nutrients and accumulation of toxic products can occur in cultures containing large numbers of actively growing colonies. Several observations support this possibility: (1) in overcrowded cultures of granulocytic and macrophage colonies, colony size can actually be smaller than in less crowded cultures even using the same concentrations of the stimulating factor, (2) in crowded cultures of B-lymphocyte colonies, catastrophic death of colonies can occur suddenly at about the 7th day of incubation, a phenomenon not seen in less crowded cultures, and (3) in cultures containing suboptimal FCS, colony growth can cease prematurely, but those colony cells which are present appear to differentiate to normal end cells.

It is generally true that colony formation by hemopoietic cells in agar has proved that hemopoietic cells have a much greater capacity for proliferation than was envisaged in models based on analysis of labeling data in vivo. However, it would be unwise to accept the present types of colony as necessarily reflecting the maximum capacity of these cells for proliferation. Even the best culture system now in use may be grossly suboptimal, and future improvements may show that these cells, under better conditions, can have an even higher capacity for proliferation. Furthermore, few attempts have so far been made to repassage or reclone colony cells in fresh medium, procedures which might also reveal a capacity for further proliferation than is normally observed.

Two comments need to be made regarding models of hemopoiesis. It is generally assumed in such models that cells of a particular differentiation stage, e.g., colony-forming cells or myeloblasts, have a uniform and limited capacity for proliferation. Casual inspection of a single culture dish of marrow cells makes this assumption untenable since no two colonies have exactly the same size, and this size variability persists regardless of the stimulating or culture conditions. Finally, the amount of proliferation exhibited by individual cells can be varied enormously by altering the culture conditions and the concentration of the stimulating factor. Estimates made in vivo on the capacity of certain cells to proliferate suffer two severe restrictions: (1) a mean, or average, answer is being obtained from a population of known heterogeneity, and (2) the proliferative capacity is being assessed under one set of conditions and could well alter in response to changing circumstances. Observations on in vitro cultures have forcibly emphasized the heterogeneity of hemopoietic cells and the great flexibility of their proliferative capacity according to regulatory influences.

K. Autopotentiation of Colony Growth and Nonspecific Growth Factors

It is generally true of hemopoietic colonies growing in agar that the more crowded the culture the larger the average size of each colony. There is, however, a limit to this crowding effect, and when cultures become overcrowded, although initial proliferative activity may be high, it is usual to have premature and often very sudden death of all cells in the culture dish, presumably due either to depletion of essential metabolites or the production by the cells of lethal levels of toxic metabolites.

Potentiation of colony growth by crowding can be a very striking phenomenon. Equally striking is the capacity of certain batches of FCS or other sera either to support the formation of very large colonies or, at the other extreme, to actually inhibit colony formation. Both phenomena seem to have confused some workers regarding the difference between essential specific growth factors and equally essential, but nonspecific, growth factors.

It must be restated that in the absence of the specific growth factor, e.g., GM-CSF, no amount of cell crowding and no variation in the medium or serum used will result in the formation of a single hemopoietic colony. This statement holds true for all normal hemopoietic colonies. As shall be seen later, it is possible by culturing certain types of hemopoietic populations to actively produce specific factors in the culture dish. Under such conditions, apparently autonomous colony formation is observed. So far, analysis has shown, however, that in each case, colony formation still depended on the specific factor which was being produced endogenously within the culture dish.

Because colony counting is based on an arbitrary predetermined lower size limit for colonies (usually 50 cells), a phenomenon in which cell crowding affects colony size could theoretically result in nonlinearity between the number of cells cultured and the number of colonies developing. When very few cells are cultured, colonies developing may be too small to be classified as colonies, and conversely in crowded cultures, unusually good colony growth may permit some clusters to reach a sufficiently large size to be scored as colonies. As shall be seen, nonlinearity of colony formation is striking with B-lymphocyte colony formation and has been described for megakaryocyte colony formation. Fortunately, methods are available for minimizing this nonlinearity, which permits cultures to be used with more confidence to enumerate the frequency of colony-forming cells.

The addition of marrow or lymphoid cell suspensions to cultures has increased the size and number of colonies of such diverse types as granulocytic and macrophage, B-lymphocyte, and plasmacytoma cells. Because such cell suspensions contain a variety of different cells, it cannot be concluded that one cell type or its products is responsible for the potentiation of these different types of colony. Indeed, it is probable that a number of quite different biological processes could be occurring in different types of cultures or even in a single culture dish. Thus, in the case of granulocyte and macrophage colony formation, addition of marrow or lymphoid cells increases the size and to a lesser extent the number of colonies developing. Both marrow and lymphoid populations have been shown to be able to produce the specific regulator GM-CSF, and in some experimental designs, additional production of GM-CSF is certainly responsible for the potentiation observed. In other experimental designs where adequate levels of GM-CSF have already been added, the addition of even killed marrow or lymphoid cells can potentiate colony growth. It has been shown that the added marrow or lymphoid cells can provide nuclear material which is reutilized by the dividing colony cells, and this may be one mechanism responsible for the observed potentiation in this latter situation.

When the potentiating effects of crowding on colony formation were first observed, it was not clear whether the potentiation was coming from adjacent colony cells (autopotentiation) or from nonproliferating cells in the surrounding medium. Analysis showed that both occurred although, as just pointed out, the mechanisms involved may be very different.

It must be admitted that there are certain aspects of the influence of crowding or serum on colony formation which are difficult to explain in relation to the action of specific growth factors. For example, it is easy to show that the poor granulocyte and macrophage colony growth achieved in sparsely seeded cultures can be increased simply by increasing the concentration of the specific regulator GM-CSF. Similarly, with at least some batches of FCS that are apparently capable only of supporting poor colony growth, large colonies will develop if high GM-CSF concentrations are used. Do these observations imply that crowding effects are entirely mediated by GM-CSF? It may be, but other more complex explanations seem possible.

The old concept of feeder layers was based on the hypothesis that a multiplicity of essential metabolites leaked out of cells placed in culture medium. If sufficient cells were crowded together, an equilibrium was established between the entry and exit of such metabolites which maintained a sufficiently high intracellular level to permit survival and proliferation. Where cloning experiments necessitated the culture of only a single fibroblast, irradiated nonproliferating feeder layers were introduced to provide the necessary concentrations of intracellular metabolites.

In retrospect, one must now question the nature and specificity of these postulated metabolites. It is now possible to grow a colony from a single cultured granulocyte-macrophage colony-forming cell if GM-CSF is added to the culture medium. The implication is strong that the concept of general metabolite traffic was wrong and that what the feeder layers were in fact doing, in supporting growth by single cells, was producing a variety of specific regulators, one of which was the specific regulator needed by the cloned fibroblast. It may also be, however, that tissue culture media are not perfectly designed and can often be improved by a watery extract of living or dying cells. If so, there may well be some occasions on which additional cells or feeder layers improve the general nutrient levels in the medium used.

L. Serum Effects on Colony Formation

The variable effects of serum on hemopoietic colony formation in vitro can be seen even with a single type of colony formation if different sources of specific stimulating factor are used. In the example given in Table 4, GM-colony counts are listed for mouse bone marrow cultures grown in medium using FCS or one of a number of different human sera as the sole serum

Table 4. Influence of serum used in culture medium on capacity of two different GM-CSF-containing preparations to stimulate granulocyte and macrophage colony formation by mouse bone marrow cells

Serum used in preparation of medium	Mean number of colonies	
	Mouse lymphocyte-conditioned medium	Human placental-conditioned medium
FCS	20	0
Human serum No. 1	76	34
2	37	0
3	0	76
4	0	0
5	16	82
6	70	17
7	0	0
8	0	8
9	0	1
10	5	11
11	2	0
12	38	4
13	70	23
14	54	34
15	58	38
16	0	0

All cultures contained 75,000 C_{57}BL marrow cells. All media contained 20% FCS or human serum. GM-colony formation was stimulated by the addition of 0.1 ml of mouse lymphocyte-conditioned medium or human placental-conditioned medium containing GM-CSF. Colony counts were performed on day 7.

source. In this experiment, colony formation was stimulated by the addition either of mouse lymphocyte GM-CSF or human placental GM-CSF. It will be seen that almost every possible combination of results was obtained. Note that with the FCS (the standard culture system), it would have been concluded that human placental GM-CSF was without activity on mouse target cells, yet in cultures prepared using a number of the human sera, the results show clearly that this is not the case.

At present, the influence of the serum used in the medium on colony formation can rarely be predicted or explained and must always be checked carefully when each new experimental system is developed. Inability to control this serum variable presents problems for all the cloning techniques to be discussed and is the most common practical difficulty in performing such cultures.

M. Comment

Regardless of the cell type involved, hemopoietic colony formation by normal cells exhibits certain common characteristics which have been briefly reviewed. These colonies are characterized by the spectacular clonal purity of cell populations but at the same time striking heterogeneity in onset of proliferation, in colony size, and in the pattern of differentiation in individual colonies. The overall flexibility in the capacity of hemopoietic populations for proliferation has been clearly demonstrated by studies on colony growth and cannot be overemphasized.

The technical capacity which now exists to stimulate the formation of hemopoietic colonies using specific, chemically defined regulators offers hematologists and cell biologists in general an almost incredibly versatile series of culture systems capable of solving a wide variety of general questions regarding mammalian cells. The availability of morphological, surface, and radioisotopic markers for various hemopoietic cells confers on hemopoietic populations great advantages over the traditionally-used fibroblast for studies on many aspects of cell biology.

From the specific point of view of normal and abnormal hemopoiesis, the heterogeneity and complexity of agar cultures is at once a reassurance and a problem. Hemopoiesis in the intact animal is obviously a complex process, involving many differentiation stages of multiple but interrelated cell populations. Any culture system which purports to be able to duplicate such proliferative activity in vitro must of necessity reproduce much of the underlying complexity. The average agar culture of bone marrow cells certainly exhibits a high degree of complexity and heterogeneity but not a bewildering picture. The clonal nature of proliferating colonies provides a rare signpost through the complexity.

Since the cultures are simple to prepare in large numbers and are so highly responsive to added stimulating factors, it is clear that such cultures can be used to dissect the complexities of hemopoiesis. To do this successfully, the basic characteristics and limitations of the techniques must be clearly understood, and these have been presented in the foregoing discussion.

Chapter 5

Neutrophil and Macrophage Colony Formation by Normal Cells

This section will discuss mainly the formation by mouse cells of neutrophilic granulocytic and macrophage colonies, the first cloning system developed and the one about which most is known. Formation of granulocytic colonies by normal human cells will also be described. Techniques have been developed for obtaining comparable colony formation by monkey, dog, rat, rabbit, hamster, cat, and chicken marrow cells, but these will not be discussed in detail. For convenience hereafter "neutrophilic granulocytes" will be referred to simply as "granulocytes." Formation of eosinophilic colonies will be discussed in Chapter 8.

A. Origin, Location and Frequency of GM-Colony-Forming Cells (GM-CFC)

In the mouse, cells forming granulocytic and/or macrophage colonies (GM-CFC) are first detectable in the 8-day yolk sac. By the 10th day of gestation, GM-CFCs are demonstrable in the developing fetal liver, and as this organ rapidly increases in size, the number of GM-CFCs rises sharply, reaching maximum levels by days 13–14 [96, 30]. Despite the relatively large numbers of GM-CFCs in yolk sac and liver, it is of interest that the formation of mature granulocytes and monocytes is minimal in these organs during this period [97]. With the development of the spleen and bone marrow on days 16–18 of gestation, GM-CFCs appear in these organs and levels rise progressively.

Culture of intact embryos with or without attached yolk sac showed that the appearance of GM-CFCs was dependent on migration into the embryo of CFUs and/or GM-CFCs from the yolk sac [96]. Since there is strong evidence that all hemopoietic tissues in embryonic and adult life are derived from the stem cells (CFUs) of the yolk sac, it can be presumed that the appearance of GM-CFCs in the bone marrow and spleen is dependent on a similar migration into these anlagen of CFUs and possibly GM-CFCs. It is likely that most of these are derived from the large pool of cells in the fetal liver, but no direct evidence exists to support this possibility. As shall be discussed later, there is now some evidence to suggest that the GM-CFCs in the yolk sac and early fetal liver may represent a distinct, primitive generation population not directly related to the cells in the late fetal liver or present in adult tissues.

Following birth, liver GM-CFCs fall rapidly to undetectable levels at 2 weeks of age. GM-CFCs rise progressively in the spleen and bone marrow reaching stable adult levels by 2–4 weeks of age. In the normal adult animal, GM-CFCs are restricted to the marrow and spleen, and small numbers are present also in the peripheral blood.

Although the adult liver lacks GM-CFCs, recent studies have shown that following injury, e.g., irradiation or partial resection, GM-CFCs can reappear temporarily in this organ together with other hemopoietic cells [98, 99].

In the adult $C_{57}BL$ mouse, the frequency of GM-CFCs, as assessed in standard cultures containing excess levels of GM-CSF, is 100–200 per 10^5 bone marrow cells, one to ten per 10^5

spleen cells, and about one per 10^5 nucleated cells in the peripheral blood. In cultures supplemented by red cells, considerably higher frequencies have been reported—up to $1000/10^5$ bone marrow cells, $100/10^5$ spleen cells, $100/10^5$ peripheral blood cells [65, 100].

Depending on the type of stimulus used, the frequency of GM-cluster-forming cells in unpotentiated cultures is 5–10 times that of colony-forming cells. It has not been clearly documented what is the frequency of cluster-forming cells in cultures potentiated by red cells, and it seems possible that many of the clusters in standard cultures increase in size and are scored as colonies in potentiated cultures. Until firm data are published, a conservative estimate suggests that in cultures of mouse bone marrow, about 2% of all nucleated cells proliferate to form either colonies or clusters of granulocytic and/or macrophage cells.

Levels of GM-CFCs in the marrow of mice of different strains are reasonably similar, but wider variations occur in spleen levels [101]. The spleen is a much more reactive organ to antigenic stimulation and other influences affecting GM-CFC levels. Calculations show that approximately 98% of all GM-CFCs in the mouse are located in the bone marrow. However, in a mouse maximally stimulated by antigens or endotoxin, up to 30–40% of GM-CFCs can be located in the spleen.

Maximum marrow GM-CFC levels have not been firmly established in other species, but the frequency of these cells appears to be somewhat lower than in the mouse, e.g., in the human marrow, 50–100 per 10^5 nucleated cells (Table 5).

B. Formation of Granulocytic and Macrophage Colonies (GM-Colonies) by Mouse Bone Marrow Cells

In cultures of mouse bone marrow stimulated by high concentrations of GM-CSF, proliferation of GM-CFCs commences asynchronously after a minimum lag of 16 h [82]. It should be noted that in this study, aggregates of three or more cells were being analyzed, requiring a minimum of two divisions. For this reason, the lag to the first division may be very short for a small minority of the cells. The developing colonies are initially tight aggregates of relatively undifferentiated cells with ring-shaped nuclei. Commencing at 3 days of incubation, the colonies begin to deviate in morphological appearance. Some remain compact and develop initially into large balls of tightly packed cells which remain relatively undifferentiated. In other colonies, differentiation of some cells occurs to metamyelocytes and polymorphs, and this is associated with the early development of an outer mantle of loosely dispersed cells containing the more mature cells. At this time, most colonies begin to develop

Table 5. Frequency of GM-CFCs per 10^5 nucleated cells in mouse and human tissue

Tissue	Mouse		Human
	Conventional cultures	Supplemented cultures[a]	Conventional cultures
Bone marrow	100–200	1000	50–100
Spleen	1–10	100	0–5
Blood	1	100	0–1

[a] Supplemented with red cell lysates [65, 100].

a second population of macrophages also usually located in the outer loose mantle of cells [72]. Progressive enlargement of these macrophage populations occurs by progressive transformation of primitive granulocytic cells to macrophage precursors and by proliferation of the macrophage cells [80]. The expansion of the macrophage populations is paralleled by a progressive reduction in the size of the granulocytic populations, either by transformation to macrophage precursors or by differentiation to short-lived polymorphs. Such mixed colonies terminate as globular aggregates of loosely dispersed macrophages which eventually disintegrate.

The transition of granulocytic colonies through the above sequence is markedly asynchronous. When cultures of mouse bone marrow grown in the presence of high GM-CSF concentrations are examined routinely after 7 days of incubation, a typical analysis of such a culture would show 30% pure granulocytic colonies, 50% mixed colonies, and 20% macrophage colonies. This pattern of differentiation varies with the culture medium used and the type and concentration of GM-CSF used. Indeed, as shall be discussed shortly, the pattern of colonies stimulated can be used to characterize various GM-CSFs. However, it must be emphasized that, regardless of these variables, most GM-colonies ultimately progress through the above sequence, and by 11 to 14 days of incubation, virtually all surviving colonies are composed of macrophages. The mixed appearance seen at 7 days of incubation should be regarded as a "time-gate" sample of a continuous process and not necessarily indicating the ultimate composition of such colonies.

While approximately 80–90% of GM-colonies pass through the granulocyte to macrophage sequence, the remainder include two types of colony which do not transform to macrophages but instead terminate as populations of mature polymorphs. The first type consists of single colonies which are initially tight but which then develop a loose outer mantle of mature polymorphs, and these colonies end as loosely dispersed aggregates of polymorphs. It is rather characteristic of these polymorph colonies that the sequence of proliferation and maturation tends to be completed early in the incubation period, and such colonies tend to achieve only a small size and may even have disintegrated by 7 days of incubation. The second type of pure granulocytic colony comprising about 10% of all GM-colonies is only detectable using very high GM-CSF concentrations since the cells are relatively unresponsive to stimulation. These colonies develop as multicentric aggregates of 5–15 irregularly shaped, tight aggregates of granulocytes. Maturation of these cells is usually delayed until after 7 days of incubation, and as a consequence these colonies can achieve a very large size before undergoing terminal differentiation to polymorphs. These latter colonies are termed "multiple granulocytic colonies." There are characteristic strain variations in the frequency of multiple granulocytic colonies, the cells forming these colonies being frequent in the marrow and spleen of NZB and SJL mice but essentially absent from the marrows of CBA and BALB/c mice [102].

So far, there has been no convincing evidence for the development of pure macrophage colonies in cultures of mouse bone marrow cells, i.e., colonies which from the onset are composed solely of macrophages. This statement is true for cultures initiated by cells taken directly from bone marrow, spleen, or peripheral blood and cultured for up to 2 weeks in agar. There are three situations, however, in which pure macrophage colonies can be grown in agar either from macrophages or more likely from some type of macrophage precursor cell not exactly equivalent to a GM-CFC. Such colonies develop in: (1) cultures of peritoneal cells taken from mice injected with various agents, if the cultures are maintained for 2–4 weeks [103], (2) recultured cells harvested from aging GM-colonies, and (3) cultures of yolk-sac cells after preliminary organ culture of the yolk sac for 2 weeks [104]. While these systems are potentially interesting, each appears to involve some type of in vitro adaptation or alteration on the part of the macrophage-forming cells. The cells involved may therefore not be strictly analogous with GM-CFCs as they occur in vivo and will not be further discussed in this chapter.

The above description of GM-colony formation by mouse cells essentially applies also to GM-colony formation by marrow, spleen, or blood cells from other species, e.g., human, monkey, guinea pig, rabbit, etc. There are certain species differences which often allow such cultures to be identified from the pattern of colony formation, but space does not permit a full discussion of such differences. The major comment which needs to be made is that in human cultures, the transformation of granulocytes to macrophages is much slower than for mouse cultures. Thus at 7–10 days of incubation, although colonies exhibit a similar heterogeneity in size and shape to colonies in cultures of mouse cells, in fact most colonies at this stage are composed wholly of granulocytes. Macrophage transformation in cultures of normal human marrow cells does not occur until the 3rd week of culture, and it seems likely that a much higher proportion of colonies terminates as pure populations of polymorphs than is seen in cultures of mouse marrow cells. This question has not yet been studied exhaustively, due mainly to the technical difficulty that human polymorphs survive much longer in agar than do mouse polymorphs, giving a higher "background noise" of cells surviving from the original population of cultured cells. When progressive dispersion of colony cells occurs following maturation, these colony cells are not readily identifiable against the background of mature cells surviving from the original cultured population.

C. Properties of GM-Colony-Forming Cells (GM-CFC) and Relation to Cluster-Forming Cells

As stated earlier, only one cell in 100–1000 mouse marrow cells is capable of forming a GM-colony, and the frequency of these cells is even lower in other organs and in the marrows from other species. While some of the properties of the GM-CFCs can be deduced from analytical experiments, identification of such cells requires enrichment of GM-CFC populations by cell separation methods.

Studies have shown that mouse marrow GM-CFCs have the following properties:

1. Most are in active cell cycle, and exposure to high concentrations of ^{3}HTdR or hydroxurea kills 30–50% of them [105, 106, 84]. In conditions of active regeneration, e.g., following irradiation or cytotoxic drugs, this proportion rises to 70–80% [107].
2. Most GM-CFCs exhibit active adherence to glass bead columns [32].
3. The buoyant density of mouse GM-CFCs is heterogeneous [32, 108] although in cultures stimulated by one type of GM-CSF, a peak of GM-CFCs was observed with a modal density of 1.074 g/cm^3 [108]. If the cultures were supplemented by red cell lysates, an additional peak of light density GM-CFCs was observed, indicating the probable existence of distinct subpopulations of GM-CFCs.
4. On velocity sedimentation separation, GM-CFCs segregate as a single peak (sedimentation velocity 4.3 mm/h) with a skewed distribution and a tail of more rapidly sedimenting (larger) cells [36] (Fig. 11). This, together with the density data, indicates that most mouse GM-CFCs probably have a diameter of 7–10μ.
5. GM-CFCs are highly radiosensitive (D_0 160 rads) [109] and are also sensitive to cytotoxic drugs and cortisone [110, 111, 112, 113].

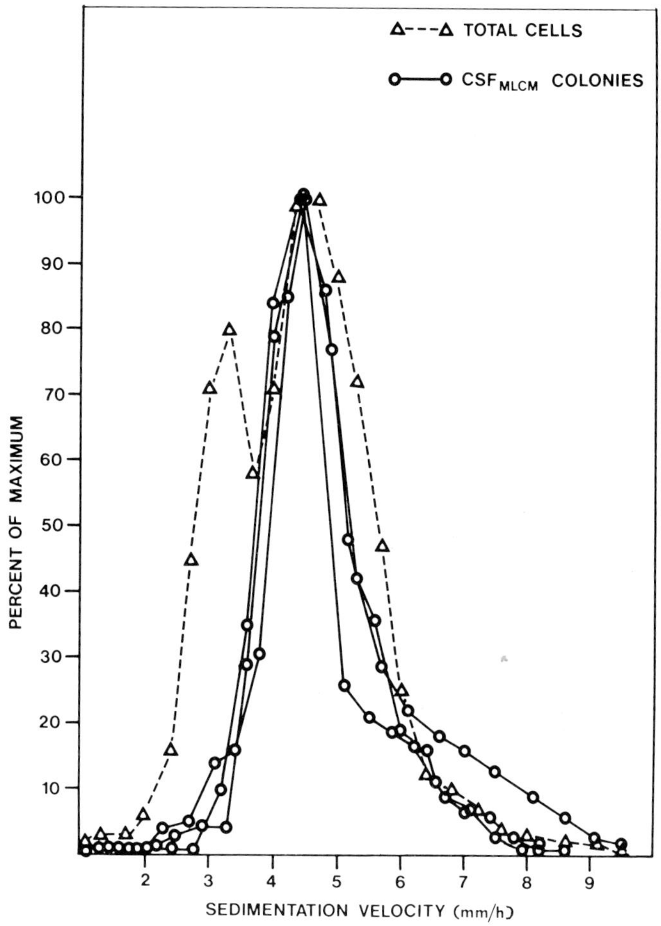

Fig. 11. Distribution of GM-colony-forming cells in C_{57}BL mouse marrow cells separated by velocity sedimentation. Broken line indicates distribution of nucleated cells. Unbroken lines are distribution of GM-CFCs in three separate experiments using mouse lung-conditioned medium GM-CSF. (From METCALF and MACDONALD, [36]. Reproduced with permission from J. Cellular Physiology)

6. GM-CFCs appear to have little or no capacity for self-replication. Evidence on this point is incomplete, but most studies on agar colonies have failed to reveal colony-forming cells within the colony population. However, liquid cultures of mouse marrow cells do generate increased numbers of GM-CFCs in the presence of CSF [114, 115, 116] (Fig. 12). While this rise in GM-CFCs is dependent on GM-CSF, cell separation studies indicated that most of the cells generating these GM-CFCs are a smaller size than GM-CFCs and have a distribution similar to CFUs [117]. It must be appreciated, however, that since some GM-CFCs can generate colonies of 2000 or more, such GM-CFCs could divide at least 4 times and each of the 16 progeny so generated still could be able to form a colony of 50 or more cells (the definition of a colony). Thus, it can be expected that in some experimental designs, unless colony size is carefully considered, GM-CFCs might be demonstrable as

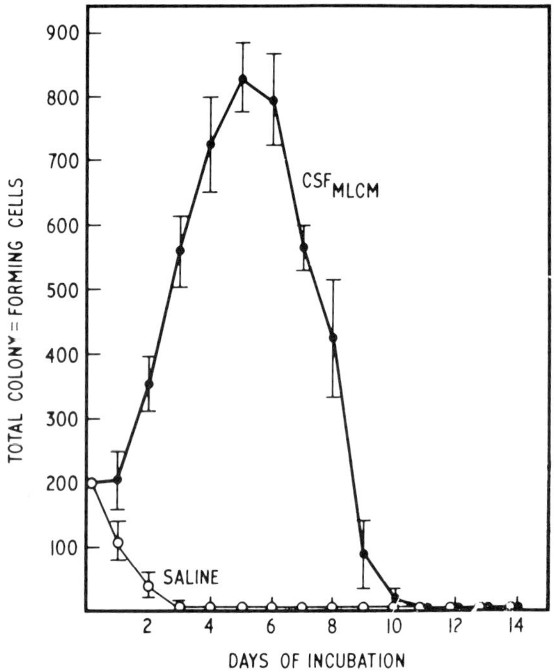

Fig. 12. Liquid cultures of mouse bone marrow cells showing rise in GM-CFCs in cultures containing mouse lung-conditioned medium GM-CSF, but progressive fall in control cultures containing saline

being able to "self-replicate" for four or five sequential divisions. Such self-replication would be wholly GM-CSF dependent and this appears to be the case in the liquid culture experiments referred to above.

Since the definition of a GM-CFC is rather loose in terms of proliferative capacity, it is perhaps quibbling to object to such evidence of self-replication. However, if GM-CFCs are capable by such a definition of a limited degree of "self"-replication, this should not be confused with the extensive capacity (about 80 times) of CFUs for self-replication [30]. More importantly, the evidence that the liquid culture type of self-replication is CSF dependent tells us nothing about the factors controlling production of new GM-CFCs from CFUs.

In monkey bone marrow labeled in vitro with ^{3}HTdR, GM-CFCs were enriched by buoyant density separation in continuous albumin gradients. GM-CFCs segregated as a single peak in which about 30% of the cells were colony-forming cells [43]. Examination of these cells using autoradiography indicated that the majority of GM-CFCs were mononuclear cells, 9–11μ in diameter in smears, with a slightly excentric nucleus, and a basophilic agranular cytoplasm (Fig. 13). The data from velocity sedimentation separation of mouse marrow cells is, in general, consistent with these observations although the mouse GM-CFCs may be slightly smaller in size.

In combined light and electronmicrograph studies on cells from monkey and human marrow, fractionated on discontinuous gradients, and enriched for GM-CFCs, correlation studies also suggested that GM-CFCs were of somewhat similar appearance [118]. The cells were

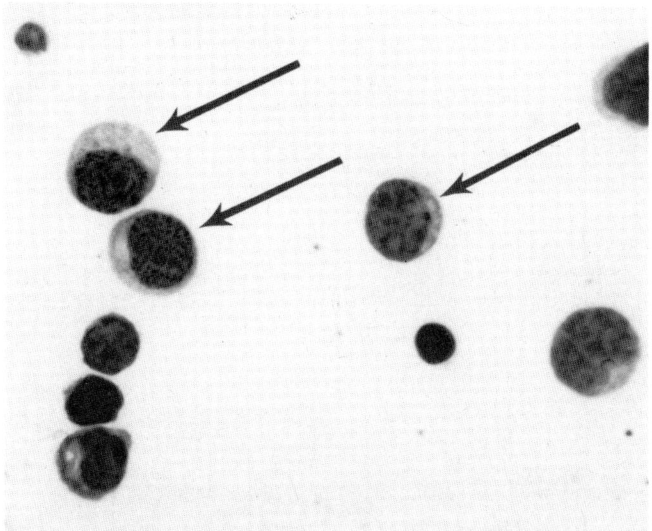

Fig. 13. Monkey bone marrow cells fractionated by buoyant density centrifugation. Cells indicated by arrows are probably cells capable of forming granulocyte and macrophage colonies in vitro

described as being round, 8–10μ in diameter, with a round or kidney-shaped nucleus, one or two prominent nucleoli, and pale blue, agranular cytoplasm.

While these studies strongly indicate that most GM-CFCs are mononuclear cells of intermediate size and unremarkable cytoplasm, it must be emphasized that GM-CFCs are heterogeneous and that not all cells have this morphology. Evidence for this comes from four types of observation:

1. Since most GM-CFCs are in active cell cycle, it is inevitable that some size heterogeneity will exist since cells double in volume before reaching G_2, preparatory to mitosis.
2. Analysis of fetal liver GM-CFCs have shown that they are of lighter density but have a much higher sedimentation velocity than GM-CFCs from adult marrow. This combination of properties indicates that GM-CFCs in fetal liver are of much larger size than corresponding cells in adult tissues [119].
3. Even within adult populations, significant size heterogeneity exists as measured by sedimentation velocity. Indeed, velocity sedimentation separation has shown that GM-CFCs are partially segregatable into subpopulations with distinctive properties. The most rapidly sedimenting (largest) GM-CFCs tend to be highly responsive to GM-CSF and to form colonies which transform early to macrophages (Figs. 14 and 15). Conversely, the most slowly sedimenting (smallest) GM-CFCs require high concentrations of GM-CSF to stimulate proliferation and produce a high proportion of multiple granulocytic and granulocytic colonies [36]. Combination of in vitro suiciding using ^{3}HTdR and velocity sedimentation separation has indicated that this heterogeneity is not based on cell cycle status at the time of velocity sedimentation separation.
4. Following the injection of endotoxin or whole body irradiation, a major size shift occurs in GM-CFC populations as indicated by an increase in sedimentation velocity unaccom-

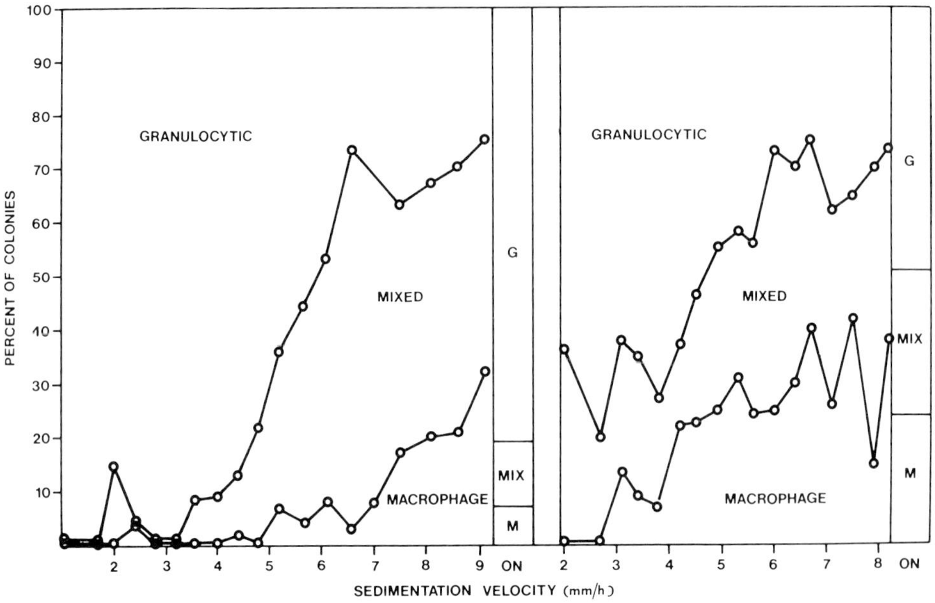

Fig. 14. Two separate experiments showing morphology at 7 days of colonies formed by $C_{57}BL$ marrow cells fractionated by velocity sedimentation. Colonies formed by unfractionated marrow cells shown in column (ON). Proportion of various colonies produced by cells from each fraction expressed as a percentage of total colonies in culture dish. (From METCALF and MACDONALD, [36]. Reproduced with permission from J. Cellular Physiology)

panied by a change in buoyant density [120, 121]. Since infections and consequent exposure to endotoxin occur frequently in normal life, this type of size variability can also be expected to be encountered in examining GM-CFC populations, particularly in animals or patients with relevant diseases.

In general, the reported properties of GM-CFCs in human marrow populations are reasonably similar to those of mouse GM-CFCs. In addition to the similar morphology just discussed, most human GM-CFCs are also in cycle [85] and are sensitive to irradiation (D_0 120–130 rads) [109, 122] and cytotoxic drugs [123]. Their buoyant density is somewhat less heterogeneous than that of mouse GM-CFCs, the cells forming a single major peak in the 1.067–1.069 g/cm^3 region [85]. Human GM-CFCs are not notably adherent, and this forms the basis for the separation of colony-stimulating (adherent) from colony-forming (nonadherent) cells, using either glass dishes or carbonyl iron [45].

A number of lines of evidence indicate that GM-colony-forming cells are the specific progenitor cells of granulocytic and macrophage populations, i.e., cells that have been committed irreversibly to a granulocytic-macrophage pathway of differentiation although not yet showing morphological evidence of this precommitment:

1. In marrow cultures known to be able to support granulocyte and macrophage, eosinophil and megakaryocyte proliferation, no eosinophils or megakaryocytes develop within granulocytic-macrophage colonies.

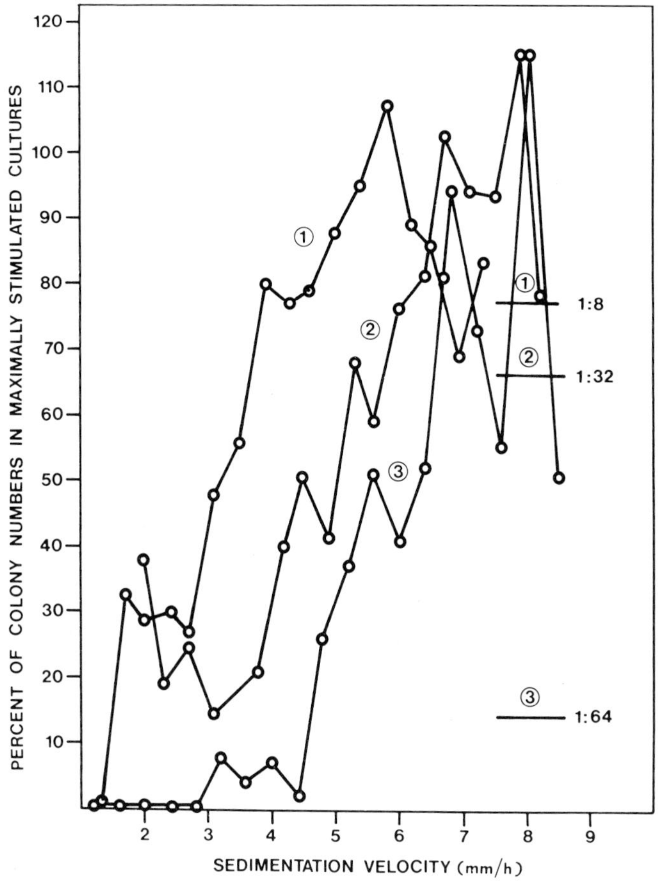

Fig. 15. Responsiveness of GM-colony-forming cells in various velocity sedimentation fractions of $C_{57}BL$ marrow to stimulation by various concentrations of mouse lung-conditioned medium GM-CSF. Replicate cultures contained (1) GM-CSF diluted 1:8, (2) GM-CSF diluted 1:32, (3) GM-CSF diluted 1:64. Colony counts expressed as percentage of colony counts in maximally stimulated cultures. Counts in cultures of unfractionated marrow cells indicated by horizontal bars. (From METCALF and MACDONALD, [36]. Reproduced with permission from J. Cellular Physiology)

2. In cultures capable of supporting erythropoiesis and granulocytic-macrophage colony formation, again no erythropoietic cells develop in granulocytic-macrophage colonies.
3. In spleen colonies generated by the injection into irradiated mice of CFUs, the level of GM-CFCs is slightly higher in granulocytic colonies than in colonies which contain predominantly erythropoietic cells [30].
4. In studies on marrow populations regenerating after irradiation, drug-induced damage, or antiserum-induced cell depletion, the temporal pattern of restoration of GM-CFC levels correlates closely with the reappearance of morphologically identifiable granulopoietic cells such as myeloblasts and myelocytes [124, 125].
5. Finally, and most compelling, GM-CFCs are capable of giving rise to large populations of cells clearly identifiable as polymorphs and macrophages.

One of the important findings emerging from the early work on granulocyte-macrophage colony formation was the clear indication from the high frequency of mixed colonies that neutrophils and macrophages probably shared the same ancestral cell, the GM-colony-forming cell. This was formally proved by cloning experiments involving micromanipulated individual GM-CFCs in which it was shown that a single GM-CFC could give rise to a colony containing both neutrophils and macrophages [43]. It is more difficult to determine whether *all* granulocytes and *all* macrophages necessarily originate from GM-CFCs. There have been numerous reports that lymphocyte populations can give rise to macrophages. However, this has never been observed in lymphocyte colonies grown in vitro. Similarly, granulocytes and macrophages have never been observed in erythropoietic, eosinophilic, or megakaryocytic colonies, and it now seems highly probable that GM-CFCs are the only immediate ancestors for these two cell populations. The studies of LIN and STEWART [103] have indicated that macrophages can have a more substantial capacity for proliferation than was formerly believed. For this reason, macrophage populations in some organs may not necessarily be recent descendants of GM-CFCs.

D. Cluster-Forming Cells

As mentioned above, cluster-forming cells outnumber colony-forming cells by five or ten to one. Clusters, like colonies, are composed of granulocytes and/or macrophages although in most situations macrophage clusters are far the more common. The ratio of cluster-forming cells to colony-forming cells varies and is low when GM-CFC levels are low and most GM-CFCs are in a noncycling state, e.g., as is seen in the normal C_{57}BL spleen [101]. Conversely, where GM-CFC levels are elevated and most cells are in active cycle, the cluster to colony ratio tends to be high [101]. In one special situation, 3–4 days after whole body irradiation, cluster to colony ratios rise to extremely high levels.

Although cluster-forming cells share many of the properties of colony-forming cells, e.g., organ distribution, cell cycle status, and buoyant density, there are certain procedures which can partially segregate the two populations. Cluster-forming cells are more adherent than colony-forming cells on glass bead columns [32], and cluster-forming cells have a higher sedimentation velocity than colony-forming cells, suggesting strongly that they are larger cells [36].

Because of the asynchronous onset of proliferation in colony-forming cells, some clusters may actually be colonies which were initiated late in the incubation period. However, continued incubation of cultures does not lead to progressive enlargement of most clusters and if anything accentuates the size discrepancy between colonies and clusters. This should not be confused with the capacity of some potentiating agents, e.g., red cell lysates, to so increase the growth of colonies and clusters that clusters exceed the minimum size for colonies (50 cells) and are then scorable as colonies. In this latter situation, a clear size difference persists between what would have been colonies and clusters. An alternative view of clusters is to interpret them as colonies whose progressive growth was prematurely interrupted by stochastic events leading to differentiation of colony cells to nondividing end cells. While this may in fact account for some clusters, the capacity of some separation methods to partially segregate cluster-forming cells from colony-forming cells makes it unlikely that these two populations are identical.

The most logical interpretation of cluster-forming cells is that they represent the immediate progeny of colony-forming cells and are simply exhibiting in agar a capacity to proliferate

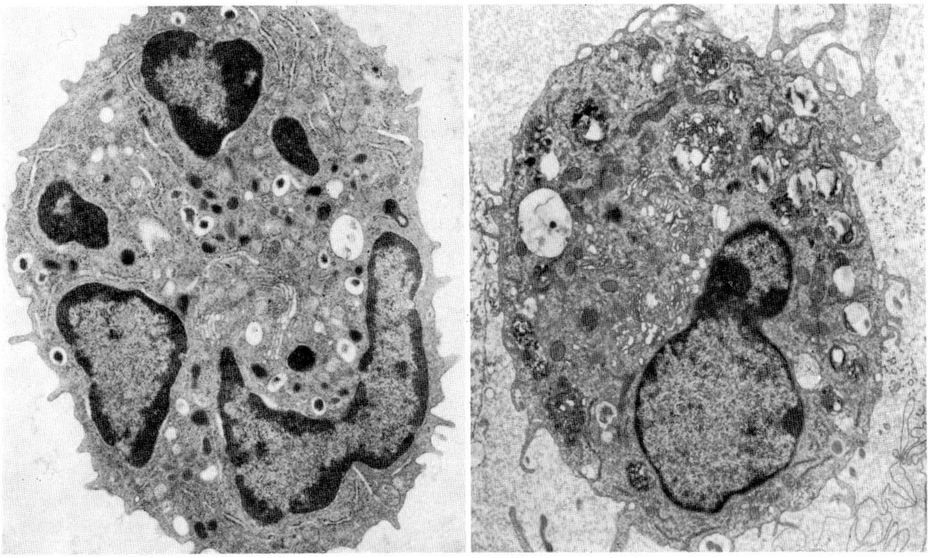

Fig. 16. Electronmicrographs of a typical colony neutrophil ×12,000 (left) and macrophage ×7000 (right) from 7-day colonies grown from mouse bone marrow cells. (Photographs by courtesy of Dr. T. Mandel)

equivalent to that shown by progeny of colony-forming cells within colonies developing in agar. On this basis, the larger size of cluster-forming cells would be expected since these cells would be expected to be intermediate in size between colony-forming cells and the larger myeloblasts and myelocytes.

It must be emphasized that while this interpretation of the significance of cluster-forming cells appears to be valid for normal populations, cluster formation by abnormal, e.g., leukemic, cells does not necessarily denote a comparable degree of maturation. Thus, if human acute myeloid leukemic cells form clusters in vitro as shall be discussed later, this does not imply that these leukemic cells are more differentiated than the cells from patients with chronic myeloid leukemia that form colonies. In the latter situation, alternative explanations such as an inability to proliferate under the culture conditions used are more tenable.

E. Differentiation in Colony Cells

As discussed earlier, GM-CFCs generate maturing populations of neutrophils and macrophages. This maturation has been documented by light and electronmicroscopy (Fig. 16) with histochemistry [75, 86, 31] and by the development of receptors for the Fc portion of IgG_{2a} and for C3 [87, 74]. In the case of macrophages these cells also acquire the capacity for active phagocytosis. By these criteria, colony cells at least qualitatively mature in a normal fashion.

However, there appears to be some impairment in the degree of differentiation achieved in colony populations. In the electronmicroscope, the number of specific granules in neutrophils is usually subnormal and many cells do not seem to progress far beyond the band stage in neutrophil maturation [31]. This situation is not unique to GM-colonies and similar deficiencies are seen in eosinophil, megakaryocyte, and lymphocytic colony cells.

F. Relation of GM-CFCs to CFUs

This question will be dealt with here in some detail as the evidence and arguments involved hold for other types of colony-forming cells, and the conclusions reached apply equally to these other cells.

When granulocytic and macrophage colonies were first grown in agar, it was felt by some that the colony-forming cells were multipotential stem cells (CFU) as previously detected by colony formation in the spleen of irradiated mice [71]. Linear relationships were observed between the number of CFUs and agar colony-forming cells in unfractionated and fractionated mouse marrow populations, and CFUs were detected in harvested agar colonies. In other studies [126], a correlation was observed in spleen colonies between CFU and agar colony-forming cell content. However, most workers have now concluded that the majority of GM colonies in vitro are not formed by CFUs but by cells which are the progeny of CFUs and are in fact precommitted progenitors in the GM-pathway. Conversely, there is considerable evidence to indicate that most CFUs are incapable of forming colonies in agar. This still leaves open a possibility that some GM-colonies might be generated by some CFUs that still have stem cell properties, particularly in cultures using fibroblast underlayers or fibroblast-conditioned media which appear capable of altering the proliferative activity of CFUs [127]. It must be emphasized, however, that if some colonies are generated by CFUs these colonies must be a minority only of GM-colonies developing in a culture dish.

The evidence that CFUs are not GM-CFCs is as follows:

1. Most CFUs behave as nonadherent cells on filtration through glass bead columns [32].
2. Although the density distribution profiles of CFUs and GM-CFCs from adult mouse marrow overlap to a considerable degree, a clear separation of the two cell classes can be achieved using marrow cells from animals preinjected with Freund's adjuvant [113] or marrow cells harvested from mice previously subjected to irradiation [93].
3. In marrow cell populations separated by velocity sedimentation, CFUs behave as a more slowly sedimenting cell with a peak sedimentation velocity of 3.8–4.0 mm/h compared with a value of 4.5 mm/h for GM-CFCs [128].
4. Most CFUs in normal mouse marrow are not in cell cycle and less than 10% are killed following in vitro incubation with ^{3}HTdR, whereas 30–50% of GM-CFCs are killed in the same suspension [105, 106].
5. Antisera raised against mouse brain tissue are cytotoxic for mouse marrow CFUs but do not deplete GM-CFC levels [38].
6. CFUs are activated into cell cycle by incubation with isoproterenol but GM-CFCs are not. Conversely, GM-CSF activates noncycling GM-CFCs into cycle but does not affect the cell cycle status of CFUs [93].
7. In liquid cultures of mouse marrow cells, GM-CFC levels rose five to sevenfold above starting levels, but CFU levels showed a progressive depletion [116].
8. In WW^V mutant mice with genetically-determined anemia, CFU levels are grossly subnormal, but GM-CFC levels are approximately normal [129].
9. The radiation sensitivities of the two cells are significantly different (D_0 CFU = 94 rads; D_0 GM-CFC = 160 rads) [130].

10. The locations of CFUs and GM-CFCs in the mouse marrow appear to differ. CFU concentrations were highest in the peripheral regions of the marrow next to the bone surface, but peak concentrations of GM-CFC were observed in the region about three-quarters of the distance from the central axis to the bone surface [131].

From these observations, it can be concluded that although the two cell populations have a similar developmental origin, occur in the same adult tissues, occur together in spleen colonies, and react similarly to radiation, cytotoxic drugs, and antigenic stimulation, the two cell populations are not identical. Clearly, the two populations are associated with one another, and the most likely interrelationship was indicated in experiments by HASKILL et al. [113]. In these experiments, mouse marrow cells surviving from vinblastine treatment were fractionated by buoyant density separation on continuous albumin gradients. Fractions were cultured in agar and also assayed in irradiated animals for CFU content. Certain fractions were found that contained no GM-CFCs but were capable of generating spleen colonies. Cultures of the cells from these spleen colonies developed high numbers of GM-colonies. These experiments indicated that CFUs were not capable of colony formation in agar but were capable in vivo of generating large numbers of GM-CFCs.

In other studies, fractionated mouse marrow populations were cultured in liquid, then these cultures were analyzed for their content of GM-CFCs. Slowly sedimenting fractions containing the highest frequency of CFUs were found to be the ones generating the highest numbers of GM-CFCs [117].

The conclusion from this evidence is that CFUs are the ancestors of GM-CFCs. Since the progeny of a single CFU can be shown to be capable of repopulating the hemopoietic tissues of an entire animal, it can be assumed that such a CFU can generate the various subpopulations of GM-CFCs referred to above. Preliminary studies on developing spleen colonies generated by individual CFUs suggest a great variability in the frequency and type of GM-CFCs appearing in individual colonies between day 7 and day 14. Some colonies have been shown to contain all types of GM-CFCs, but it is not known whether all such colonies ultimately generate all types of GM-CFCs (JOHNSON, G. and METCALF, D., unpublished data).

Although the data are less extensive, the same types of experiments as discussed above have led to the conclusion that the cells forming eosinophil, megakaryocyte, erythroid, and lymphoid colonies in vitro are also not CFUs but the progeny of CFUs.

G. Role of GM-Colony-Stimulating Factor (GM-CSF)

An adequate concentration of the specific glycoprotein, GM-colony-stimulating factor (GM-CSF), is required for GM-colony formation by mouse marrow cells in vitro. In cultures of marrow cells from other species, a limited degree of "spontaneous" GM-colony formation can occur without the deliberate addition of an exogenous source of GM-CSF [42]. Analysis of this phenomenon of spontaneous colony formation has shown that the GM-CFCs in other species are no more capable of proliferating in the absence of GM-CSF than are mouse cells. The apparent species difference is due to the fact that significant numbers of GM-CSF-producing cells are present in marrow cell suspensions from most species but not the mouse. If sufficiently large numbers of marrow cells are placed in a culture dish, these cells release sufficient GM-CSF to endogenously stimulate low levels of colony formation. Spontaneous colony formation can be prevented either by culturing marrow cells at low cell density (usually below 50,000 per ml) [42] or by preliminary removal of GM-CSF producing cells by adherence separation [45], or density centrifugation [42, 44], the GM-CSF-producing cells being relatively dense and adherent cells.

Thus, the requirement for GM-CSF appears to be absolute for GM-colony formation by cells from all species. GM-CSF is not simply a trigger for the first cell division but is required continuously throughout colony growth. Transfer of developing colonies to cultures lacking GM-CSF causes immediate cessation of colony growth followed rapidly by death of colony cells [78, 79].

GM-CSF is also required for survival of GM-CFC (or survival of their proliferative capacity) in both agar or liquid [83, 115]. This has raised the possibility that GM-CSF is not a stimulus so much as a factor permitting survival, the proliferation following as an automatic consequence due to some intrinsic intracellular stimulus to proliferate. This situation in which target cell survival in vitro depends on the presence of the regulator is not unique for GM-CSF and holds also for erythropoietin and NGF and survival of their respective target cells in vitro.

The survival factor interpretation is unlikely to be correct because of a number of observations:

1. Injected GM-CSF stimulates granulopoiesis and monocyte formation in vivo [132].
2. Preincubation in vitro with GM-CSF forces noncycling GM-CFCs to enter the S phase of the cell cycle within 3 h, an experimental system not involving cell death regardless of whether or not GM-CSF is present [93].
3. GM-CSF has a concentration-dependent effect on the mean length of the cell cycle of dividing colony cells [81], on the lag phase before initiation of proliferation in GM-CFCs [83], and on the growth rate of individual colonies [95].
4. GM-CSF initiates RNA synthesis in granulocytic cells within 10 min in an action which appears to be specific for granulocytic and macrophage cells [91].

None of these aspects of GM-CSF is consistent with the interpretation that GM-CSF is simply a survival factor, and it is reasonable to conclude that GM-CSF is a genuine proliferative stimulus.

Tests on a wide range of cells capable of colony formation in agar, including precursors of normal erythropoietic cells, cells forming eosinophilic, magakaryocytic, B-lymphocytic, fibroblastic, and neoplastic lymphoid, plasmacytoma and reticulum cell sarcoma cells have shown that GM-CSF is highly specific in its action on target cells stimulating only granulocytic and monocyte-macrophage proliferation. Conversely, neither purified NGF nor relatively pure erythropoietin is able to stimulate GM-colony formation. The only other cell types stimulated to proliferate in vitro by GM-CSF are neoplastic granulocytic and monocytic cells from the same lineage as GM-CFCs. Target cell specificity in vivo has been less completely analyzed, but injected human urine GM-CSF had no measurable effect on erythropoiesis, lymphopoiesis, or mitotic activity in kidney or liver cells in recipient mice [132].

When mouse bone marrow cells are cultured in the presence of high concentrations of GM-CSF, most colonies stimulated are granulocytic or mixed when analyzed after 7 days of incubation. Conversely, the few colonies developing in cultures containing very low GM-CSF concentrations are usually mainly or wholly composed of macrophages [81, 133] (Table 6). On the assumptions that all GM-CFCs were essentially similar and that these cells were the ancestors of both granulocytes and macrophages, this correlation between GM-CSF concentration and colony morphology led to the conclusion that the concentration of GM-CSF determined which of the two alternative pathways of differentiation colony cells enter as

Table 6. Effect of varying the concentration of purified $GM\text{-}CSF_{MLCM}$ on the frequency and morphological type of colonies developing

$GM\text{-}CSF_{MLCM}$ dilution	Mean No. of colonies	% Colonies		
		Granulocytic	Mixed granulocytic and macrophage	Macrophage
1:1	127	51	35	14
1:2	124	50	38	12
1:4	97	45	23	32
1:8	83	33	26	41
1:16	66	42	21	37
1:32	49	19	28	53
1:64	27	10	21	69
1:128	9	0	15	85
1:256	4	0	0	100

Cultures contained 75,000 $C_{57}BL$ marrow cells. Colonies analyzed on day 7 of incubation. 45 sequential colonies examined from cultures containing each $GM\text{-}CSF_{MLCM}$ dilution.

the colony increases in size. GM-CSF was envisaged as operating a switch mechanism affecting cellular differentiation, directing cells either to granulocytic or macrophage differentiation according to the GM-CSF concentration [133, 134].

However, cell separation studies using velocity sedimentation showed that rapidly sedimenting GM-CFCs tended to form macrophage colonies and were responsive to stimulation by low GM-CSF concentrations. Conversely, slowly sedimenting GM-CFCs tended to form granulocytic colonies and were only capable of being stimulated by high GM-CSF concentrations [36]. These observations suggested a simpler mechanism of action of GM-CSF in which the molecule acts solely as a proliferative stimulus. The apparent influence of GM-CSF on colony differentiation can then be explained by selective activation of various CFCs, each preprogrammed to form either granulocytic or macrophage colonies. It should be noted, as discussed earlier, that a 7-day "time gate" is used in the routine scoring of cultures at 7 days of incubation. The differences in differentiation of colonies mean, in most cases, differences in the time interval required for transformation from granulocytic to macrophage populations since most colonies eventually undergo this transformation.

Additional aspects of GM-CSF action on colony differentiation will be discussed in Chapter 6 describing the growth of myeloid leukemic cells in vitro.

With the availability of purified GM-CSF, it has become possible to begin studies on other aspects of the action of GM-CSF on target cells. It has been shown that, within 10 min, GM-CSF stimulates a detectable increase in RNA synthesis in mouse bone marrow cells [91]. Rates of RNA synthesis fell progressively in marrow cells incubated in vitro in the absence of GM-CSF, but in cultures containing GM-CSF, rates were maintained so that the maximum effect of GM-CSF was seen at 10 h (Fig. 17). Cell death was equivalent in cultures with or without GM-CSF in the first 24 h.

The magnitude of the stimulation of RNA synthesis was dependent on the concentration of GM-CSF used, and the phenomenon was restricted to tissues containing granulopoietic and macrophage-forming populations.

Autoradiographic analysis of RNA synthesis in cells preincubated with GM-CSF revealed a surprising phenomenon. The cells exhibiting the greatest increase in RNA synthesis were postmitotic metamyelocytes and polymorphs [91].

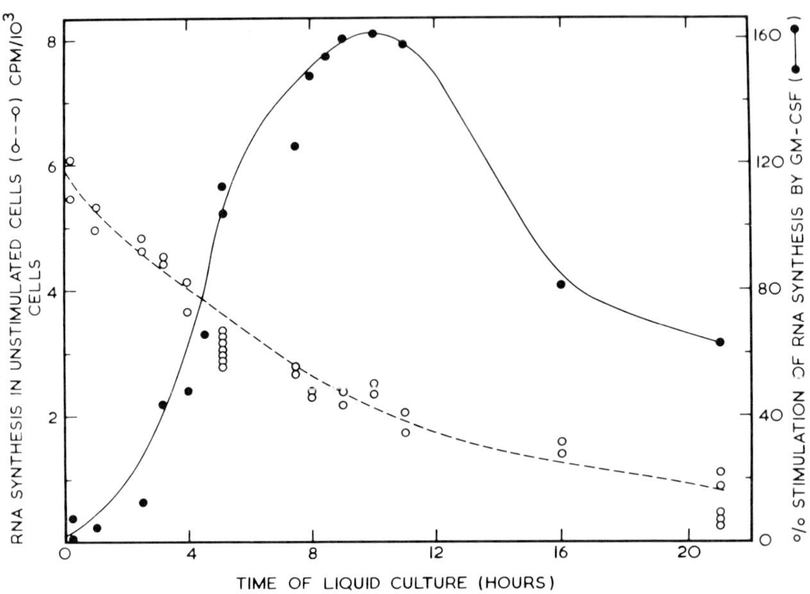

Fig. 17. Stimulation of RNA synthesis in liquid cultures of mouse bone marrow cells by addition of purified GM-CSF. Note maximum response at 10–12 h and progressive fall in RNA synthesis in unstimulated cultures although no cell death occurred. (From BURGESS and METCALF, [91]. Reproduced with permission from J. Cellular Physiology)

Two conclusions of some general importance can be drawn from these observations:

1. GM-CSF, like erythropoietin, appears to have a dual action on target cells, not only stimulating cell proliferation but also RNA, and presumably protein synthesis in postmitotic cells. In the case of erythropoietin, the protein synthesized is well-known (hemoglobin); in the case of GM-CSF, the protein or proteins have yet to be identified. In both cases, the dual action is difficult to ascribe to a single sequence of biochemical events, and the observations imply that the regulators may have at least two sites of action in the target cells.
2. The observed activation by GM-CSF of RNA synthesis in end-cell polymorphs raises the interesting possibility that GM-CSF may be able to induce heightened functional activity in preformed polymorphs and macrophages. The important role of macrophage activation in the early response to infections is well-known (see review by NELSON, 135), and the possibility that this could be mediated by GM-CSF requires careful investigation.

One final aspect of GM-CSF action has not been fully resolved at present. The more rapid growth rates of colonies developing in the presence of high concentrations of GM-CSF cannot really be ascribed solely to earlier onset of proliferation and/or shorter cell cycle times since the size differences involved are much too large.

A more important factor in determining the rate at which a colony population increases in size is the proportion of daughter cells of preceding divisions which remain capable of further divisions. It is possible that GM-CSF may have an influence on the pattern of end-cell maturation, high concentrations forcing daughter cells to remain immature and capable of further divisions. A simple analysis of this proposition has now been made much more difficult with the recognition of the extreme degree of heterogeneity between GM-CFCs and the differing responsiveness of these cells to GM-CSF. This question is of much more than academic interest. The fundamental abnormality in cancer or leukemia involves the proportion of daughter cells remaining capable of division and thereby ensuring progressive increase in the tumor population size. As will be shown in Chapter 6, myeloid leukemias are as dependent on GM-CSF as are normal cells for proliferation. GM-CSF could therefore be a major factor in determining the progressive enlargement of a population of myeloid leukemic cells if indeed it is capable of influencing the proportion of daughter cells differentiating to nondividing end cells.

H. Sources of GM-CSF (Synonyms: CSA, MG-Inducer Protein)

Cultures of marrow cells have proved to be a superlative system for bioassaying GM-CSF concentrations because of the sigmoid dose-response curve between GM-CSF concentrations and the number of colonies developing. Despite the availability of a satisfactory assay system capable of measuring molar concentrations as low as 10^{-11}, the purification and characterization of GM-CSF has proved to be a difficult problem.

Apart from purely technical problems involved with separative protein chemistry and the stability of highly purified proteins in low concentrations, two major factors have made these studies difficult: (1) the low starting concentrations of GM-CSF in most potential source materials, and (2) the fact that GM-CSF occurs in more than one molecular form.

In the mouse, GM-CSF is extractable from all tissues in concentrations higher than those present in the serum [136]. Primary cultures of cells from many tissues (and initially containing mixed populations of cells) can also produce and/or release GM-CSF [7, 137, 138]. Similarly, cultures of some cloned or uncloned normal or neoplastic cells adapted to continuous growth in vitro are able to produce GM-CSF [139, 140]. Finally, GM-CSF is present in the serum and urine [95, 141, 52].

These results suggest either that many different cells can produce or store GM-CSF, or alternatively that one cell type present in all tissues, e.g., fibroblasts, macrophages, endothelial, or lymphoid cells, is the source of GM-CSF. In this context, human vascular endothelial cells have been shown to be able to produce material stimulating GM-colony formation by human marrow cells [142]. The data from tissue culture-adapted cell lines would appear to show that many different cells can produce GM-CSF, but this data must be accepted with reservation since these cells are not entirely normal and genetic derepression may have permitted a functional activity not normally engaged in by that cell in vivo.

The richest sources of GM-CSF using organ extraction methods are the salivary gland, lung, thymus, kidney, and spleen [136]. Tissues effective in producing large amounts of GM-CSF in vitro are lung, heart and bone stromal tissue [50, 143, 20]. Early evidence suggested that monocytes and macrophages were the only cell types capable of releasing GM-CSF in culture. Thus, studies with fractionated marrow or peripheral blood cells from mouse, human, or monkey sources indicated that fractions containing monocytes were the most effective in feeder layers or in conditioning medium [42, 144, 145, 44, 146, 339, 426]. Studies on patients and dogs with cyclic fluctuations in neutrophil, monocyte, and CSF levels were consistent with this hypothesis [147, 148, 134, 149]. However, these experiments were performed under culture conditions that only permitted survival of monocytes and macrophages. The same reservation applies to the analysis of autostimulating cells in cultures, e.g., of human marrow, where again analysis has shown that the cells involved are probably monocytes and macrophages [42]

Furthermore, the early appearance of GM-CSF in macrophage culture medium after the addition of endotoxin [150] is not blocked by inhibitors of protein synthesis unlike the situation with the production of GM-CSF by mouse lung tissue [151]. Studies using ^{125}I-labeled GM-CSF has shown that macrophages actively ingest CSF (BURGESS, A. W. and METCALF, D., unpublished data). While studies on continuous macrophage cultures have made it clear that these cells can actively synthesize GM-CSF, much of the GM-CSF released by macrophages in culture could conceivably represent material taken up by these cells in vivo.

When lymphocytes are cultured under conditions permitting survival and proliferation (i.e., in the presence of mitogens) these cells in fact produce large amounts of GM-CSF. Thus, in mixed leucocyte cultures or cultures containing mercaptoethanol, PHA, pokeweed mitogen, endotoxin, BCG, or concanavalin A, large amounts of GM-CSF were produced [17, 18, 152, 20, 153, 154, 155]. As shall be discussed in following chapters, lymphocyte-conditioned media are valuable sources of other factors stimulating eosinophil and megakaryocyte proliferation.

These observations have provided several methods for producing large amounts of GM-CSF that have been used as source materials to characterize GM-CSF. The most commonly used source materials are: (1) pregnant uterus and embryo extracts or conditioned medium [138], (2) L-cell: conditioned medium [140], (3) mouse lung-conditioned medium [50], and (4) mouse lymphocyte-conditioned medium [20].

In studies on the regeneration of marrow GM-CFCs following irradiation, fluctuations were observed in the capacity of bone stromal cells to produce GM-CSF which corresponded well in timing with the subsequent wave of regeneration of granulopoietic tissues [156]. Corresponding fluctuations were not observed in spleen, lung, or serum GM-CSF levels. This has suggested that local production of GM-CSF within the marrow itself may be a major regulatory factor in controlling marrow granulopoiesis, but other control systems have certainly not been excluded.

This question of the origin of GM-CSF has been made more complex by the observation that, even within the same inbred mouse, GM-CSFs extracted from different organs differ in physical properties and antigenic reactivity [157, 158, 159]. It is conceivable that the different molecular forms of GM-CSF are interrelated in some precursor—active form—breakdown product relationship, but all have roughly comparable biological activity in stimulating granulocytic and macrophage colony formation in vitro. However, the recent demonstration that some subsets of GM-CFCs respond preferentially or only to certain types of GM-CSF [36, 108] suggests that more than one metabolically active form of GM-CSF may exist in vivo and have genuine functional activity.

Further complications have arisen from the observation that the type of GM-CSF produced by a tissue can change in response to stimulation. For example, following injection of endotoxin, not only do tissue and serum GM-CSF levels rise sharply [49, 157] but the type of GM-CSF present in the salivary gland is demonstrably different from that present in the salivary gland of unstimulated mice [157].

Part of the very large apparent rise in serum GM-CSF levels following the injection of endotoxin is an in vitro artifact due to parallel rises in another serum factor potentiating CSF action [48, 64]. Furthermore, part of the observed rise in serum colony-stimulating activity may be due to a fall in the level of serum inhibitors [160]. Despite this, GM-CSF levels do rise substantially, and it might be wondered what functional purpose is served by such apparently excessive rises. The demonstration that some GM-CFCs can only be triggered by GM-CSF levels 25-fold in excess of those activating other GM-CFCs provides a possible explanation of the functional purpose of such rises. This suggests that under some abnormal circumstances, it is advantageous to produce certain types of granulocytes, e.g., the progeny of multiple GM-CFCs, and the function of these cells must therefore differ in some way from the more common forms generated by other GM-CFCs.

Another aspect of this problem is whether GM-CSF produced by neoplastic hemopoietic cells is exactly the same as that produced by, or present in, normal cells. This question will be discussed further in Chapter 6.

At the present stage, it is not possible to be dogmatic about the location of GM-CSF production in the body nor about the cell types involved in its production. Hemopoietic populations and stromal elements are good candidates for the production of significant amounts of GM-CSF, a process made more important by the juxtaposition of GM-CSF source and target cells. However, it seems evident that GM-CSF must also be produced elsewhere in the body, from whence it may reach the marrow via the circulation. Under abnormal circumstances, it is conceivable that other cells in other sites may become important sources of this regulator.

I. Nature of GM-CSF

Several forms of GM-CSF with activity on mouse marrow cells have been studied in some detail. GM-CSF has been purified from human urine and shown to be a neuraminic acid-containing glycoprotein of 45,000 mol wt [161, 162, 163]. The neuraminic acid is removable by neuraminidase and is not necessary for biological activity in vitro [164, 165]. Human urine GM-CSF binds to Concanavalin A-Sepharose [165, 166], has an α-postalbumin electrophoretic mobility [161], is relatively resistant to proteolytic enzymes [164], and is biologically active at 10^{-11}M concentrations, stimulating both granulocytic and macrophage colony formation [162, 166]. However, it is relatively ineffective in stimulating colony formation by the slowly sedimenting mouse GM-CFCs (i.e., the cells forming granulocytic and multiple granulocytic colonies), [36].

Table 7. Purification of GM-CSF from mouse lung conditioned medium

Purification procedure	Volume ml	Total protein mg	Specific activity colonies × 10^{-6}/mg	Yield
Conditioned medium	3600	4800	0.02	100%
Calcium phosphate gel	42	620	0.14	87%
DEAE Cellulose	17	60	0.9	52%
Concanavalin A-Sepharose	22	13	2.0	25%
Ultrogel AcA44	7	0.7	34	23%
Preparative gel electrophoresis	2	0.12	70	8%

Specific activity calculated from linear portion of dose-response curve using 1 ml cultures containing 75,000 C_{57}BL marrow cells and expressed as calculated total colonies/mg protein.

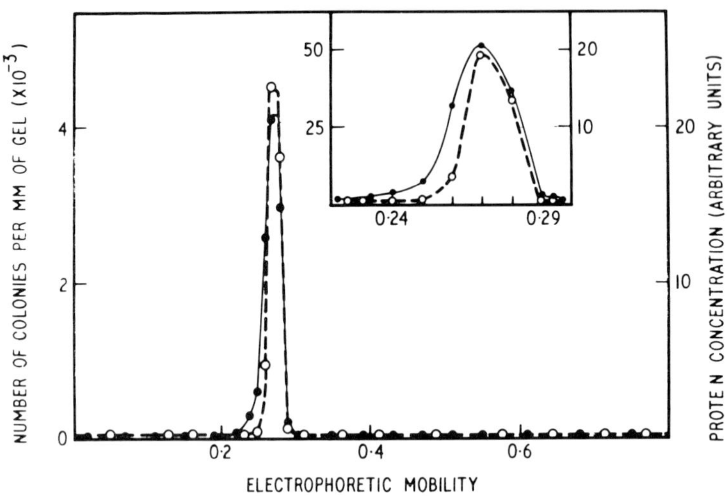

Fig. 18. Electrophoresis in polyacrylamide gel of purified GM-CSF from mouse lung-conditioned medium. Note coincidence of colony-stimulating activity ○—○ with single band of Coomassie blue-staining material ●—●. (BURGESS, A. W. and METCALF, D., unpublished data)

Subsequent work succeeded in purifying the GM-CSF produced in vitro by lung tissue from mice previously injected with endotoxin [158, 167, 94] (Table 7, Fig. 18). Based on the change in electrophoretic mobility of this type of GM-CSF following pretreatment with neuraminidase [158] and its selective binding to, and elution from, Concanavalin A-Sepharose [94], this form is also a neuraminic acid-containing glycoprotein although the mol wt is only 20,000–30,000. This form of GM-CSF is more susceptible to digestion by proteolytic enzymes, has an α-postalbumin electrophoretic mobility, and is also active at molar concentrations of approximately 10^{-11} [158, 94]. Purified GM-CSF of this type is capable of stimulating all types of GM-CFCs so far detected [36].

The form of GM-CSF produced in vitro by mouse L-cells [140] has also been purified (168, STANLEY, E. R., personal communication). Although this type of GM-CSF is again a glycoprotein, the content of carbohydrate in the molecule, as judged by the proportion of molecules binding to Concanavalin A-Sepharose, falls if the culture conditions for the L-cells become suboptimal. The mol wt of this GM-CSF is 65,000, and after mercaptoethanol treatment, two fragments of 17,000 and 35,000 have been recovered, both apparently lacking biological activity. The GM-CSF produced by L-cells has been shown to be identical with macrophage growth factor (MGF) [168], a molecule previously described as being able to stimulate to proliferation in vitro of mouse peritoneal macrophages [169, 170, 171].

The nature of a somewhat similar type of GM-CSF (macrophage and granulocyte inducer, MGI) produced by a cloned mouse embryo cell line was analyzed by GUEZ and SACHS [139]. Although the mol wt was also 65,000–70,000, no carbohydrate was detected in the active factor. This material was reported to have the peculiar requirement that the culture medium needed to be supplemented by adenine-containing nucleotides before colony formation was stimulated [172]. This material is the only GM-CSF reported not to contain carbohydrate and may be exhibiting an extreme form of the variability in carbohydrate content of GM-CSFs produced by cells in vitro. Alternatively, the material analyzed may not have been as highly purified as was believed, and the absence of carbohydrate from contaminating molecules may have been what was observed. The requirement for supplemented adenine-containing compounds has not been observed for other forms of GM-CSF and might reflect differences in the culture medium used.

The in vivo half-life of GM-CSF in the mouse has been estimated using selective antisera (for human urine GM-CSF) and ^{125}I-labeled GM-CSF (for mouse lung-conditioned medium). The estimates were 2.9 h for human urine GM-CSF [173] and 6.4 h in syngeneic mice for GM-CSF derived from mouse lung-conditioned medium [174]. The metabolic fate of injected GM-CSF is not known. There is some evidence to suggest that the GM-CSF in the urine is not simply filtered from the plasma but is either a metabolically degraded form or may actually be a product of renal or urinary tract tissue [175, 174]. Although a number of organs, e.g., salivary gland, developed high levels of radioactivity following the injection of ^{125}I-GM-CSF, it has not been established whether this is due to native GM-CSF, degraded products of the labeled molecule, or indeed iodine itself.

GM-CSFs from mouse or human sources are antigenic in the rabbit and antisera have been prepared against GM-CSF from human urine [176], mouse lung-conditioned medium [158], and L-cell-conditioned medium [159]. The results emphasize the heterogeneity of GM-CSFs but also demonstrate that some antigenic cross-reactivity exists between the different GM-CSFs. In part, the complex pattern of cross-reactions seems to depend on the individual rabbit generating the antisera. Antisera against mouse lung-conditioned medium GM-CSF cross-neutralized human urine GM-CSF and endotoxin serum but, surprisingly, were inactive against a number of preparations of GM-CSFs extracted directly from various organs in mice of the same strain [158]. However, the antisera inhibited the activity of a number of types of GM-CSF produced in vitro by cells and tissues from mice of this strain. A similar complex pattern was seen with an anti-L-cell GM-CSF serum. This was highly inhibitory for endotoxin serum and human urine GM-CSF, moderately active against a number of GM-CSF preparations extracted directly from mouse tissues or produced in vitro by mouse cells, but was inactive against mouse lung-conditioned medium GM-CSF [159]. This same antiserum was effective in inhibiting the GM-CSF in human placental-conditioned medium when assayed on mouse target cells but not when assayed on human cells (METCALF, D., unpublished data), the crude conditioned medium apparently containing two different GM-CSFs.

Considerably less information exists on the biochemical nature of GM-CSFs with activity on human marrow cells. Studies in this area have been hampered by a lack of suitable starting material in large quantities, with high biological activity, and a low starting protein content. A number of studies have used media conditioned by normal or leukemic leukocytes [56, 177]. Separation of this material by column chromatography yielded three types of GM-CSFs with approximate mol wt of 93,000, 36,500, and 14,700 [177]. Biological activity was lost after digestion with several peptidases but not after treatment with neuraminidase. In parallel studies, peripheral blood leukocytes were solubilized with sodium dodecyl sulphate. The major part of the colony-stimulating activity extractable from these cells was membrane associated [178]. On gel filtration, again three molecular species of material with colony-stimulating activity were observed.

The above conditioned media were prepared using unfractionated peripheral blood cells and the cellular source of the active material was not established.

The active colony-stimulating material in human placental-conditioned medium has been shown to be macromolecular in nature and to have a mol wt of approximately 30,000 [57].

Material of a quite different nature has been reported to be extractable from medium conditioned by human leukocytes and to have a weak capacity to stimulate colony formation

Table 8. Classification of mouse GM-CSFs into those capable of stimulating granulocytic colonies and those stimulating mainly macrophage colonies

Granulocytic colonies	Macrophage colonies
Mouse lung-conditioned medium	Normal serum
Postendotoxin serum	Human urine
Lymphocyte-conditioned medium	Yolk sac-conditioned medium
Bone-conditioned medium	Mouse embryo-conditioned medium
Organ extracts	

by human marrow cells. The active material was readily extractable by chloroform and on gel filtration had a mol wt of approximately 1300 [179]. In an extension of this work, differences were noted between low molecular weight "CSAs" produced by blood cells from different types of leukemic patients [180]. Iodinated low molecular weight CSA was reported to bind to GM-CFCs and, through radiation damage, to reduce the frequency of these cells. No specificity controls of other hemopoietic cells were included in this study.

The extraction from human sera of chloroform-soluble material with colony-stimulating activity for human marrow but not mouse marrow cells has now been reported (ROBINSON, W. A., personal communication). It is uncertain whether this material is of the same general type as the low molecular weight CSA described in white cell-conditioned medium. Chloroform extraction does not remove all colony-stimulating activity from human sera and the nonextractable material is active in cultures of both human and mouse marrow cells. It remains to be determined whether one type or other of the active materials fluctuates significantly in various disease states. It has been known for some time that there is frequently poor agreement between assays for colony-stimulating activity of human sera performed on human and mouse marrow cells [181, 182]. The presence of two different types of GM-CSF in human sera, only one of which is active on mouse cells, is a possible explanation of this discrepancy and further information is urgently needed on the occurrence and levels of chloroform-soluble active material in human sera.

In the mouse, GM-CSFs appear to fall into two broad groups: (1) those capable of stimulating a high proportion of granulocytic colonies if used in high concentrations, and (2) those capable of stimulating mainly macrophage colonies, regardless of the concentration used. The various GM-CSFs have been classified in Table 8. It is probably an oversimplification to attempt to place all GM-CSFs into only two categories; nevertheless, some functional interrelationship may exist between members of each group.

At the present time, the only summary which can be made regarding the macromolecular GM-CSFs so far purified and analyzed is that they appear to be glycoproteins with certain features in common, some sharing of antigenicity, and some possible interrelationships.

Despite the differences between different GM-CSFs, no reports have been made of semipurified GM-CSF having any other biological activity and it must be emphasized that granulopoiesis in vitro is wholly dependent on specific stimulation by GM-CSF, a family of glycoproteins having no other known biological activity. Tissue culture studies have discredited earlier suggestions based on in vivo studies that a miscellany of materials could stimulate granulopoiesis. It is now apparent that, when an agent like endotoxin or an antigen is injected into an animal and stimulates granulopoiesis, this response is probably mediated by the stimulation of high tissue and serum levels of GM-CSF. None of these agents is capable of direct stimulation of granulopoiesis in vitro (if the cultured populations are first freed of endogenous GM-CSF producing cells).

J. GM-Colony Formation by Fetal Cells

During fetal development, it is known that a distinctive fetal population of erythropoietic cells of yolk sac origin exists which is subsequently displaced by an unrelated population that then persists throughout adult life. It has not previously been suggested that a similar situation may exist for granulopoietic populations, but certain observations have raised this as a distinct possibility.

GM-CFCs are demonstrable in the mouse yolk sac and later accumulate in large numbers in the fetal liver although in both locations very few morphologically identifiable granulocytes are produced [97]. Formation of granulocytic populations only occurs late in fetal life, at which time granulopoietic populations are localizing in the developing spleen and bone marrow.

Despite the minimal evidence of granulopoiesis as assessed by the formation of mature end cells, analysis has shown that the early mouse fetal liver contains a high frequency of GM-CFCs—indeed, the frequency is approximately twice that in the adult marrow. However, a peculiarity of such cells is that the majority in the early (e.g., 12-day) fetal liver tend to form macrophage colonies regardless of the GM-CSF concentration used [183, 119]. These colonies have a characteristic morphology, being broken into fragments of relatively tightly packed macrophages. In late fetal life, there is a progressive rise in the frequency of GM-CFCs in the liver capable of forming granulocytic and mixed colonies, and the general appearance of such cultures does not differ from that of adult marrow cultures.

It has been reported that premature transformation of granulocytes to macrophages is seen also in cultures of human and monkey fetal liver [183]. The GM-CFCs in the fetal liver of species with a long gestation period—guinea pig, lamb, calf, monkey, and human—show a curious phenomenon in the middle third of the gestation period in that the majority of the cells enter a noncycling state [183]. This persists until the development of the spleen and bone marrow signals commencement of a large expansion in granulopoietic and macrophage-forming populations.

Early fetal liver GM-CFCs are of unusually light buoyant density, but late in fetal life, the buoyant density approaches that of adult cells [184]. GM-CFCs in monkey and human fetal liver are also of much lighter buoyant density than corresponding cells in adult marrow. Separation of early fetal liver cells by velocity sedimentation indicates that these cells have an unusually high sedimentation velocity, two peaks being noted at 7.7 and 9.4 mm/h (adult value 4.5 mm/h) [185, 119] (Fig. 19).

Taken together, the density and velocity sedimentation data indicate that early fetal liver GM-CFCs must differ markedly in appearance from corresponding cells in late fetal or adult life in that the early fetal GM-CFCs must be very large. The early fetal population is not entirely homogeneous as sedimentation separation studies indicate that a heterogeneity of responsiveness to GM-CSF similar to that seen in adult GM-CFCs is also seen in fetal liver populations, the most rapidly sedimenting cells being the most responsive to stimulation [119].

In a study of possible fetal sources of GM-CSF, it was shown that the yolk sac cells, fetal cells (excluding liver), and peripheral blood cells all have the capacity to stimulate colony

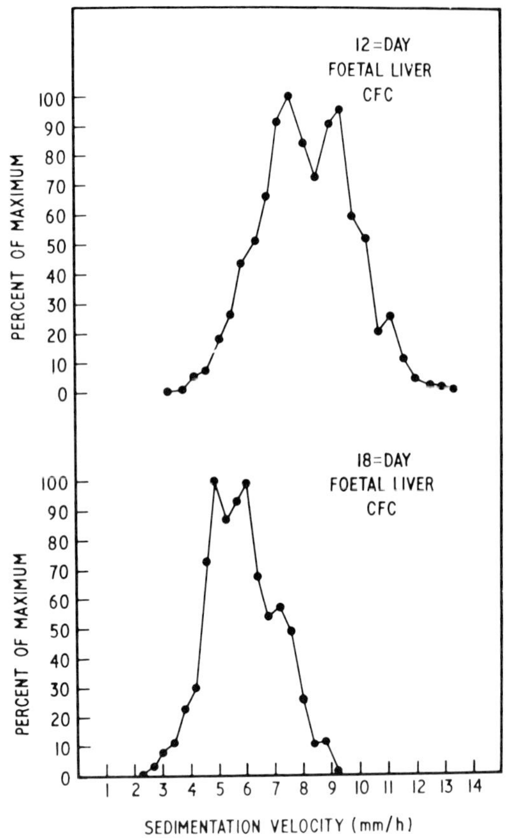

Fig. 19. Velocity sedimentation profiles of GM-CFCs from 12-day and 18-day mouse fetal livers. Note the much lower sedimentation velocity of GM-CFCs in late fetal liver populations. (JOHNSON, G. R. and METCALF, D., unpublished data)

formation by adult marrow cells (JOHNSON, G. and METCALF, D., unpublished data). A curious feature of these colonies was that the majority were macrophage in type. The yolk sac appeared to be outstanding in its capacity to produce GM-CSF in conditioned medium. Studies on partially fractionated GM-CSF from yolk sac-conditioned medium have shown that even in concentrations stimulating maximum colony numbers, the colonies formed by adult marrow cells were mainly macrophage in type (Table 9). Yolk sac GM-CSF is also curious in that fetal liver GM-CFCs respond relatively poorly to the stimulus compared with adult marrow GM-CFCs.

It has yet to be established whether any maternal GM-CSF can reach the fetus via the placenta. If it does not, then the yolk sac type GM-CSF may represent the only GM-CSF available to the fetus. The peculiarity of this stimulus, coupled with the relative unresponsiveness of early fetal GM-CFCs to the stimulus, may explain the virtual absence of granulopoiesis in the early fetus and why those progeny that do appear are monocytes and macrophages.

Further work is required to determine whether early fetal liver and late fetal GM-CFC populations are members of the same lineage or represent two separate populations. Spleen colonies generated in irradiated mice by early fetal liver stem cells seem to contain adult type GM-CFCs (JOHNSON, G. and METCALF, D., unpublished data), but this does not resolve the problem of the identity or otherwise of the two fetal GM-CFC populations.

K. Factors Modifying GM-CFC Levels in Mouse Tissues

The age-related fluctuations in GM-CFC levels in the various tissues have been described earlier. In general, these fluctuations are paralleled by changes in the number of morphologically identifiable granulopoietic cells, i.e., myeloblasts, myelocytes, and metamyelocytes. The exceptions to this are (1) the yolk sac and early fetal liver, where there are relatively large numbers of GM-CFCs but little granulopoiesis, and (2) the peripheral blood, where an occasional GM-CFC is present but no granulopoiesis.

GM-CFCs are absent from the thymus and the various lymph nodes. Where lymph nodes are draining sites of active infection or tumors, it is common to find a large number of granulocytes and macrophages in the lymph nodes. It might be anticipated that such lymph nodes would have some GM-CFCs or at least some cluster-forming cells. However, a careful search in mice using a number of model systems has failed to find such a situation. Mixing experiments in vitro in which lymph node or thymus cells are cocultured with marrow GM-CFCs has not revealed any inhibition of colony formation. On the contrary, if suboptimal culture systems are used, it is quite easy to show that added viable or killed lymphoid cells potentiate colony growth. The colony cells actively reutilize DNA from the disintegrating lymphoid cells [66].

Despite the absence of GM-CFCs from lymphoid tissues, or the sites of infection or tumors, many studies have shown that antigens and other microbial products have a profound influence on GM-CFC and cluster-forming cell levels in hemopoietic tissues. It is quite apparent from these observations that the functional activity of GM-CFCs and cluster-forming cells together with their eventual progeny of neutrophils and macrophages is chiefly

Table 9. Effect of dilution on stimulation of bone marrow colony formation by yolk sac GM-CSF

Yolk sac GM-CSF dilution	Mean No. colonies	% Colonies		
		Granulocytic	Mixed	Macrophage
1:1	61	3	27	70
1:2	81	21	17	62
1:4	113	3	7	90
1:8	120	7	10	83
1:16	145	0	7	93
1:32	144	4	0	96
1:64	71	0	0	100
1:128	19	0	0	100
1:256	1	0	0	100

Cultures contained 40,000 syngeneic CBA bone marrow cells. Colonies scored on day 7. Yolk sac GM-CSF semipurified from 13–14-day mouse yolk sac-conditioned medium.

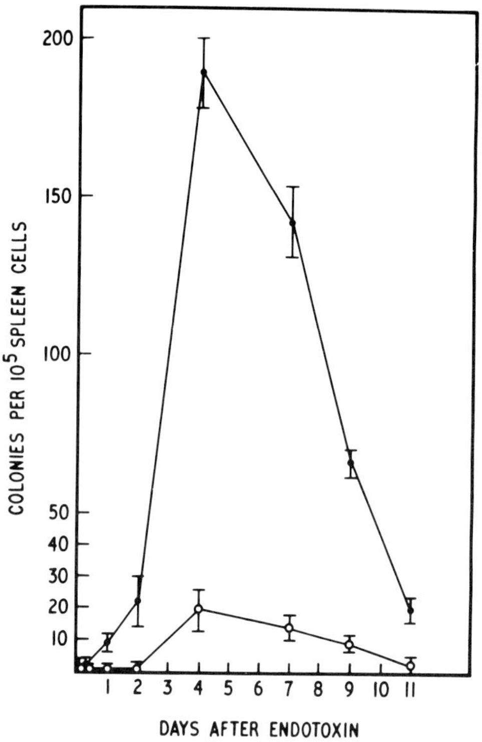

Fig. 20. Rise in spleen levels of GM-CFCs in $C_{57}BL$ mice after the intravenous injection of 5 μg endotoxin ●—●. Control mice injected with saline ○—○. Mean data from three mice at each timepoint ± standard deviations. (METCALF, D., unpublished data)

concerned with responses to antigens and microbial products. The magnitude of the changes induced in granulopoietic and macrophage-forming populations often exceeds comparable responses in lymphoid and plasma cell populations.

In the mouse, antigen-induced changes are usually not notable in the bone marrow where there are space limitations and where normally granulocytic cells comprise almost 50% of the marrow population, a situation providing little scope for population expansion. Thus, after the injection of the bacterial antigen polymerized flagellin or endotoxin, only slight rises occur in marrow levels of GM-CFCs although the ratio of clusters to colonies often rises [186]. One exception to this apparent unresponsiveness is observed following the injection of Freund's complete adjuvant when the marrow rapidly becomes composed of 80% granulocytic cells and GM-CFC levels rise three to fourfold [187].

While levels of GM-CFCs in the marrow do not normally rise dramatically after antigenic stimulation, it cannot be concluded that this tissue is unresponsive since the possibility exists that responses may be obscured by a corresponding increase in the release of GM-CFCs to the circulation with subsequent localization of these cells in the spleen. Studies have shown that GM-CFC levels rise 20-fold in the blood within 30 min of the injection of polymerized flagellin and that there is a simultaneous rise in spleen GM-CFC levels, consistent with seeding of these cells in this organ [188, 101].

After the injection of bacterial-derived antigens, endotoxin, or sheep red cells, spleen GM-CFCs rise progressively, reaching peak levels 4–7 days after injection, depending on the antigen used (Fig. 20). At peak responses, the spleen can contain 100–200 times the normal number of GM-CFCs, and there is an even greater rise in the number of cluster-forming cells [101, 189]. After peak responses, levels decline towards preinjection values, reaching them by 2–3 weeks.

A somewhat similar pattern of GM-CFC responses has been observed in mice bearing syngeneic progressively growing tumors, viral-induced but regressing tumors and mice carrying allogeneic tumors (190, METCALF, D., unpublished data). It is not clear whether the responses observed are due solely to tumor-specific transplantation antigens or partly to material from microorganisms contaminating the tumors.

The magnitude of splenic responses to antigens and endotoxin has been shown to be determined by the genetic makeup of the animal, the highest responses being exhibited by C_{57}BL mice. Colony-forming responses are reduced in mice at the extremes of age [191]. One very useful mouse strain is the C3H/HeJ which is unresponsive to endotoxin. When injected with endotoxin, mice of this strain fail to develop elevated GM-CSF levels and do not develop a rise in spleen GM-CFC levels [192, 193].

It is a characteristic feature of granulopoietic and macrophage responses to antigenic stimulation that, on secondary challenge, the responses are not increased but depressed or absent. This is the converse of the situation with lymphoid populations. Thus, in mice preinjected with polymerized flagellin, a challenge injection does not cause the rise in GM-CFCs in the peripheral blood and little change in spleen GM-CFC levels [188]. A similar pattern has been observed in mice injected and then challenged with endotoxin [120].

The converse of the response to antigens or endotoxin is seen in adult germfree mice. Although bone marrow levels of GM-CFCs and cluster-forming cells are near normal, spleen levels are notably subnormal [101]. However, such mice respond normally following challenge with antigens.

Not so much information exists on GM-CFC responses during the more complex situation of an actual bacterial or viral infection. However, in an extensive study by TRUDGETT et al. [194] mice were infected with *S. typhimurium*. In this model, 55% of the mice died within 14 days and the remainder had a persistent infection. During the observation period, femur GM-CFC levels remained fairly constant at 2–3 times normal levels. Spleen GM-CFC levels rose progressively during the infection reaching levels 20–50-fold above normal levels. These responses and the consequent leukocytosis were able to be maintained even in animals with overwhelming infections. A comparable study of the response of C_{57}BL mice to an *E. coli* septicemia documented similar changes in spleen GM-CFC levels (METCALF, D., and GLAUSER, J., unpublished data).

ITURRIZA and SEIDEL [195] observed similar changes in CBA mice infected with Rauscher leukemia virus. A progressive rise was observed in spleen CFU and GM-CFC levels reaching levels 20-fold above normal by 42 days after infection. Femur levels of GM-CFCs remained unaltered. However, this is a potentially very complex model in which the simple effects of a virus infection are complicated not only by the fact that the virus probably infects granulopoietic cells but also induces leukemia development. Because of this, part of the observed response might be viral-driven proliferation of granulopoietic cells or responses to the tumor-bearing state.

KURNICK and ROBINSON [196] reported a tenfold elevation of GM-CFC levels in the blood of patients in the acute stages of infectious mononucleosis and other viral infections. Most workers culturing marrow specimens from hematology clinics have cultured occasional specimens from patients with severe acute infections, e.g., septicemias. In most of these, GM-CFC levels have been high or very high.

There is a clear need for further studies on patients with acute infections to document whether some types of infections are characterized by abnormally high or low GM-CFC responses.

The conclusion from these observations is that splenic GM-CFC levels are almost wholly determined by current levels of exposure to microbial antigens and products, the considerable variability in spleen GM-CFC levels in conventional mice of a single strain reflecting varying recent exposure to such products.

While these conclusions appear to be true for adult animals, factors regulating spleen GM-CFC levels in fetal and embryonic mice may well differ. Neonatal spleens of germfree mice contain normal levels of GM-CFCs, and levels in both germfree and conventional neonatal spleens were much higher than those in adult animals [101]. It may be that these populations in fetal and neonatal animals are controlled by microenvironmental (tissue) factors that regulate the enlargement of these developing organs, but the nature of these influences has yet to be examined.

A number of studies have investigated the influence of macrophage numbers and functional activity in modifying spleen GM-CFC responses, a factor which might also be of relevance in determining the different response pattern between neonatal and adult spleens.

Pluznik et al. [189] showed that spleen GM-CFC levels rose in mice following the injection of sheep red cells, the height of the response being proportional to the concentration of red cells injected. Blockade of the reticuloendothelial system by saturation with particulate material can be achieved by the injection of colloidal carbon or horse red cells. While these procedures suppressed immune responses to sheep red cells, the blockading procedures themselves provoked a similar increase in spleen GM-CFC levels to that observed following the injection of sheep red cells alone [197]. One suggestion for interpreting these results is that stimulation of the phagocytic activity of spleen macrophages by particulate material [198] might block the inhibitory influence normally exerted by macrophages on GM-CFC numbers and proliferation [199]. In this context, addition of normal macrophages to cultures of GM-CFCs substantially inhibited colony formation stimulated by mouse embryo fibroblast GM-CSF. However, addition of macrophages which had ingested colloidal carbon or sheep red cells had a reduced inhibitory effect [200].

As discussed earlier, there is extensive evidence that macrophages can release and probably synthesize GM-CSF. If macrophages can also inhibit GM-CSF-induced cell proliferation under other circumstances, it is likely that some extremely complex interrelationships may exist between macrophages and GM-CFC populations during a biological process as intricate as an infection. To this must be added the likelihood that functionally different subpopulations of macrophages may exist [201] and play different roles in these interactions. For these reasons, there is an urgent need to miniaturize the assay systems so that macrophages from individual GM-colonies can be assessed for their functional activity.

Granulopoietic tissue is not distributed uniformly in the adult mouse spleen and tends to be restricted to regions under the capsule and the peripheral regions of the fibrous septae. The phenomenon of colony formation by hemopoietic cells in the spleen and the tendency for such granulocytic colonies to be subcapsular also indicates that the formation of morphologically identifiable granulopoietic populations depends on local tissue influences which are not distributed uniformly throughout the organ.

The nonrandom distribution of granulopoietic cells need not necessarily be paralleled by a corresponding distribution of GM-CFCs since such cells might be distributed uniformly but only be capable of proliferation in certain tissue locations. However, culture of cells from spleens divided into fragments also has shown a nonrandom distribution of GM-CFCs [101]. Many factors might account for this observation, e.g., a nonrandom distribution of CFUs, nonrandom distribution of microenvironments inducing CFUs to generate GM-CFCs, or nonrandom distribution of antigens and bacterial products.

The distribution pattern of GM-CFCs in marrow populations is more difficult to investigate because it is more difficult to get access to the undisturbed total population and because of the high level of GM-CFCs and their apparent unresponsiveness to antigens. Despite this, evidence has been produced that GM-CFCs are not distributed at random in the marrow population. Using controlled jets of fluid to selectively flush out more central and more peripherally located populations of cells, LORD et al. [131] demonstrated that the peak frequency of GM-CFCs occurs about three-quarters of the distance from the central axis to the surrounding bone, a distribution unlike that of CFUs which tend to be more peripherally located. As is the case for the spleen, this observation clearly indicates the importance of local control factors in determining GM-CFC levels, but again it cannot yet discriminate between the selective generation of GM-CFCs from CFUs or a selective build-up of GM-CFCs by accumulation, self-replication, or failure to proliferate.

Many of these questions may not be soluble until purified populations of the various precursor cells are available and simple three-dimensional matrices containing cells can be devised for an in vitro analysis of these problems under controlled conditions.

Two mouse strains, the NZB and SJL exhibit unusually high levels of GM-CFCs. Observations have not been made on levels in germfree mice of these strains, and the origin of the high levels has not been determined. NZB mice suffer from progressive autoimmune hemolytic anemia which raises the possibility that continuous antigenic stimulation may be a factor. The SJL mouse is noted for its capacity to develop myeloid leukemia following irradiation and for its spontaneous development of a high incidence of Hodgkin's-like lymphomas. It is thus a potentially very interesting mouse strain for extensive studies on GM-CFC populations.

One factor found to alter the frequency of GM-CFCs is the level of erythropoiesis in the mouse. If mice are rendered anemic by bleeding or phenylhydrazine, there is a fall in the frequency of GM-CFCs in the marrow, but oddly, a rise in GM-CFC levels in the spleen [202, 203, 204]. Conversely, hypertransfusion causes a regular increase in the frequency of marrow GM-CFCs.

These observations suggest that many erythropoietic progenitor cells and GM-CFCs may share a common ancestral cell, but it is unknown what is the mechanism underlying the apparent funneling of cells either into granulopoiesis or erythropoiesis according to demand.

As mentioned earlier, GM-CFCs are sensitive to irradiation and cortisone, and the sequence of regenerative changes has been observed following damage to these populations by either agent. No observations appear to have been made on responses to dietary or vitamin restrictions. Neither splenectomy or thymectomy in adult life has a significant influence on GM-CFC levels. Splenic GM-CFC levels are often abnormally high in young adult nude (congenitally athymic) mice, but this almost certainly is a consequence of their heightened susceptibility to infections and not to a direct effect of the absence of T-lymphocytes (METCALF, D., unpublished data).

Information on the distribution and level of GM-CFCs in other species including man is fragmentary. In all species, the relative frequency of GM-CFCs in the marrow, spleen, and blood is essentially similar to that described in detail for the mouse, but no detailed studies have been made on distribution patterns within organs or population changes following antigens, irradiation, drugs, etc. It is unlikely that, in principle, the situation in man or other animals will differ significantly from that in the mouse.

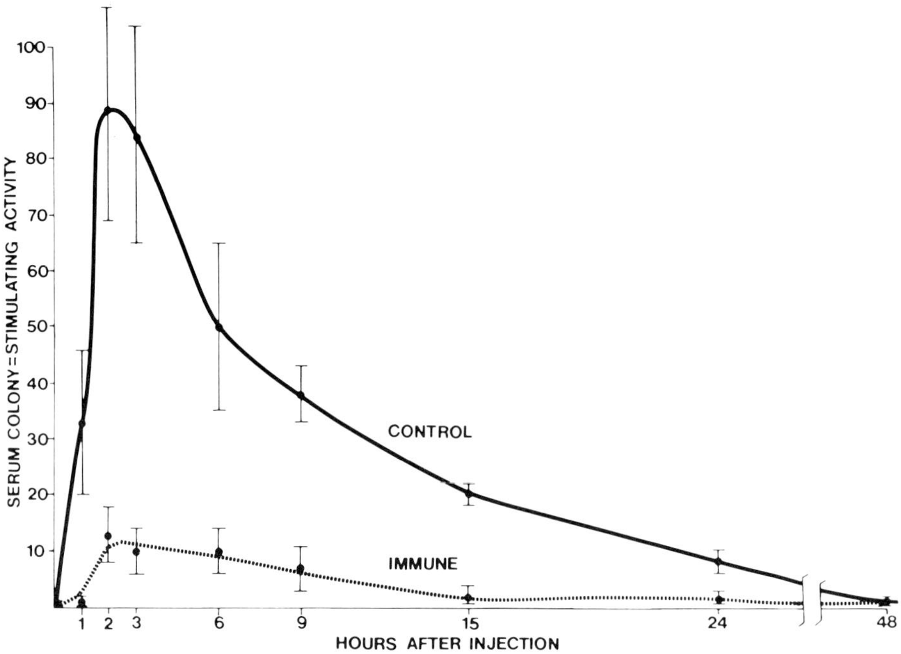

Fig. 21. Serum GM-CSF levels in $C_{57}BL$ mice after challenge with an intravenous injection of 10 μg of SL871 polymerized flagellin. Control mice had been injected 1 week earlier with saline ●—●, immune mice had been injected 1 week earlier with 20 μg SL871 polymerized flagellin. (Data redrawn from METCALF, 188)

L. Factors Modifying GM-CSF Levels

In the normal adult mouse the major factor influencing serum GM-CSF levels appears to be the same as that influencing GM-CFC levels in the spleen, namely, exposure to bacterial antigens and other microbial products.

Following the injection of polymerized flagellin or endotoxin, tissue levels of GM-CSF commence rising within 30 min and reach peak levels in 3–6 h [157]. This is paralleled by rises in serum GM-CSF levels which at 3–6 h reach levels 50–100-fold higher than in normal serum [49, 205] (Fig. 21). It should be recalled, as mentioned earlier, that serum GM-CSF levels tend to be overestimated because of a parallel rise in serum levels of a factor potentiating GM-CSF action in vitro [48, 64]. Some of the rise in serum CSF levels may be due to release of GM-CSF from tissue cells, a phenomenon which has been documented in vitro following the addition of endotoxin to macrophages [150, 151]. However, analysis of the GM-CSF present in tissues and serum after the injection of endotoxin has shown that much of it differs chemically from normal CSF and probably represents newly synthesized CSF [157]. Following achievement of peak levels at 6 h, tissue and serum levels fall progressively to preinjection values by 24–48 h. With other antigens and agents like Freund's adjuvant, serum GM-CSF levels become elevated more slowly and rises are more sustained [187].

An essentially similar response to endotoxin injection has been observed in humans [206].

Serum colony-stimulating activity for human marrow cultures rose to a maximum 1 h after injection and remained elevated for at least 3 h.

In mice preinjected with the same antigen or endotoxin, challenge injections induce very little rise in GM-CSF levels [49, 188, 207]. Unresponsiveness following a priming injection begins to be demonstrable within 24 h of the first injection and persists for at least 3–6 months. The basic GM-CSF response to antigens or endotoxin is radioresistant and is still demonstrable after 1500 rads of whole body irradiation [49]. It is also not dependent on T-lymphocytes since nude (congenitally hypothymic) mice exhibit normal responses. In preinjected unresponsive mice, whole body irradiation is capable of partially breaking the unresponsive state, and some rise in GM-CSF levels then occurs following challenge [188]. Depressed responsiveness can be transferred to normal mice by injection of serum from preimmunized mice prior to challenge injection.

The simplest, though not necessarily correct, interpretation of this data is that in preimmunized mice, small amounts of circulating antibody rapidly eliminate injected antigen or endotoxin thus preventing it from reaching target cells and provoking GM-CSF production and/or release. One problem with this type of explanation is in accounting for the fact that sequestered antigen-antibody complexes would be removed by macrophages, one of the cells involved in GM-CSF release following contact with antigen. It would need to be postulated that antigen-antibody complexes are presented to these cells in a manner not provoking GM-CSF release or that the antibody covers the active site on the endotoxin or antigen molecules.

Studies by PLUZNIK and his colleagues have shown that the lipid A portion of the endotoxin molecule is the active moiety in provoking GM-CSF rises and this portion of the molecule is also responsible for a number of the other biological actions of endotoxin [208].

APTE and PLUZNIK [192] have also demonstrated that C3H/He mice are unresponsive to endotoxin in terms of rises in serum GM-CSF and spleen GM-CFC levels. A genetic analysis of this situation using crosses and back crosses of responsive (C3H/eB) and unresponsive (C3H/He) mice has shown that serum GM-CSF responsiveness is determined by a single dominant gene; however, the splenic GM-CFC response appeared to be under polygenic control. In this work a notable linkage was observed between GM-CSF levels and spleen GM-CFC levels in individual mice providing strong indirect evidence that GM-CSF is biologically active in vivo. It is of interest that C3H/He mice are also unresponsive to endotoxin in terms of lymphocyte stimulation, a point of some potential interest in view of the known capacity of stimulated lymphocytes to produce GM-CSF. The GM-CFCs from nonresponder mice appear to be as responsive to GM-CSF in endotoxin sera as are GM-CFCs from responder mice [193].

Addition of antigens, endotoxin, or synthetic double-stranded polyribonucleotides directly to cultures of marrow cells does not stimulate GM-colony formation. However, in cultures containing low levels of GM-CSF, addition of such materials potentiates colony formation [209, 210, 186]. It is doubtful whether this potentiation results from a direct action of antigens on colony-forming or colony cells, and there is in fact some evidence that the antigens provoke a moderate release or production of GM-CSF within the culture dish thus indirectly stimulating colony formation [186]. A similar antigen-induced rise in GM-CSF production can be observed in cultures of normal or presensitized lymphoid cells [211].

A number of observers have shown that whole body irradiation provokes not only an immediate rise in serum CSF levels but also a delayed rise appearing up to several days later [212, 213]. In both cases, the magnitude of the rises is related to the dose of irradiation. It is probable that the delayed rise in GM-CSF levels is not a direct effect of irradiation but is due to secondary endotoxemia. It has been shown that germfree mice have very low serum GM-

CSF levels [214]. Whole body irradiation of germfree animals fails to elicit a serum rise in GM-CSF levels [215], and this only occurs if the animals are subsequently contaminated by gram-negative organisms [216].

Indirect in vivo evidence for a rise in serum and/or tissue fluid levels of granulopoietic factors has been obtained from an analysis of colony formation in agar contained in diffusion chambers [70, 217]. Colony formation was increased if the chambers were placed in preirradiated or cyclophosphamide-treated animals, suggesting that irradiation caused a rise in some diffusible factor, probably GM-CSF.

As discussed earlier, it has also been shown that whole body irradiation increases the capacity of radioresistant cells firmly adherent to the walls of the marrow cavity to produce GM-CSF in vitro [156]. After a dose of 250 rads, this capacity rose above normal at 7 days, 3 days before substantial regeneration of GM-CFCs occurred. CSF-producing capacity returned to normal levels when marrow granulopiesis was restored to preirradiation levels. This rising capacity to produce GM-CSF was preceded by a fall in serum levels of the lipoproteins capable of inhibiting granulocyte and macrophage colony formation in vitro. This association may indicate some relationship between serum inhibitor levels and either GM-CSF production or its capacity to stimulate target cells in the marrow.

As might be anticipated from the response of GM-CSF levels to bacterial antigens, serum and urine GM-CSF levels are elevated in most mice and patients in the acute stages of viral, bacterial, or protozoal infections [194, 218, 219, 220, 221, 222, 223]. Such elevated levels can be sustained for many days in contrast to the brief elevation and subsequent unresponsiveness following an injection of bacterial antigens or products. The reason why grossly elevated levels can be sustained almost indefinitely during natural infections has not yet been explained. It may be that, during a natural infection, the body is stimulated by a succession of active but unrelated antigens or possibly adjuvent-like effects might produce more sustained levels. Conceivably also, if sufficient organisms persist in the lesions, circulating antibody might be bound and permit the circulation of excess antigens or other products, so providing a continuous stimulus for GM-CSF production. Following natural or antibiotic-induced resolution of the infection, GM-CSF levels fall rapidly to normal levels.

Moderate elevations of GM-CSF levels have been observed in mice and humans with leukemia and other tumors, and the question of GM-CSF levels in leukemia will be discussed in Chapter 6. The mechanisms causing elevated GM-CSF levels in mice with spontaneous or transplanted tumors have not been investigated [16, 190]. Conceivably, they may result from stimulation by tumor-specific antigens although stimulation by allogeneic cells or foreign proteins has not been observed to cause an acute elevation (3–6 h) of GM-CSF levels. It is more likely that, as in the case of irradiation, the GM-CSF responses are triggered by low levels of bacterial products arising from intercurrent infections in these animals. A similar explanation probably is true for the moderate elevations of GM-CSF levels observed in F_1 hybrid mice injected with parental strain lymphoid cells and exhibiting mild graft-versus-host disease (Hibberd, A. D., unpublished data).

Elevations of serum and urine GM-CSF levels have been observed in patients with a variety of solid tumors. In one study, serum GM-CSF levels correlated with white cell levels in the patients [224]. In an analysis of serum and urine GM-CSF levels in patients with lymphoma, marked rises in levels were observed after chemotherapy [225].

Serum GM-CSF levels were observed to fall in mice following the injection of cortisol [110]. This was associated with a diuresis and the appearance of increased levels of GM-CSF in the urine [226]. The mechanism of action of the cortisone is unknown. While nephrectomy or ureteral ligation causes a rise in serum GM-CSF [226, 227], these procedures do not prevent the fall in serum GM-CSF levels which follows an endotoxin-induced rise [175], and there is other evidence to suggest that urine GM-CSF is not simply GM-CSF filtered from the plasma [175, 174].

Elevations of serum and urine colony-stimulating activity were observed in patients on lithium carbonate, a substance capable of provoking a granulocytosis [228, 229]. Two types of cyclic fluctuation in serum and/or urine GM-CSF levels have been observed in man and dogs: (1) a diurnal fluctuation has been observed in man in the urine output of GM-CSF [52] and (2) cyclic fluctuations of 2–3 weeks periodicity have been observed in patients and gray collie dogs with cyclic neutropenia [147, 149, 230, 134]. The association of these cycles with out-of-phase cycles of granulopiesis is strong evidence for an in vivo function of GM-CSF.

One situation in which it might be expected to observe alterations in GM-CSF levels is in experimentally induced neutropenia or in patients with neutropenia. While this should be similar to the well-known inverse relationship between hematocrit and erythropoietin levels, the situation is made much more difficult to interpret by the fact that neutropenia increases susceptibility to infections which, as discussed above, have a strong influence on GM-CSF levels.

In mice made neutropenic by the injection of antineutrophil serum, increased GM-CSF levels were observed [231]. On the other hand, no increases in serum or urine GM-CSF levels were observed in patients with chronic neutropenia of more than 1 year's duration [232] or in children with severe congenital neutropenia [233].

Further correlative studies are needed in neutropenic patients to determine the exact situation. Ideally, such studies should examine both chloroform-extractable and nonextractable material, and assays should be performed both in human and mouse marrow cultures. Because human serum is capable of potentiating colony formation in the presence of low concentrations of GM-CSF [48, 234], such assays may even need to be performed using fractionated sera.

M. Inhibitors of Granulocyte-Macrophage Colony Formation

It is generally agreed that, for the control of proliferating mammalian cells, the optimal system would be a balanced set of stimulating and inhibitory factors. Little concrete evidence exists to support this widely accepted notion, and it may be nothing more than a model builder's dream. However, the in vitro cloning systems should be ideal for the detection of such inhibitors if they exist. So far, efforts to detect such inhibitors have been restricted almost entirely to inhibitors of granulocyte-macrophage colony formation. The general subject of humoral inhibitors of granulopoiesis has been extensively reviewed by VOGLER and WINTON [235].

Three general types of inhibitory factors for granulocyte-macrophage colony formation have been demonstrated by various workers: (1) serum inhibitors, (2) granulocyte-derived inhibitors ("chalones"), and (3) uncharacterized low molecular weight inhibitors.

1. Serum Inhibitors.

In some of the earliest work on GM-colonies, colony formation was stimulated by normal or leukemic mouse sera [95, 236, 237]. It was soon recognized that the addition of 0.1 or 0.2 ml of undiluted mouse serum to a culture dish frequently stimulated the formation of fewer and smaller colonies than did smaller serum doses. The plates characteristically had a scum on the surface, often pseudocrystalline in appearance, most cells in the dish appeared to be pyknotic, and those colonies that did develop were invariably composed of macrophages with bulky opaque cytoplasm. If the plates were not well-mixed, some colony formation could occur in parts of the plate obviously containing lower serum concentrations. Investigation of this phenomenon showed that the serum inhibitors were heat labile [237, 238], poorly diffusible in agar, and could be removed by ether or chloroform extraction [239, 222] or by dialysis of the serum against water [238]. The inhibitory material did not pass through the dialysis bag but precipitated out of the dialyzed serum and could be removed by centrifugation, then redissolved in phosphate buffered saline [238, 239].

Parallel studies showed that the two most efficient methods for removing serum inhibitors were either chloroform extraction [222] or floatation centrifugation over sodium chloride gradients [222, 102] where the majority of the inhibitory material was recovered in the very light density fractions (Fig. 22).

From the very low buoyant density of the inhibitors and their removal by chloroform, it can be concluded that they contain lipid. Fractionation procedures using Sephadex chromatography suggested that the inhibitors in BALB/c serum had an apparent mol wt of 250,000 [102]. Treatment of human serum with a specific antihuman β-lipoprotein serum removed most of the inhibitory activity [222]. These serum inhibitors are frequently referred to as "lipoproteins," but they have not been purified, and no formal tests have been performed using peptidases to demonstrate their peptide content. At present therefore the lipoprotein nature of these inhibitors remains unproven.

To be satisfactory candidates for selective inhibitory factors for GM-CSF, these serum inhibitors should exhibit the same high degree of specificity of target cell action as shown by GM-CSF. However, studies on semipurified serum inhibitors have shown them to be equally inhibitory for colony formation in agar by eosinophils, B-lymphocytes, lymphoid leukemic

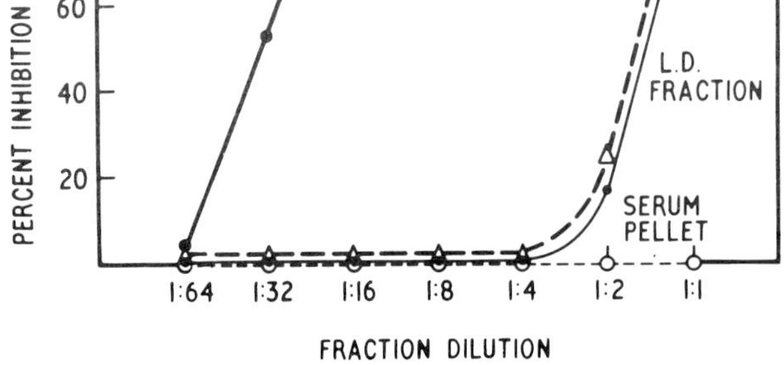

Fig. 22. Inhibitory activity for GM-colony formation by $C_{57}BL$ marrow cells of BALB/c serum, very light density fraction (VLD), light density fraction (LD), and serum pellet from BALB/c serum. GM-CSF source was endotoxin serum. (From METCALF and RUSSELL, [102]. Reproduced with permission from Experimental Hematology)

cells, mastocytoma, and plasmacytoma cells [102]. While it must be emphasized that the preparations tested had not been purified to a single molecular species, the apparent complete lack of target cell specificity is not encouraging.

One argument in favor of the possibility that serum inhibitors may represent a balancing system for GM-CSF is that, in the presence of moderate concentrations of inhibitors, colony formation can be achieved by increasing the concentration of GM-CSF [102]. This raises the possibility that inhibitors might complex with GM-CSF extracellularly or compete with membrane receptors for these molecules. However, if inhibitory serum containing GM-CSF is placed in an 0.5% agar underlayer, the CSF readily diffuses into the target cell overlayer. The inhibitors have essentially no capacity for diffusion through agar of this concentration and are retained in the underlayers [239]. This suggests that if such inhibitor-GM-CSF complexes exist in serum, they must readily be dissociable.

A puzzling aspect of serum inhibitors is the fact that, as assayed in vitro, serum levels of inhibitory activity appear to be extremely high. Indeed, if equivalent concentrations of inhibitors are used to duplicate levels present in the serum, no concentration of GM-CSF is sufficiently high to be able to compete and stimulate colony formation [102] (or else the material is completely cytotoxic). This forces the conclusion that if these inhibitors function in vivo as they do in vitro, some sort of shielding system or microenvironment would be necessary to permit granulopoiesis.

There are characteristic strain differences in inhibitor levels, C_{57}BL mice uniformly exhibiting the lowest levels [102]. Indeed, there are some interesting correlations to be observed in comparing different strains of mice. As pointed out first by McNeill and Fleming [240] and confirmed in this laboratory [102], GM-CFCs from different mouse strains vary in their responsiveness to GM-CSF, cells from C_{57}BL mice being the most responsive while cells from BALB/c and CBA mice (mice with the highest serum inhibitor levels) are relatively unresponsive (Fig. 23). In cultures containing GM-CSF from mouse lung-conditioned medium or endotoxin serum, cells from C_{57}BL mice tend to produce mainly granulocytic or mixed colonies, whereas BALB/c and CBA cells produce a higher proportion of macrophage colonies. Chan [238] observed that the preincubation of C_{57}BL marrow cells with serum inhibitors, followed by washing of the cells, altered the subsequent behavior of these cells in culture, and they produced a higher than normal proportion of macrophage colonies. In an extension of this work, this basic observation was confirmed and preincubation with BALB/c serum inhibitors was shown to render C_{57}BL cells less responsive than normal to GM-CSF [102]. In other words, the characteristic growth pattern of BALB/c or CBA marrow cells could be duplicated in cultures of C_{57}BL marrow cells if the cells were first preincubated with low concentrations of inhibitor preparations from BALB/c mice.

These observations certainly raise a strong possibility that serum inhibitors may somehow be involved in the regulation in vivo of granulopoiesis and monocyte formation. Conflicting evidence on this question can be summarized as follows:

1. Serum inhibitors can be reduced by prior starvation [160], or within minutes by the intravenous injection of heparin (Chan, S. H., unpublished data). However, neither procedure seems likely to have a significant influence on granulopoiesis.
2. It has been claimed that higher net colony-stimulating activity of sera from patients with acute infections is not due to elevated GM-CSF levels but to a fall in serum inhibitor levels [222]. A similar fall in inhibitor levels was noted in mouse sera 2–8 h following the injection of endotoxin (Granstrom, M., M.D. Thesis, 1974). However, analysis of serum inhibitor levels in BALB/c mice showed no significant falls in inhibitor levels at 3 and 6 h after the injection of endotoxin (Russell, S. and Metcalf, D., unpublished data).

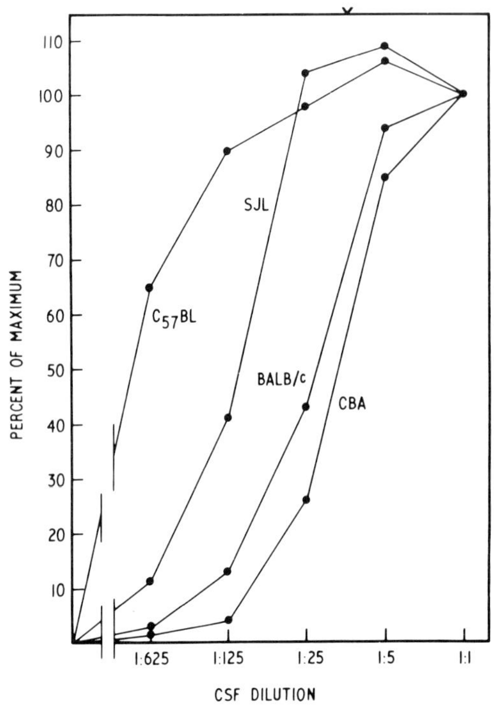

Fig. 23. Relative responsiveness of GM-CFCs from mice of different strains to stimulation by varying concentrations of GM-CSF. (From METCALF and RUSSELL, [102]. Reproduced with permission from Experimental Hematology)

Similarly, removal of inhibitors using chloroform did not alter the colony-stimulating activity of post endotoxin sera from responding and nonresponding C3H mice [193].

3. Serum inhibitor levels fell in mice bearing advanced myelomonocytic leukemias, and in a small series of control experiments, this effect was not seen in mice bearing plasma cell tumors or a fibrosarcoma [238].
4. Serum inhibitor levels in irradiated C_{57}BL and BALB/c mice fell abruptly a few days prior to an increase in the bone stromal capacity to produce GM-CSF in vitro and the simultaneous onset of regeneration of granulopoietic populations [156]. Serum inhibitor levels returned to normal at the same time as restoration of full marrow cellularity. The suggestion from these studies was strong that serum inhibitor levels normally might partially suppress GM-CSF production in the marrow and that release from this suppression permitted the onset of regeneration. Such an effect has been demonstrated in vitro using serum inhibitors to suppress bone stromal production of GM-CSF by tissues from irradiated mice [241].
5. Serum inhibitor levels were undetectable or abnormally low in about half the serum samples tested from patients with AML in cultures of mouse bone marrow cells [242, 223]. This was not seen with sera from other types of leukemia. No correlation was observed between serum inhibitor levels and the relapse-remission status of the patient, but some correlation was observed between low serum inhibitor levels and a short survival time in the patients. However, parallel studies by GRANSTROM et al. [243] failed to confirm the presence of low inhibitor levels in sera from patients with acute leukemia.

These serum inhibitors are somewhat unsatisfactory candidates for specific GM-CSF inhibitors. There is so far no evidence of specificity, they have proved refractory to purification using standard techniques of separative protein chemistry, and they fluctuate in response to nonspecific procedures such as starvation. Despite these unpromising aspects, there are sufficiently intriguing correlations between changes in inhibitor levels and granulopoiesis to force them to be retained as candidates for specific inhibitors. A resolution of this dilemma will almost certainly require purification of the inhibitors and subsequent stringent tests for their specificity of target cell action.

2. Granulocyte and Macrophage-Derived Inhibitors (Chalones)

The chalone concept postulates that proliferating cell systems can be specifically inhibited by products from the most mature elements in the sequence. Frequently added provisos are that the inhibition be reversible and that the inhibitors, while tissue-specific, need not be species-specific. Application of this concept to granulopoiesis and macrophage formation would propose that polymorphs and/or macrophages should be able to specifically inhibit granulopoiesis and macrophage formation.

While the chalone concept has an immediate appeal to logic, it suffers from forcing an unlikely simplicity onto clearly complex biological systems and to be rigidly proved demands technical expertise beyond the level so far attained in any laboratory. As a consequence, many papers have been written purporting to work with granulocytic chalones in which the experimental procedures in no way fulfilled the requirements of a purified starting population of end cells as source material and usually made little effort to document specificity.

Use of the term "chalone" usually seems to have a polarizing effect, splitting any scientific group into the disciples and the unbelievers. This is unfortunate since there is quite a lot of evidence that various inhibitory factors can be derived from polymorphs and macrophages. Rather than enter the fruitless controversies surrounding chalones, these will be discussed as granulocytic and macrophage-derived inhibitors.

RYTOMAA and KIVINIEMI [244] reported studies on serum of normal and leukophoresed rats and extracts of blood and peritoneal exudate cells. The active material from these sources was claimed to be granulocyte-derived, although this was not proved, and was shown to inhibit the uptake of tritiated thymidine by marrow cells. Autoradiographic analysis suggested that the observed depression was due mainly to inhibition of granulocytic cells [245]. Analysis of the active fractions suggested a mol wt of approximately 4000.

Inhibitory material for granulocyte and macrophage colony formation was noted by SHADDUCK [246] and MACVITTIE and MCCARTHY [247] in incubates containing a high proportion of granulocytes although the exact cellular origin and chemical nature of the inhibitory material were not established. PARAN et al. [248] also described inhibition of granulocyte and macrophage colony formation by granulocyte-conditioned medium, the active material being nondialyzable.

A superficially similar inhibitory influence ascribed to granulocytes was noted in cultures of human marrow cells [249]. Analysis of this type of culture has supported the likelihood that the polymorphs are indeed the source of the inhibitory material, but the mechanism of action appears to be via a suppression of colony-stimulating cells (cells producing GM-CSF in the feeder layer and/or target layers), rather than a direct inhibitory effect on target granulopoietic cells. In fact, if exogenous GM-CSF is used to stimulate the cultures, no inhibition of granulocyte colony formation is observed [46].

The influence of polymorphs on colony formation by human cells appears to be dose related. At high cell concentrations, polymorphs inhibited colony formation but at low concentrations quite strongly potentiated colony formation [425].

LORD et al. [250, 251] analyzed the effects of saline extracts of granulocytes on marrow populations or cultured granulopoietic cells, inhibition being measured by determination of the structuredness of the cytoplasm, an indirect measure of the cell cycle status of the cells. The active inhibitory material in such extracts appeared to be of 500–2000 mol wt and was reasonably specific in that it did not inhibit parallel cultures of fetal liver erythropoietic cells or PHA-stimulated lymphocytes.

PAUKOVITS [252, 253] also reported the extraction of a low molecular weight inhibitor from calf serum and the supernatant of granulocyte-rich ascites fluid. The assay method was inhibition of tritiated thymidine uptake into unfractionated bone marrow cells, but no data were presented to support the claim either that the inhibitor really was of granulocytic origin or that the inhibition was restricted to granulopoietic cells.

Although these experiments leave much to be desired, collectively they do suggest that relatively specific inhibitors may be released or extracted from polymorphs. These inhibitors may not only block GM-CSF synthesis but also inhibit the proliferation of granulocytes and macrophages. One feature of many of these experiments is worthy of comment. The duration of the period during which the polymorphs "conditioned" the medium was often extremely short, i.e., under 1 h. Often this represented merely a washing of the cells. No valid evidence has been presented that such inhibitory material is actually synthesized by the polymorphs, and a possibility exists that in fact the inhibitory material might have originated elsewhere in the body and have been bound to the membranes of the polymorphs. If so, it is not surprising that some selectivity of action against granulocytes might be demonstrable.

3. *Miscellaneous Inhibitors*

In earlier studies it was shown that many normal and neoplastic cells in culture release low molecular weight material into the medium which inhibits colony formation in granulocyte and macrophage cultures [254]. No specificity of cell origin was able to be documented nor was there any evidence for specificity of target cell inhibition. These low molecular weight inhibitors might well be toxic metabolites of trivial importance.

On a possibly more significant plane, it has been reported that macrophages release relatively large amounts of prostaglandin E, particularly after stimulation by GM-CSF and that this low molecular weight substance is a potent inhibitor of colony formation [255]. It is tempting to speculate that prostaglandin E might represent a negative feedback inhibitory loop by which mature macrophages inhibit granulopoiesis and macrophage formation. However, at the same concentrations, prostaglandin E is inhibitory for colony formation by unrelated B-lymphocytes and various tumor cell lines [255]. Lack of adequate selectivity in inhibitory action again appears to mar prostaglandin E as a genuine candidate for an inhibitor in the granulopoietic system.

LOZZIO and LOZZIO [256] isolated a low molecular weight (less than 1000) substance from human and bovine spleen which was cytotoxic for granulocytic and macrophage colonies in agar.

Finally, interferon has been shown to be capable of inhibiting granulocyte and macrophage colony formation [257, 258]. However, interferon is inhibitory for a wide range of normal and neoplastic cells in vitro and it is again difficult to accept this substance as a significant specific regulator of granulopoiesis in vivo.

For none of these miscellaneous inhibitors has a strong case been made for consideration as a specific inhibitory regulator of granulopoiesis. Progress will only be made in this field by a willingness to use all of the available hemopoietic cloning systems in elementary tests of target cell specificity and a much more stringent attempt to free starting populations of contaminating cells of other types. It is not satisfactory to use populations of only 80 or 90% purity. Work with inhibitors is acknowledged to be fraught with the hazard that irrelevant in vitro artifacts will be detected. Minimum prerequisites before extensive studies are undertaken should be that there is clear evidence (1) for the occurrence of the inhibitor in the serum or relevant tissue, and (2) that inhibitor levels fluctuate in circumstances where fluctuations in granulopoiesis are occurring. Unless both conditions are met, the likelihood of the phenomenon being an in vitro artifact must be recognized as being very high.

N. Evidence for the in vivo Function of GM-CSF

Evidence of two types has been produced to indicate that GM-CSF probably functions in vivo as a major regulator of granulocytic and monocyte-macrophage formation: (1) indirect studies on correlations between GM-CSF levels and GM-CFC levels or other parameters of granulopoiesis, and (2) observations on the in vivo effects of injected GM-CSF.

Related fluctuations in serum and/or urine GM-CSF levels on the one hand and granulopoiesis on the other have been observed in: (1) cyclic neutropenia in dogs and man [147, 149, 134], (2) cyclic neutropenia in patients with CML [148], (3) following injection of endotoxin in mice and man [186, 49, 187, 101], (4) in acute viral and bacterial infections in mice [194, 221], and (5) in regeneration following irradiation or the injection of antigranulocytic antisera [156, 231].

As mentioned earlier, the parallel failure of GM-CSF and GM-CFC levels to rise following the injection of endotoxin in refractory C3H/He mice [193] or mice preimmunized by prior injection of endotoxin [188, 120] are of particular interest in this context.

Observations on the effects of injections of purified GM-CSF are the only real method for determining GM-CSF action in vivo. Purified $GM\text{-}CSF_{MLCM}$ has a half-life of 5–7 h in syngeneic mice [174] and human urine GM-CSF a half-life of approximately 3 h [173]. No studies have yet been performed on mice injected with purified GM-CSF, but some observations have been made on mice injected with partially purified human urine GM-CSF or crude mouse embryo-conditioned medium and mouse lung-conditioned medium. Following the injection of crude GM-CSF, no immediate rise in blood GM-CFC levels occurred indicating that this factor does not cause release of GM-CFCs to the circulation [188]. This agrees with correlative studies indicating that GM-CSF and the leukocytosis inducing (releasing) factor (LIF) are not identical [259]. Minor rises in marrow GM-CFC levels were observed following a single injection of human urine GM-CSF in adult mice. Rises in cluster-forming cell levels were also observed and labeling studies with ^{3}HTdR indicated an increased production of neutrophils and monocytes, blood levels peaking at 48 h following injection [132]. Of some interest, in view of the action of GM-CSF in vitro in shortening the lag time before initiation of proliferation, was the observation that GM-CFCs from mice injected 24 h previously with GM-CSF showed a comparable reduction in the lag period before proliferation commenced after these cells were placed in culture. Control injections of urine fractions containing no GM-CSF did not produce this effect.

Earlier studies on the effects of crude GM-CSF from mouse embryo-conditioned medium indicated that repeated injections over a 6-day period could induce a substantial rise in spleen and blood GM-CFC levels with some rise in peripheral blood neutrophil levels [260]. Injections of control (inactive) thymus-conditioned medium did not produce these effects.

O. Comparison of Agar Cultures with Other Methods for Assessing Granulopoiesis and Monocyte-Macrophage Formation in vivo

The assessment of the level of granulopoiesis or monocyte-macrophage formation in a patient or animal is a difficult technical problem. Unlike the situation with erythropoiesis where red cell and reticulocyte levels in the peripheral blood are valuable parameters, blood levels of neutrophils and monocytes can be quite misleading measures of the rate or magnitude of production of these cells [261].

Marrow biopsies can provide at best a representative sample of the marrow population, but in humans total cell numbers can only be guessed at from the apparent cellularity of the specimen. Since no specific isotopic markers exist for either cell population, whole body scanning can only give a rough approximation of total marrow cells. This usually involves an assumption, e.g., that the labeled cells have a constant frequency in relation to neutrophilic and monocytic cells.

The alternative procedure is to perform an autoradiographic analysis of marrow and blood populations following in vivo labeling with ^{3}HTdR. This procedure can provide accurate estimates of transit times between various relatively mature compartments in these related populations but has a number of disadvantages: (1) it is a time-consuming and expensive procedure only available to highly specialized laboratories, (2) it involves multiple sampling of marrow and blood populations, (3) it can provide no information on granulopoietic and monocytic progenitor populations since these cannot be identified morphologically, and (4) data produced must be interpreted on the assumption that cells of a particular morphological category are uniform populations with similar proliferative capacity and a similar capacity for differentiation. Work on agar cultures has shown that this last assumption is quite incorrect, as granulopoietic populations are extremely heterogeneous, and in any disease state or experimental manipulation not all subpopulations can be assumed to respond uniformly.

Agar cultures of neutrophilic and macrophage colonies cannot supply some of the information obtained from isotopic labeling methods, but they offer several advantages which make them irreplaceable in the assessment of granulopoiesis and monocyte-macrophage formation both in patients and experimental animals: (1) the technique is relatively simple and inexpensive, (2) the information is generated by a single biopsy specimen, (3) the technique permits the enumeration of progenitor cells and an assessment of their proliferative capacity, information which cannot be obtained by any other method, (4) the technique permits studies on the heterogeneous subpopulations of progenitor cells, again a unique virtue of cloning techniques. Because of the high plating efficiency of the technique, agar cultures give an accurate estimate of the frequency of progenitor (colony-forming) cells and their individual proliferative capacity (colony size). A more detailed analysis of the pattern of cluster and colony formation in the culture dish provides an instantaneous representation of the general pattern of proliferation exhibited by these cells in the marrow at the time the sample was taken. For example, if cultures contain only colonies but no clusters, it can be concluded that in vivo the GM-CFCs were either not proliferating or that the progeny were destroyed or matured abnormally rapidly. Conversely, a high cluster to colony ratio indicates usually the existence of active proliferation in these populations.

Agar cultures of human marrow populations have the same limitations as other methods in that the *frequency* but not the total number of cells is being enumerated. Furthermore, the possibility of a variable degree of dilution by blood cannot readily be excluded. To correct this latter possibility, some workers have related the frequency of GM-CFCs to marrow cells exclusive of polymorphs and/or lymphocytes, but this is not a wholly satisfactory procedure

since at least some of both cell types are genuine members of the marrow population.
For experimental animals, where total marrow cell counts can be performed, agar cultures give highly reproducible data on granulopoiesis and monocyte-macrophage formation subject only to the provision that possible fluctuations in culture media or incubating conditions are controlled by the parallel culture of reference populations of cultured cells, e.g. pooled marrow cells from the standard animal being used or reference populations kept in liquid nitrogen.
Few parallel studies have yet been performed to compare assessments of granulopoiesis by agar culture and labeling methods, but there is sufficient general information from experimental animals to make it probable that the two methods of assessment would usually be in good agreement. In one study, GM-CFC levels in patients with myeloid hyperplasia were elevated above normal and in patients with myeloid hypoplasia were less than half normal levels [262]. Similarly, in patients with idiopathic or drug-induced granulocytopenia or aplastic anemia, reduced levels of GM-CFCs were observed in the marrow [263]. It is quite conceivable, however, that in certain disease states the two methods may give apparently inconsistent answers, e.g., granulopoiesis may be documentable in the apparent absence of GM-CFCs, etc. Provided that these discrepancies are not due to simple technical faults, the inconsistencies are more likely to provide important clues as to the nature of the underlying abnormalities rather than to indicate the unreliability of agar cultures. One possible example of this type of situation is the report [264] that GM-CFC levels in patients with genetic neutropenia were not depressed and in fact were about twice normal levels. A similar finding was made in children with congenital neutropenia [233]. This might reflect an attempt at compensatory hyperplasia in the presence of some maturation defect leading to premature loss of maturing cells.
In the special case of granulopoiesis in AML, as shall be discussed in Chapter 6, agar cultures have provided dramatic evidence of the inherent proliferative abnormalities in the leukemic cells and their abnormal responsiveness to stimulating factors, observations which could never have been deduced from in vivo labeling studies.

P. Summary

Cells forming neutrophilic and macrophage colonies (GM-colony-forming cells, GM-CFC) are the progeny of multipotential stem cells (CFU) and the ancestors of the cells forming clusters of neutrophils or macrophages in vitro. In the adult, the GM-CFCs are mainly located in the bone marrow, with small numbers also present in the spleen and blood.
The proliferation of GM-CFCs to form colonies is under the control of a specific glycoprotein, GM-colony-stimulating factor (GM-CSF). GM-CSF occurs in more than one molecular form varying in size from 23,000 to 100,000 daltons. The heterogeneity of GM-CSFs is matched to some extent by a corresponding heterogeneity of GM-CFCs since distinct and partially separable subpopulations of these cells exist which vary in their responsiveness to different types of GM-CSF. GM-CSF is required continuously and is active at molar concentrations of 10^{-11}. It can force noncycling GM-CFCs into cycle, shorten the cell cycle time of dividing cells, and influence the rate of maturation of colony cells.
Direct and indirect evidence indicates that GM-CSF functions in vivo in a comparable manner to regulate neutrophil and monocyte-macrophage formation.
The major factor influencing GM-CSF and GM-CFC levels in normal life is exposure to microbial antigens, but GM-CSF levels are altered in a number of disease states affecting

granulopoiesis and monocyte formation and by experimental procedures affecting these populations.

Agar cultures permit the determination of the number of granulocytic and monocyte progenitor cells in tissues, the assessment of their proliferative capacity or activity, the measurement of GM-CSF levels, and the detection of other factors influencing the action of GM-CSF on granulopoietic and macrophage-forming cells.

Chapter 6

Colony Formation by Myeloid Leukemic Cells

Following the demonstration that normal progenitor cells of neutrophils and monocyte-macrophages could be cloned in semisolid cultures, extensive studies have been made on the capacity of the neoplastic equivalents of these cells to proliferate in agar.

A. Colony Formation by Mouse Myeloid and Myelomonocytic Leukemic Cells

Although the first successful demonstrations of the capacity of myeloid and myelomonocytic leukemic cells to proliferate in agar were made using transplanted mouse tumors [14, 15, 16], subsequent studies have shown that most mouse myeloid leukemias are in fact unable to proliferate in the type of culture system being used at present. As shall be discussed later, the situation is quite different with human myeloid leukemic cells where cells from the vast majority of patients can be cultured successfully.

Most information on the behavior of mouse myeloid leukemic cells has come from studies by ICHIKAWA, SACHS, and their colleagues on a myeloid leukemia in SD mice and from studies by METCALF and colleagues on two transplantable myelomonocytic leukemias in BALB/c mice. While the data are extensive, the conclusions must be accepted with the reservation that only a small number of individual leukemias has been investigated, and the results may not necessarily be applicable to all myeloid leukemias in mice. This type of reservation does not apply to the studies on human myeloid leukemias where many hundreds of patients have been examined.

ICHIKAWA [14] demonstrated that cells from a spontaneously arising transplantable myeloid leukemia of SL mice (Ml) could be grown in liquid suspension cultures as uniform blast cells exhibiting little sign of differentiation. When such cells were cultured in semisolid agar, they formed compact colonies composed of the same type of relatively undifferentiated cells. However, when the cultures contained medium conditioned by normal secondary mouse embryo cells, increased numbers of colonies formed, and in a high proportion of these colonies maturing granulocytes and monocytes developed. Increasing the concentration of conditioned medium increased the proportion of differentiating colonies, and active conditioned media were obtained using a number of other normal tissues. Medium conditioned by the leukemic cells themselves had some capacity to induce differentiation in agar colony cells but did not stimulate granulocyte or macrophage colony formation by normal cells.

In further studies, it was shown that preincubation of leukemic cells for 48 or 72 h in the absence of conditioned medium led to a loss of colony-forming ability [15]. Based on differential heat lability, it was suggested that two factors were present in the conditioned media: (1) a heat-labile factor affecting differentiation of colony cells, and (2) a relatively heat-stable growth-stimulating factor affecting the number of colonies formed by the leukemic cells. Ultrafiltration using diaflow membranes indicated that both activities were due to molecules probably larger than 10,000 mol wt although some growth stimulation was observed with the filtrates, suggesting the presence of active material of lower molecular weight [265].

Exposure of cultured cells to 5-bromodeoxyuridine (BUdR) has been found to suppress differentiation in various cells although not interfering with cell replication [266, 267, 268]. Preincubation of the M1 leukemic cells with BUdR had a similar effect in suppressing their capacity to differentiate to phagocytic macrophages [265].

One important aspect of the differentiation induced in these leukemic cells by incubation with conditioned medium was the loss, or marked reduction, of the capacity to produce leukemia on reimplantation of the cells in syngeneic recipients. Thus all mice injected with 10^5 control cultured leukemic cells died of leukemia, whereas injection of 10^6 cells from cultures containing conditioned medium failed to produce leukemia [15].

Subsequent extensive studies on this line of murine myeloid leukemic cells were made by FIBACH, SACHS, and their colleagues. Addition of medium conditioned by mouse fibroblasts increased colony numbers produced by the leukemic cells and induced maturation to nondividing granulocytes and macrophages. Similar results were obtained with 600-fold purified macrophage-granulocyte inducer (MGI) from such conditioned medium [269]. MGI is probably equivalent to GM-CSF although, as noted in Chapter 5, the Israeli investigators have not observed carbohydrate in the molecule and have found that, in their culture system, addition of adenine-containing compounds is necessary for colony formation by normal cells [172]. However, with the myeloid leukemic cells, this cofactor was not required for colony formation or the differentiation of colony cells [269].

Further studies showed that clones could be derived from this leukemia which were capable of being induced to differentiate to granulocytes and macrophages (D+) and clones which were not (D−). D+ clones were able to segregate some D− progeny and vice versa. Apparently normal differentiation could be induced by MGI even when the cells were aneuploid [270, 271]. Sera from mice of many strains injected with endotoxin [272] and mouse lung-conditioned medium [273] were also able to increase cloning efficiency and to induce differentiation in D+ but not D− cells. Normal serum from the same mouse strains was able to stimulate colony formation by D+ cells but not to induce maturation of the colony cells.

The centrifugal migration of cells from D+ leukemic colonies and the maturation to granulocytes and macrophages stimulated by the conditioned medium or endotoxin serum could be mimicked by a number of agents blocking cell division, e.g., cytosine arabinoside, hydroxyurea, and mitomycin C [274]. Analysis of the membranes of differentiating D+ cloned cells showed that they acquired receptors for the Fc portion of immunoglobulin and complement receptors similar in nature to those developing on normal granulocytic and macrophage colony cells. (IR+D+ cells) [275]. Receptors were also able to be induced on D+ cells by prednisolone, cytosine arabinoside, 5-iododeoxyuridine and actinomycin D, receptor development requiring protein synthesis. Further analysis of D− cells showed that some could be induced to develop receptors (IR+D− cells) although not to undergo morphological differentiation to mature cells. The steroid hormones prednisolone, dexamethazone, and estradiol were able to induce IR+D+ cells to develop receptors for complement but not Fc [276], but progesterone, testosterone, and cortisone were inactive and in fact inhibited induction of the receptors by the other hormones.

Comparative analysis of IR+D+, IR+D− cells after preincubation with mouse lung-conditioned medium showed that only the IR+D+ cells failed to produce leukemia after reinjection into syngeneic mice. Thus, loss of leukemic potential in terms of capacity for progressive proliferation in vivo was correlated with morphological differentiation to mature

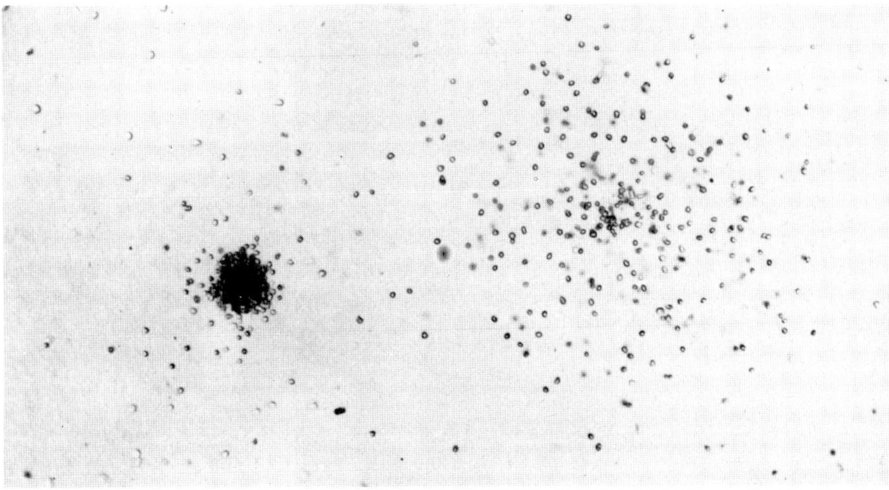

Fig. 24. Two colonies in an unstained culture of spleen cells from a BALB/c mouse with transplanted WEHI-3 myelomonocytic leukemia. Left, compact WEHI-3 leukemic colony; right, loose normal macrophage colony. (From METCALF et al. [16]. Reproduced with permission from Journal of the National Cancer Institute)

granulocytes and macrophages rather than simply the acquisition of Fc or C3 membrane receptors characteristic of normal differentiated cells [273].

A parallel series of experiments has been performed by METCALF and colleagues on two transplantable myelomonocytic leukemias of BALB/c mice (WEHI-3 and WEHI-265). The etiological origin of both is uncertain—WEHI-3 arising in a BALB/c mouse subjected to the regime of multiple injections of mineral oil for plasmacytoma induction and WEHI-265 in a BALB/c mouse injected with cells exposed in vitro to the Abelson virus. Both tumors are myelomonocytic leukemias exhibiting evidence in vivo of a capacity to differentiate to macrophages although in two sublines derived from WEHI-3, a capacity for granulocytic differentiation was also clearly exhibited [277].

Cells from one of the sublines of WEHI-3 (WEHI-3B) were found to be capable of colony formation in agar [16] (Fig. 24) although the cells from the other three sublines usually were not. In this context, it should be repeated that many unsuccessful attempts have been made in this and other laboratories to obtain colony formation in vitro by cells from a number of transplantable myeloid leukemias, particularly in SJL mice, and a complete inability to proliferate would seem to be more typical than the capacity for colony formation being discussed.

Colonies were able to be formed in vitro by WEHI-3 cells without the use of underlayers or conditioned medium. However, addition of human urine GM-CSF or medium conditioned by mouse kidney cells increased colony numbers and growth rates [16]. The colonies were identified as being derived from the leukemic population by a karyotypic marker and, on reimplantation to the spleen of BALB/c mice, individual colonies were able to produce progressively growing transplanted leukemias derived from the implanted colony cells (Fig. 25). Thus, in the case of both the MI and WEHI-3 leukemias, the colony-forming cells have been shown to be equivalent to leukemic stem cells and capable of generating leukemic populations with the capacity of indefinite proliferation in vivo and exhibiting all the characteristics of the original leukemic populations.

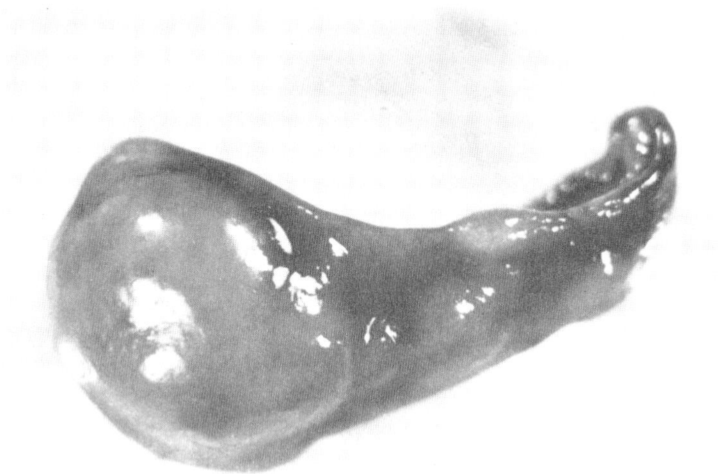

Fig. 25. Tumour mass in BALB/c mouse spleen 3 weeks after implantation with a single colony of WEHI-3 leukemic cells grown in agar. (From METCALF et al., [16]. Reproduced with permission from the Journal of the National Cancer Institute)

While this formal proof that leukemic colony-forming cells are the equivalent of leukemic stem cells is possible when using leukemias of inbred mice, similar tests to determine the significance of human leukemic colony-forming cells obviously cannot be made. In the case of CML, to be discussed shortly, it is tempting by analogy to equate colony-forming cells with stem cells, but while this is a reasonable working assumption, it must be emphasized that the assumption is currently unproved.

Cells of the more recently investigated WEHI-265 myelomonocytic leukemia also have the capacity to form colonies in agar without stimulation. However, such spontaneous colony formation is markedly density-dependent, and no colony formation occurs in cultures containing fewer than 5000 cells. Addition of mouse lung-conditioned medium, endotoxin serum, or human urine GM-CSF all strongly stimulated both the number and growth rate of colonies developing and permitted linearity of colony formation with cell numbers cultured down to very low limits (Fig. 26). With this latter tumor, it has been demonstrated that colony formation is also able to be stimulated by purified GM-CSF derived from mouse lung-conditioned medium.

The strong influence of cell density on the capacity of murine myelomonocytic leukemic cells to proliferate in agar together with the demonstration that such cells are responsive to stimulation by purified GM-CSF (or MGI) makes it likely that the cells resemble normal cells in their dependency on GM-CSF. The apparent inconsistency in these two types of observations would be eliminated if the leukemic cells could be shown to themselves produce GM-CSF (or MGI). This is in fact readily demonstrable in the case of WEHI-3 cells which not only have the capacity to produce GM-CSF-stimulating neutrophil and macrophage colony formation by normal marrow cells [16] but also have the unusual capacity to produce the specific forms of CSF required to stimulate eosinophil and megakaryocyte colony formation [16, 30, 19]. Mice bearing WEHI-3 leukemias also exhibited elevated serum GM-CSF levels although these were not notably higher than in mice with spontaneous or transplanted tumors of other types [16].

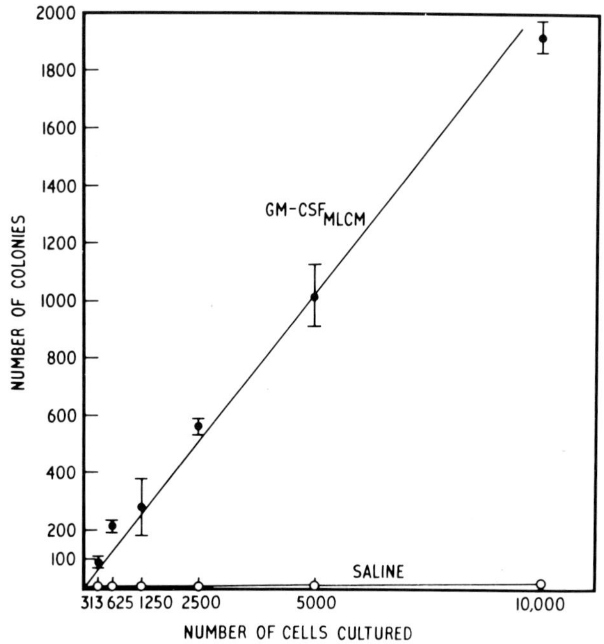

Fig. 26. Formation of colonies in agar by WEHI-265 myelomonocytic leukemic cells in cultures containing added saline or GM-CSF purified from mouse lung-conditioned medium. Note almost complete dependence of leukemic cells on GM-CSF. (METCALF, D., unpublished data)

Studies on mice with transplanted WEHI-3 leukemia documented an interesting situation with respect to the frequency of stem cells in the leukemic population, as assessed by the frequency of colony-forming cells. Colony-forming cell levels were low in tumor masses in the subcutaneous tissues or peritoneal cavity but were very high in apparently similar deposits in the spleen [278]. Randomly selected colonies grown in agar from spleen deposits were reimplanted under the spleen or kidney capsule or in the subcutaneous tissues. In all three locations, the colonies produced apparently similar tumor masses growing at the same rate. However, the spleen tumors again contained higher frequencies of GM-CFCs, while the kidney and subcutaneous tumors contained low numbers. Similar differences were noted between colonics implanted in subcutaneous spleen-versus-thymus grafts. Repassage of spleen tumor masses to other sites produced tumor masses with again a low frequency of colony-forming cells. It is apparent that the frequency of stem cells in this leukemic population is not a constant, genetically determined trait of the population but is largely influenced by the microenvironment in which the leukemic tissue is resident.

As in the case of MI colonies, growth of WEHI-3 colonies in the presence of GM-CSF induced differentiation in the leukemic population. However, not all colony cells differentiated, and in the case of the granulocytic cells, the differentiation was notably incomplete and the morphology of those cells which did attempt differentiation was clearly abnormal [16]. Furthermore, although colony cells did acquire Fc receptors and many became capable of phagocytosis, studies using immunoglobulin fragments showed that the Fc receptors failed to exhibit the normal subclass specificity [279].

An additional potentially useful model of mouse myeloid leukemia has been described by NOOTER and BENTVELSEN [280]. In this model, myeloid leukemia is induced in BALB/c mice by the Soule myeloid leukemia virus. Although no proof was offered that the GM colonies developing were in fact leukemic colonies, they had unusual growth characteristics. The responsiveness of these cells to GM-CSF was normal, but unlike normal GM-CFCs, they were able to form colonies with the use of much lower serum concentrations in the medium than were normal cells. This characteristic has yet to be explored with human myeloid leukemic cells.

The principles emerging from the clonal analysis of the mouse myeloid and myelomonocytic leukemias that could be grown in vitro are:

1. Colony-forming cells can function as leukemic stem cells in vivo.
2. The frequency of such cells in a leukemic population is not constant but is subject to modification by tissue microenvironmental factors.
3. The proliferation of the leukemic cells is responsive to, and probably dependent on, the same GM-CSF molecules that control equivalent normal cells.
4. Leukemic cells themselves have the capacity to produce GM-CSF.
5. Some, but not all, leukemic colony-forming cells can generate progeny capable of maturation to nondividing cells. These cells sometimes, but not always, were morphologically and functionally normal and were then no longer capable of proliferation in vivo to produce transplantable tumors.

The two key issues raised by these mouse studies were : (1) the continued dependency of leukemic cells on stimulation by a normal regulator, and (2) the possible capacity of leukemic cells for reversion or maturation to functionally normal populations. Both questions will be rediscussed following the description of the behaviour in vitro of human myeloid and myelomonocytic leukemic cells.

B. Growth of Cells from Patients with Chronic Myeloid Leukemia (CML)

Following the development by PIKE and ROBINSON [12] of a modified agar culture system capable of supporting GM-colony formation by human marrow cells, extensive studies were undertaken by a number of investigators on the growth in vitro of cells from patients with CML and AML.

There is general agreement that cells from patients with classical Ph^1-positive CML can form colonies in agar cultures when stimulated either by underlayers of peripheral blood cells or by medium conditioned by white cells or certain other tissues [54, 85, 281]. In general appearance, cultures of marrow or blood from patients with CML resemble cultures of normal human marrow. Both colonies and clusters are present, and the ratio of clusters to colonies is near normal. The colonies have the same size and shape variability as normal human granulocytic and macrophage colonies, but the leukemic origin of the colonies has been confirmed by the presence of the Ph^1 chromosomal abnormality in dividing colony cells. The cells in colonies derived from CML cells also are capable of maturation to cells resmbling normal polymorphs and macrophages although macrophage transformation may occur slightly earlier than in normal colonies [85].

Despite the superficially normal appearance of cultures of cells from patients with CML, the colony-forming cells in these patients show a number of abnormalities:

1. The frequency of colony-forming cells is greatly elevated in comparison with levels in

Table 10. Frequency of colony-forming and cluster-forming cells in normal humans and pretreatment patients with CML

Tissue	Colony-forming cells per 10^5 cells	Cluster-forming cells per 10^5 cells	% Colony-forming cells of lighter density than 1.062 g/cm^3
Normal marrow	28	195	6
Normal blood	0.2	2	3
CML marrow	230	895	61
CML blood	510	1050	74

Mean data from 27 pretreatment patients. Cultures stimulated by underlayers of 1×10^6 peripheral blood cells and scored on day 7.

normal subjects. In a comparative study of untreated CML patients and patients without hematological disease, the average frequency of GM-CFCs in the bone marrow of CML patients was almost 10 times higher than in control patients, and the average frequency in the peripheral blood was more than 2000 times higher than normal levels [85, 281, 282] (Table 10). There is in fact a striking inversion of the normal relative frequency of GM-CFCs in the bone marrow versus the peripheral blood. In normal subjects, GM-CFCs are 100 times more frequent in the marrow than in the blood, whereas in CML patients, GM-CFCs are twice as frequent in the blood as in the marrow.

2. The ratio of cluster-forming cells to colony-forming cells in CML patients is only 2:1 compared with the normal relative frequency of 7–10:1 [85].
3. A lower proportion of colony-forming cells from CML patients is in the S phase of the cell cycle than in normal subjects (less than 10% versus 30%) [85]. This implies that cell cycle times are longer for CML colony-forming cells and/or that a higher proportion of CML GM-CFCs are noncycling.
4. In continuous density gradients of BSA, colony-forming cells from patients with myeloid leukemia segregate as a single peak but this peak is significantly displaced to the light density region of the gradient [85] (Fig. 27). Using the technically simpler procedure of centrifuging cells in BSA of density 1.062 g/cm^3, 70% of CML colony-forming cells were found to be of lighter density than 1.062 g/cm^3 compared with a figure of less than 5% for normal cells [85].
5. On karyotypic analysis, dividing colony cells exhibited the Ph^1 chromosomal abnormality [283, 284, 427] although one study on individual colonies reported the presence also of some Ph^1-negative colonies. No mixed colonies were seen in this latter study [285].

On the assumption that colony-forming cells in CML patients are equivalent to those in normal subjects, the situation in a pretreatment patient with CML can be described as one of profound enlargement of the granulocytic progenitor cell compartment. While more mature cluster-forming cells and differentiating cells are also present in greatly increased numbers in CML, the degree of hyperplasia in the granulopoietic series appears to be greatest in the earliest members of the series — the GM colony-forming cells.

In one important aspect, colony-forming cells from CML patients behave in a near normal fashion. They appear to remain responsive to, and dependent on, GM-CSF for proliferative activity in vivo. Thus, in low density cultures or in cultures of cells from which endogenous colony stimulating cells have been removed by density centrifugation or adherence separation, no colony formation and essentially no proliferation occurs [85, 281]. A detailed

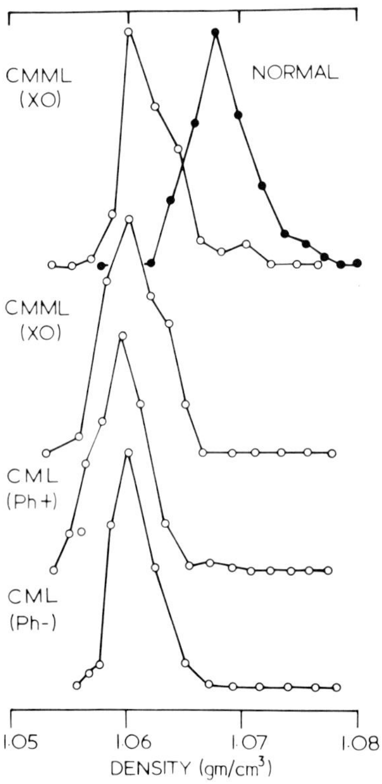

Fig. 27. Density distribution profiles of GM-CFCs from normal human marrow and typical patients with Ph^1-positive or negative CML and 45XO chronic myelomonocytic leukemia. Note in each case that the leukemic profiles are shifted towards the light density regions compared with the normal profile. (From MOORE et al., [288]. Reproduced with permission from Munksgaard)

analysis of the responsiveness of CML cells to stimulation by monkey lung-conditioned medium or human white cell-conditioned medium showed that CML cells were possibly hyporesponsive compared with normal cells (Fig. 28), but this study confirmed the absolute dependency of proliferation by CML cells on exogenous stimulation [286]. As is true for normal CFCs, CML colony-forming cells were able to be activated into the S phase of the cell cycle within 3 h of incubation with GM-CSF [93].

The low buoyant density of colony-forming cells from CML patients has allowed some of these cells to be identified morphologically [85, METCALF, D. and KOLBER, S., unpublished data]. If a peripheral blood sample is centrifuged in BSA of density 1.062 g/cm^3, the majority of the cells, being denser, form a pellet at the bottom of the tube. The small number of cells remaining in the supernatant is a highly enriched population of myeloblasts of varying sizes (Fig. 29). Culture of these cells from several patients has shown a plating efficiency of essentially 100%, every cultured cell forming either a colony or a cluster [85] (Table 2). It can be concluded from this that some colony-forming cells in CML patients must have the morphology of myeloblasts. There are, of course, many colony-forming cells in the pelleted cells in such an experiment, but while this population tends to be depleted of myeloblasts, some are present. From this type of experiment, it is not possible to say dogmatically that *all* colony-forming cells have the morphology of myeloblasts although the data from pelleted cells are not inconsistent with this conclusion.

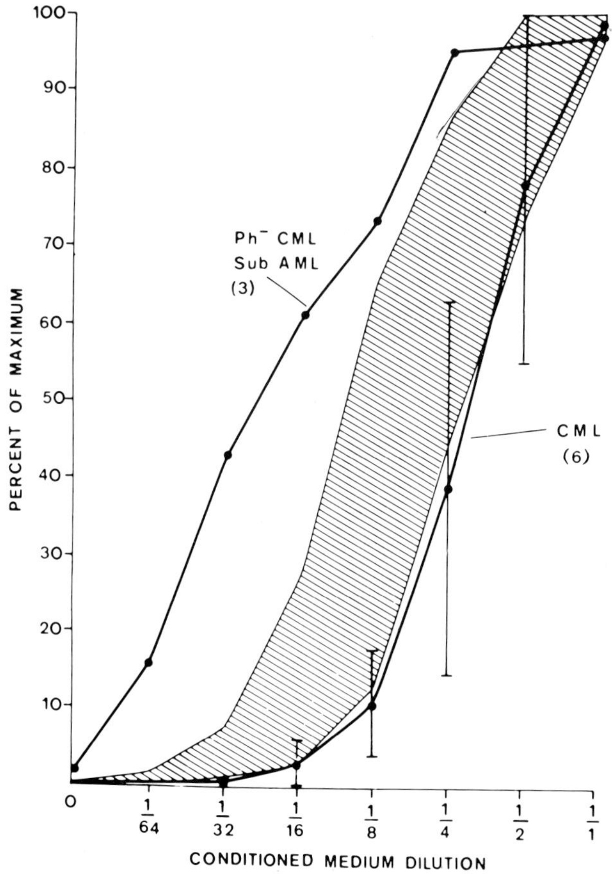

Fig. 28. Responsiveness of leukemic cells from six patients with CML and three patients with Ph$^-$ CML or subacute myeloid leukemia to stimulation by increasing concentrations of monkey lung-conditioned medium. Vertical bars are standard deviations. Hatched area represents range of the dose response curve for normal human GM-CFCs. (From METCALF et al., [286]. Reproduced with permission from Blood)

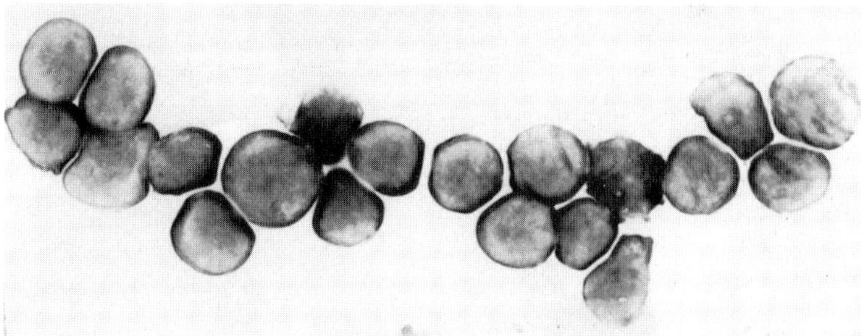

Fig. 29. Light density fraction of peripheral blood cells from an untreated patient with CML showing an almost pure population of myeloblasts of varying size. All cells from this fraction were capable of forming either colonies or clusters in agar cultures.

In view of the earlier discussion on the size heterogeneity of normal mouse GM-CFCs, it is of interest to observe the heterogeneity in size shown by the CML light density myeloblasts in Figure 29. Heterogeneity is also evident when CML cells are separated by velocity sedimentation separation. Whereas GM-CFCs from normal human marrow segregate as a single peak at 7–8 mm/h, CML GM-CFCs segregate as a double peak with an additional peak at 6–7 mm/h (JOHNSON, G. R. and METCALF, D., unpublished data). The velocity sedimentation profile of CML cells is probably displaced because of the abnormally light density of the CML GM-CFCs referred to above, and the cells are probably equal to or larger in size than normal GM-CFCs.

There may be a discrepancy between the morphology of normal and CML colony-forming cells which has not been commented upon previously. Most GM-CFCs in the monkey do not possess a strongly basophilic cytoplasm and could not be described as myeloblasts [43]. The less complete data from the mouse support this conclusion that GM-CFCs are of smaller size than myeloblasts [118]. If this is true also for the human, then the myeloblasts with typical basophilic cytoplasm shown in Figure 29 clearly are of different morphology. The significance of this possible difference in morphology cannot be assessed at present, but as discussed in the preceding chapter, a number of factors, e.g., endotoxin, can cause a major shift in the size of GM-CFCs. It should be recognised, of course, that the label "myeloblast" is a hopeful morphological classification, and it may be possible for two quite different cells to have approximately the same morphology. Most of the so-called myeloblasts in CML patients may in fact be GM-CFCs rather than genuine myeloblasts.

The striking feature of culturing cells from CML patients is the relative uniformity of the results. In our experience with more than 50 patients of this type of leukemia, the cells from only one patient with CML have ever failed to form colonies in agar. This patient was a young woman with classical Ph^1-positive CML who was also pregnant. On repeated analysis, her cells failed to grow in vitro although cell separation studies failed to document the presence of inhibitory cells in the cultured population.

The behavior of cells from Ph^1-negative cases of CML and from the XO males with chronic myelomonocytic leukemia (CMML) [287] is slightly more unpredictable than that of cells from Ph^1-positive cases, but in all cases colony formation has been obtained and the cells from several patients shown to be of abnormally light buoyant density [288, 85, 284].

After commencement of treatment on busulphan, a pronounced fall in blood GM-CFCs occurs in the first 2 weeks which precedes a significant reduction in white cell levels. On continuing therapy, GM-CFC levels in the peripheral blood are found to be within normal limits although the level of GM-CFCs in the marrow can remain higher than in normal subjects [85, 281].

Sequential analyses of CML patients progressing to the stage of acute transformation have documented a characteristic series of changes. In most, there is a progressive fall in the frequency of colony-forming cells in the blood and marrow [54, 85, 289] although colony-forming cells usually persist in the acute transformed state [290, 54]. In one study, cells from three of 36 patients examined in the stage of acute transformation failed completely to proliferate in agar. The cells from the remaining patients formed clusters similar to those produced by cells from patients with AML or generated an abnormally high ratio of clusters to colonies [85, 289] (Table 11).

One characteristic feature of clusters and colonies formed by cells from patients entering acute transformation was the abnormal differentiation exhibited by the colony and cluster cells (83% in one study, 289). As is true of cells from patients with CML, the cells forming colonies or clusters were also of abnormally light buoyant density [85].

The onset of these changes in culture pattern in patients with CML preceded changes in the

Table 11. Correlation between in vitro growth pattern and responsiveness to therapy in 36 cases of acute transformation of CML[a]

Growth pattern of leukemic cells	% of cases	% Achieving remission
No growth (single cells)	3	0
Clusters (up to 20 cells)	3	100
Clusters (up to 40 cells)	25	0
Colonies (abnormal cluster to colony ratio)	38	14
Colonies (normal cluster to colony ratio)		
High plating efficiency	14	20
Low plating efficiency	17	50

[a] Data from MOORE [289].

clinical condition or morphological changes in the marrow or blood by a period of 2–6 months.

Although studies have shown that populations in acutely transformed patients have evolved from the original CML clone, it is apparent that this evolution is associated with a profound alteration in the capacity to proliferate in agar.

It has been suggested [291], particularly from studies on terminal transferase, that some patients with acute transformation do not have AML but acute lymphoid leukemia (ALL). The culture results described above are not inconsistent with this possibility since cells from 17% of patients in acute transformation formed low numbers of colonies (see Table 11), and on analysis, these colonies still had the characteristics of CML colonies [289]. It is possible that these are nongrowing acute leukemias, and the blast cells had no granulocytic markers, did not respond to GM-CSF, and may well have been ALL. The good response to therapy of this group is consistent with this possibility. However, the cluster formation by cells from most patients with acute transformation suggests strongly that in most of these patients the acute terminal episode does involve granulocytic cells.

C. Growth of Cells from Patients with Acute Myeloid Leukemia (AML)

The growth pattern of marrow or peripheral blood cells from an untreated patient with AML or a patient in complete relapse is characterized in most cases by a complete absence of normal-sized colonies [292, 290, 293, 294, 53, 288, 85, 295, 296, 297].

In an analysis in this laboratory of the growth pattern of cells from 127 pretreatment patients with AML or acute myelomonocytic leukemia (AMML) [298], four basic types of growth pattern were observed:

1. In cultures from 12% of the patients, no colonies or clusters developed, and the cultures either contained no surviving cells or only dispersed single cells or doublets.
2. In the largest growth pattern group, cultures from 47% of patients developed no colonies but varying numbers of clusters, 3–20 cells in size.
3. Cultures from a further 24% of patients also developed only clusters, but these were of larger size ranging from 3–40 cells.
4. Finally, in cultures from 17% of patients, some colonies or clusters developed in the culture dish although in one-third of these the cultures also exhibited an extremely high ratio of clusters to colonies.

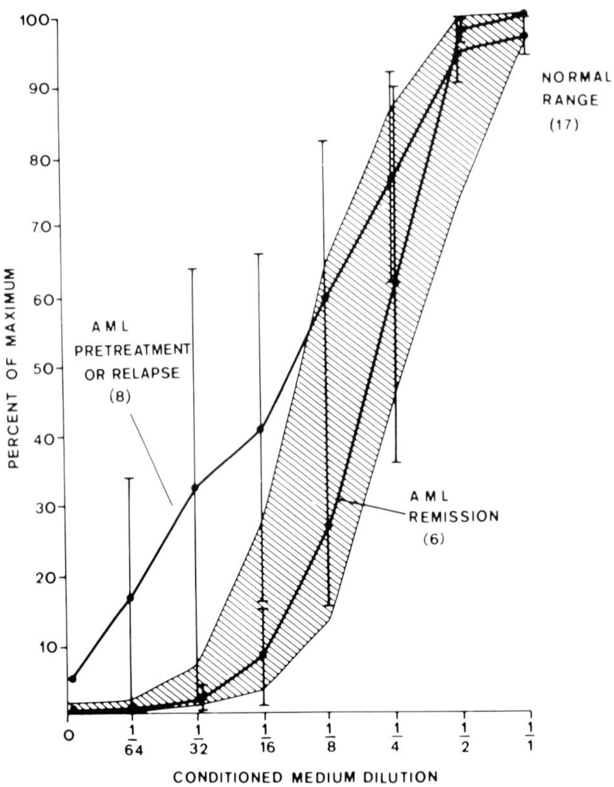

Fig. 30. Responsiveness of leukemic cells from eight patients with AML either prior to treatment or in relapse compared with response curves of normal GM-CFCs in six AML patients in remission when stimulated by increasing concentrations of monkey lung-conditioned medium. Vertical bars are standard deviations. Hatched area is the range of the dose response curve for normal human GM-CFCs. (From METCALF et al., [286]. Reproduced with permission from Blood)

These patients in group 4 were heterogeneous and may have included one or two with misdiagnosed ALL in whom some normal GM-CFCs were present or nongrowing AML with some surviving normal GM-CFCs. There were, however, some patients where the leukemic cells undoubtedly formed colonies although the clinical course of these patients would better have been described as subacute leukemia.

No correlation was observed between the morphological subtype of the leukemia, e.g., AML AMML, acute promyelocytic leukemia, acute monocytic leukemia, etc. and the growth pattern observed. There was also no age-related correlation with growth pattern. In sequential studies on AML patients, the culture pattern exhibited during subsequent relapse phases tended to be identical with the initial pretreatment pattern, and no sequence of culture patterns was observed as the disease progressed.

From the biological point of view, the most important aspect of the growth pattern of AML cells in vitro is their *absolute* dependence on GM-CSF for proliferation [54, 53, 85]. As shown in the examples in Figure 30, the shape of the titration curve can be slightly abnormal; nevertheless, the responsiveness of the cells to stimulation is clearly evident [286].

As for normal marrow cultures, if sufficiently high concentrations of unfractionated AML cells are cultured, "spontaneous" proliferation will occur. However, if colony-stimulating cells are first removed, no example has yet been reported where the leukemic cells were autonomous.

Nothing can be said regarding the small percentage of patients whose cells do not grow in conventional agar cultures. It may be that these cells are unable to survive in the present types of agar culture although on morphological grounds these acute leukemias cannot be distinguished from the majority of cases whose cells are able to proliferate. On the other hand, the leukemic cells in these patients may require stimulation by an abnormal form of GM-CSF. In the complete absence of any information, there is no reason at this stage to suppose that these cells are a GM-CSF-autonomous population.

For most patients with AML or AMML, the growth pattern of leukemic cells can be summarized as either being the formation of clusters of various sizes or an inability to proliferate. A wide variation was noted in the absolute frequency of clusters developing per 10^5 cultured cells denoting either a highly variable plating efficiency for the leukemic cells from different patients or a highly variable frequency of cluster-forming cells in different leukemic populations. In this context, the incidence of clusters was higher in cultures from patients with acute promyelocytic leukemia and AML than from patients with AMML [298]. Maturation of cluster cells to morphologically normal metamyelocytes, polymorphs, monocytes, or macrophages was observed in only 12% of cases, and even here an increased frequency of macrophages suggested the possibility of some less obvious maturation abnormalities [298]. In the majority of cultures of AML cells, obvious abnormalities of differentiation were observable. The most common abnormality was maturation arrest at the myelocyte or promyelocyte stage, but in about one-quarter of the cultures, the cluster cells had bizarre morphology and exhibited early degenerative changes. There is some disagreement in the published literature concerning the capacity of AML cells to mature with several early reports [299, 54, 294] describing normal granulocytic maturation. More recently, the consensus of opinion is that maturation defects are usual in most cultures of AML cells. It may be that the initial studies were performed on patients whose cells happened to be capable of maturation. The important alternative is that some types of medium might be capable of supporting near normal maturation. The question is extremely important to resolve as the implications are far-reaching for interpreting the nature of AML.

As was true for colony-forming cells in CML, the cells in AML populations forming clusters or colonies in agar culture are also of abnormally light buoyant density [85]. Between 50–60% of these cells were found to be lighter than 1.062 g/cm^3 regardless of the cluster or colony type generated in agar. Studies in which AML cells were preincubated in vitro with ^{3}HTdR also indicated a similar situation to that in CML. An abnormally small reduction in colony or cluster-forming cells was noted, indicating that these cells either had an abnormally prolonged cell cycle time or that an abnormally small proportion of these cells was in cycle [85]. That is in agreement with labelling studies in acute leukemic patients which have reached similar conclusions [300] regarding the blast cell population.

Information on the morphology of cluster and colony-forming cells in AML is less complete than in CML. In occasional patients whose cells formed a very high frequency of clusters, light density fractions mainly composed of myeloblasts were able to generate clusters with a very high plating efficiency. Such cells may represent typical cluster-forming cells. Alternatively, in other patients the cluster-forming cells may have a different morphology.

One point worth emphasizing is that in an untreated patient with AML or AMML, the frequencies of cluster-forming cells in the blood and marrow are usually similar. This is particularly true in patients with elevated peripheral white cell levels and a high proportion of blast cells. As shall be discussed in Chapter 7, the similarity of cluster or colony levels in blood and marrow cultures from AML patients is an important point which distinguishes leukemic from preleukemic patients.

It must be emphasized that the pattern of cluster formation described above for AML cells relates to cultures performed in agar, using white cell underlayers and scored at 7 days of incubation. The culture details should always be listed when describing culture results since they have a significant influence on the pattern of growth observed. The leukemic cells forming large clusters of up to 40 cells by day 7 are often capable of further proliferation. If these cultures are scored at 10, 14 or even 21 days as in some laboratories, these clusters will by then have exceeded the lower size limit for colonies (40 cells), and the leukemia will be described as a colony-forming leukemia. A similar change might possibly occur if cultures are supplemented by some growth-promoting additive, e.g., serum, red cell lysates, mercaptoethanol, etc. Obviously, the correlative data between growth pattern and clinical behavior that will be described shortly could not be expected to apply if the investigator has used different culture methods or a different culture interval. This rather elementary point seems to have caused some confusion to certain workers in the field. One point of interest, however, is that the small clusters formed by leukemic cells do not seem to increase in size on continued incubation, and this may indicate a genuine restriction in their capacity for proliferation.

One point alluded to earlier in this book needs to be repeated. In normal cultures, cluster-forming cells are likely to be the progeny of colony-forming cells, i.e., to be more mature cells. If one attempted to transfer these conclusions to CML and AML, the conclusion might be reached that AML cells are derived from a more mature population than CML cells. Such a conclusion may be correct, but it is more likely that the proliferative capacity of AML cells as seen in agar is not truly representative of their capacity in vivo and that no conclusions can be drawn from the in vitro growth pattern.

Relevant to this issue is the broader question of whether the leukemic stem cells in either CML or AML are being grown in the present types of agar culture. There is evidence in CML that the erythroid and megakaryocytic populations are also Ph^1-positive and could well be members of the leukemic clone [301, 302, 303, 304, 305]. Similar evidence has been produced that the erythroid population may be part of the leukemic clone in at least certain patients with AML where the leukemic clone can be identified because of an abnormal karyotype [306]. If these suggestions are correct, both AML and CML are diseases involving more than one hemopoietic family, and this implies that the cells initiating the leukemic clone must be located in the stem cell compartment. Important confirmation of this hypothesis would be obtained if it could be shown that individual colonies or clusters grown in semisolid medium contained granulocytic and erythroid or megakaryocytic cells. So far, no study has been reported on this question, but it should be technically feasible using methylcellulose cultures containing both GM-CSF and erythropoietin.

In this laboratory, a limited investigation of the multipotentiality of CML colonies has been made in cultures stimulated by placental-conditioned medium which are capable of supporting the development of both neutrophil and eosinophil colonies. A careful analysis of cultures of CML cells showed that although both types of colony developed, mixed eosinophil and neutrophil colonies were never observed (DRESCH, C. and METCALF, D., unpublished data). So far as this study goes, the implication is that the CML colony-forming cells are not multipotential since they were not able to generate eosinophil progeny. It must be emphasized, however, that no information yet exists as to whether eosinophils are in fact members of the Ph^1-positive population.

In view of the highly variable number of clusters generated by leukemic populations from different patients, it is relevant to consider whether the cells that do proliferate are a fully representative sample of the leukemic population. This question was answered in the affirmative for colonies grown in vitro from mouse myelomonocytic leukemic cells when individual colonies were retransplanted to syngeneic mice and reproduced the original subline variant from which the colonies were grown.

Such tests are not possible using human cells, and to date the only observations that have been made are at the karyotype level. In one study, cultures were analyzed from six patients with AML or AMML in whom the leukemic population exhibited karyotypic markers. Analysis of dividing cluster cells harvested from cultures of the marrow or blood from these patients revealed that the same karyotypic abnormalities were present [284]. Where more than one marker was present, the proportion of cells with the different markers in the cultured cells agreed reasonably well with the relative frequency of these markers in a direct analysis of the leukemic marrow population. Similar results were obtained by DUTTERA et al. [307] and AYE et al. [428] in an analysis of AML cells grown in methylcellulose.

In the above analysis of cultures from pretreatment patients with AML, three important correlations were observed between growth pattern and the subsequent response of these patients to chemotherapy [298]:

1. Patients whose leukemic cells formed small clusters had a much better remission rate following chemotherapy than patients whose cells either failed to grow or formed large clusters. Response to therapy was also correlated with the age of the patient (better responses in the under 40-year old group), but the correlation between growth pattern and remission rate was still seen within each age group (Table 12). It must be emphasized that the frequency of clusters generated is not important in determining the classification. Even if only a few clusters are present in a culture, it should be classified according to the size of these cultures and not scored as a nongrowing culture.
2. In the group of patients whose cells formed colonies, remission rates and survival were better if the colony-forming cells were of normal buoyant density and/or the ratio of clusters to colonies was normal (Table 13).
3. Where the frequency of clusters or colonies formed per 10^5 cultured cells was high, the remission rate was lower than in patients whose cells had a low plating efficiency.

In an extension of this study [289], these basic correlations between growth pattern and response to therapy were found to hold true in a total of 174 patients analyzed although the proportion of patients whose cells failed to grow was much smaller than in the series just described. The same basic correlations appeared to hold true also for patients with acute transformation of CML. In a series of 36 cases analyzed (Table 11), good therapeutic responses were seen only in patients whose cells formed small clusters or colonies with a normal cluster to colony ratio. The major difference between acute transformation and AML was that the cells from relatively few of the patients with acute transformation grew with a good prognosis growth pattern. This is in line with the known poor responsiveness of such patients to therapy.

The basic correlations between growth pattern and response to therapy have been confirmed [308], but no explanation is immediately apparent as to why there should be such correlations.

Two reports on the correlation between the growth of acute leukemic cells in vitro and response to therapy are in apparent disagreement with the preceding description [309, 310]. However, both were relatively small studies, and the method of classifying growth involved combinations of the above categories. The data cannot therefore be directly compared. Both studies reported a good remission rate in colony-forming leukemias, but these patients were not further analyzed in terms of cluster to colony ratios or the density of the colony-forming cells.

Table 12. Relationship between age, in vitro growth pattern of the leukemic cells and the probability of achieving a remission in 108 patients with AML

Age in years	No. achieving remission/No. in group (%)				
	Total	Small clusters	Large clusters	No growth	Colony formation
<40	22/30(73%)	16/18(89%)	1/6(17%)	0/1(0%)	5/5(100%)
40–60	13/32(41%)	8/15(53%)	1/9(11%)	2/3(67%)	2/5(40%)
>60	4/46(9%)	3/18(17%)	1/11(9%)	0/9(0%)	0/8(0%)
Total	39/108(36%)	27/51(53%)	3/26(12%)	2/13(15%)	7/18(39%)

Data from Moore et al. [298].

Table 13. Relationship between GM-CFC density, cluster to colony ratio, and response to therapy in patients with AML whose cells formed colonies in vitro

Patient No.	Type	Remission	Survival days	Cluster to colony ratio	Colonies/ 10^5 cells Marrow	Colonies/ 10^5 cells Blood	GM-CFC density %<1.062
1	Stem cell leukemia	Yes	509	3	2	16	4.2
2	Stem cell leukemia	Yes	>525	5	0	1	0.1
3	Stem cell leukemia	Yes	>247	1	0	1	9.6
4	Stem cell leukemia	Yes	> 70	6	1	0	—
5	AML	No	24	5	1	0	6.0
6	Smouldering AML	No treatment	>539	3	3	0	90
7	AMML	No treatment	89	2	10	40	41
8	AML	No	34	3	350	6	93
9	AML	Yes	>146	3	0	1	100
10	A mono L	Yes	270	17	—	15	71
11	AML	No	>130	10	1550	3	37
12	AML	Yes	>177	5	10	263	—
13	AML	No	>102	33	110	0	83
14	AMML	No	61	70	188	6	21
15	AML	No	> 39	145	1	0	—
16	Erythroleukemia	No	26	270	1	0	89
17	AML	No	69	396	20	4	45
18	AML	No	157	717	—	3	86

Data from Moore et al. [298].

The different clinical implications associated with small-versus-large cluster formation highlights the one major defect in the use of methylcellulose instead of agar in semisolid cultures, particularly in the analysis of cultures from cells from leukemic patients. Because methylcellulose is not a gel but a highly viscous liquid, clusters and colonies do not remain suspended in the three-dimensional matrix of the gel but tend to form a monolayer on the bottom of the culture dish. Embedded as these clusters and colonies are in a background of surviving single cells, it becomes impossible to count or even discern the number or size of clusters, and an analysis of the above type cannot be performed. If it is desired to use methylcellulose to allow harvesting of cultured cells, parallel agar cultures should be used to permit adequate analysis of the culture pattern.

One important technical matter needs comment. There appears to be a quite different clinical prognosis if the leukemic cells form large, rather than small, clusters. If cultures are going to be used as an adjunct in the assessment of a patient, it is absolutely essential that such cultures always have a quality control. A normal or nonleukemic marrow should always be cultured at the time of preparing the AML cultures. Unless good colony formation occurs in control cultures, the significance of cluster size or frequency in the AML cultures will be very doubtful.

It will be appreciated that the growth pattern of typical AML cells in agar does not permit leukemic colony or cluster-forming cells to be identified positively. The individual clusters or colonies do not differ in gross appearance from comparable aggregates in normal cultures. While a density cut with culture of cells lighter or denser than 1.062 g/cm^3 can, with some assurance, indicate the presence of leukemic cells, even this is vitiated if there is a low frequency of such cells in the marrow or the plating efficiency of these cells is very low. Thus, agar cultures fail to provide a method for detecting small numbers of surviving or regenerating leukemic cells in a normal population—the situation in which a discriminatory culture is most needed to aid the morphologist.

D. Colony Formation by AML Cells After Stimulation by Phytohemagglutinin

A system has been described by DICKE et al. [67, 338] based on the two-stage culture system developed for T-lymphocyte colony growth which may provide a discriminatory culture system for leukemic cells. As described in Chapter 3, marrow cells are incubated overnight in the presence of phytohemagglutinin. After washing, the cells are cultured in agar in the absence of phytohemagglutinin. Duplicate cultures of washed cells are prepared over white cell underlayers. In these cultures 14–440/10^5 marrow cells from pretreatment AML patients or patients in relapse formed tight or loose colonies. These colonies have been identified as being composed of leukemic cells on the basis of light and electronmicroscopy of colony cells and a limited amount of karyotypic analysis. It is likely that numerous clusters also arise in such cultures, but because of the high numbers of cells cultured (100,000 per ml), the background of cells surviving from the original inoculum makes scoring difficult.

Following preincubation with phytohemagglutinin, the leukemic cells in the second-step agar culture are not only able to proliferate in the absence of phytohemagglutinin (distinguishing them from T-lymphocytes) but also in the absence of peripheral blood underlayers. It is this latter feature which permits the cultures to discriminate between leukemic and nonleukemic GM-CFCs since normal GM-CFCs, even after preincubation with phytohemagglutinin, still require stimulation by GM-CSF to form colonies.

The number of colonies developing per 10^5 cultured cells in this system is low, suggesting strongly that colonies are generated by some type of leukemic stem cell. Despite the disadvantage that the detection system is relatively insensitive, the method does have the virtue of permitting the leukemic cells to positively identify themselves by exhibiting GM-CSF-independent proliferation.

The culture method has also been applied to monitor the development of acute transformation in CML patients. CML cells, like normal GM-CFCs were unable to proliferate unless stimulated by feeder layers. However, in patients with acute transformation, the leukemic cells behaved as in AML and were capable of forming colonies in the absence of GM-CSF. It was observed that some CML patients with cells capable of forming GM-CSF-independent colonies underwent clinical acute transformation within months of the demonstration of the presence of the abnormal colony-forming cells [311].

In its present form, the system is limited by two technical problems: (1) There is nonlinearity in the liquid culture phase, and unless more than a minimum concentration of cells (? leukemic) is cultured with the phytohemagglutinin, no colony formation occurs in the subsequent agar culture. The minimum number of cells is approximately 10^5, but varies from patient to patient. (2) About one-third of cultures are unsatisfactory because of PHA-induced agglutination of the cells during the liquid incubation step. The agglutinated cells cannot be redispersed adequately before reculture in agar, and this makes it almost impossible to determine whether "colonies" in such plates genuinely arose by proliferation.

From the theoretical point of view, these leukemic colonies are of considerable interest since proliferation appears to occur in the absence of added GM-CSF. Since phytohemagglutinin can provoke GM-CSF production by normal and leukemic white cells, it will need to be rigorously excluded that small amounts of GM-CSF are not being produced in the cultures even though the PHA was removed after the liquid incubation step.

A potentially similar phenomenon was described by Aye et al. [55] in which suspension cultures of cells from one patient with AML exhibited increased incorporation of tritiated thymidine when incubated with phytohemagglutinin. Some evidence was produced that a factor was released from leukemic cells after contact with phytohemagglutinin that stimulated thymidine uptake by other cells.

Regardless of the mechanism involved, this system for obtaining colony formation by AML cells potentially provides a very important method for selectively growing leukemic cells.

E. Growth of Cells from Patients with Acute Lymphoid Leukemia (ALL)

There have always been problem patients in whom, on morphological grounds, it has been difficult to decide whether the disease is AML or ALL. In view of this longstanding difficulty, it is useful to compare the growth patterns exhibited by blood or marrow cells from patients with ALL with the pattern of growth just described for cells from patients with AML.

In conventional underlayer-stimulated agar or methylcellulose cultures, no one has yet succeeded in growing colonies or clusters from the lymphoid leukemic cells. Relatively good agreement exists between the published descriptions of the results of culturing blood or marrow cells from patients with ALL [312, 313, 298, 314]. Cultures of the marrow from these patients usually show reduced or greatly reduced numbers of GM-colonies.

The GM-colonies exhibit normal size heterogeneity, normal cluster to colony ratios, and a normal pattern of differentiation in the colony cells [298]. On analysis, the colony-forming cells have been found to exhibit a normal buoyant density and normal cell cycle status. The interpretation of these findings is that the colony-forming cells are in fact normal GM-CFCs surviving in the face of a varying degree of infiltration of the marrow by lymphoid leukemic cells. In extreme cases (approximately one-quarter of pretreatment patients), the infiltration is so extensive that no GM-CFCs are detectable.

In contrast, and quite characteristically, levels of GM-CFCs are elevated 20–30-fold in the peripheral blood [298, 312, 314]. These colonies are again of normal morphology, exhibit normal differentiation, and are generated by colony-forming cells with a normal buoyant density. It seems reasonable to conclude that the elevated levels of GM-CFCs in the blood are an attempt at compensatory hyperplasia or redistribution of GM-CFCs consequent upon infiltration of their normal habitat, the bone marrow. Studies have not been made on the levels of GM-CFCs in the spleen or liver in these patients, but it is likely that elevated levels of GM-CFCs would also be demonstrable elsewhere in the body.
Following the successful induction on a remission, levels of GM-CFCs in the marrow return to normal and often rebound above normal levels [313]. These colonies often appear larger or more rapidly growing than normal colonies.

F. Growth of Marrow Cells from Patients with AML in Remission

When marrow from a patient with AML in *full* clinical and hematological remission is cultured, the pattern of growth observed is completely different from that seen in cultures of pretreatment marrow. Remission marrow cells produce a pattern of colony and cluster formation which is identical with a normal marrow culture (Fig. 31). Commonly, the frequency of clusters and colonies is higher than normal, but the ratio of clusters to colonies is normal [315, 290, 294, 316, 288, 85, 296, 297]. When the colony-forming cells were analyzed in continuous albumin gradients, the density of the cells was found to be normal [85]. Similarly, studies in which the marrow cells were preincubated in vitro with ^{3}HTdR

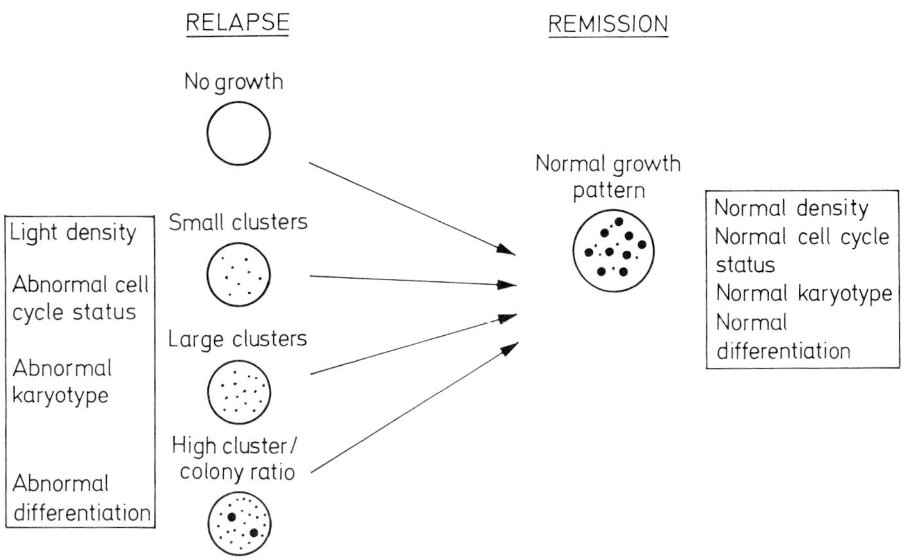

Fig. 31. Schematic summary of the change in growth pattern of cells from patients with AML after the development of a full clinical remission. By parameters used, growth pattern of remission marrow is not distinguishable from normal

indicated that the proportion of GM-CFCs or cluster-forming cells killed was at least as high as in normal marrows (35–40%), and often, if the marrow was exhibiting active regeneration, was as high as 60–70% [85].

In a few suitable patients, a karyotypic analysis of the dividing cells in remission colonies showed that the leukemic marker was not present, and the karyotypes were normal [284]. Colony and cluster cells exhibited normal differentiation to metamyelocytes and polymorphs with later monocyte and macrophage development. In cultures analyzed for eosinophil colony development, relapse cultures developed no colonies, whereas in remission cultures, eosinophil colony and cluster numbers were, if anything, higher than normal (DRESCH, C., JOHNSON, G. R., METCALF, D., unpublished data).

Cultures of peripheral blood from patients in remission either behaved as cultures of normal human peripheral blood and developed an occasional colony or exhibited elevated numbers of apparently normal colonies.

One of the major controversies in leukemia research for the last 50 years has concerned the nature of a remission in acute leukemia. When a normal-appearing population of hemopoietic cells returns to the marrow, is this the regrowth of a previously dormant population of normal cells or is it a modification of the leukemic cells that now permits them to proliferate and differentiate in a normal manner?

From the semisolid culture data, the answer seems clearly that, in the majority of these patients, remission involves the regrowth of a previously suppressed normal population of granulopoietic cells. In an occasional patient, the granulopoietic population is characterizable as having some persisting abnormalities, and in these exceptional situations, the marrow may have been repopulated by a preleukemic clone (see Chapter 7).

If the data indicate that a normal population rebounds during a remission, why are none of these cells detectable in cultures of cells from the untreated patient? The question of suppression of normal cells by leukemic cells in the culture dish will be discussed in a separate section, but such a mechanism seems unlikely to explain the quite striking absence of normal colonies. It seems more probable that suppression of the normal granulopoietic clone (or clones) by the leukemic population occurs in the body and is at a stage prior to the granulopoietic progenitor (colony-forming) cell level. Because the present cultures are unable to support colony formation by stem cells, a normal population blocked in the stem cell compartment cannot be detected in the culture dish. Possible mechanisms by which leukemic cells might achieve this suppression will be discussed shortly, but whatever reversion of this process permits the onset of a remission, this is signaled by the reappearance of colony-forming cells and shortly thereafter by obvious morphological evidence of a return to normality in the marrow.

For most patients, remissions are only of temporary duration, and the disease relapses because of the regrowth of leukemic cells surviving the original chemotherapy. As mentioned earlier, when the leukemic population regrows, it appears to be the clone originally present (or a variant of it). Indeed, the growth pattern of leukemic populations from individual patients appears to be remarkably stable throughout the duration of the disease.

It must be reiterated that agar cultures are often unable to positively identify the presence of residual leukemic cells because leukemic clusters have the same gross morphology as normal clusters. Where agar cultures have proved particularly instructive in the clinical setting has been in providing positive evidence of the reappearance of *normal* GM-CFCs in a patient under therapy.

It is fairly common to have a leukemic patient under therapy with a relatively aplastic marrow containing 5–20% of what appear to be abnormal blast cells. On morphological grounds, there is little encouragement from such a picture and therapy may even be intensified. However, on culture many such marrows can be shown to contain GM-CFCs often in very high frequency, and the likelihood in such cases is that a remission is actively in progress [317]. To assault this regenerating normal population with increased levels of chemotherapy would be undesirable. Unfortunately, the 7-day delay in obtaining the culture data is often too long to postpone a clinical decision regarding therapy, but the cumulative restrospective experience obtained from the culture analyses of such marrows may eventually lead to more accurate clinical assessments and judgments regarding therapy.

Certain evidence would appear to conflict with the conclusion that in remission a normal granulopoietic population regenerates. It has been reported that when remission marrow was cultured in liquid in the presence of medium conditioned by peripheral blood cells from certain patients (and presumably containing GM-CSF), the cultured marrow cells developed detectable abnormal reverse transcriptase and released virus-like particles. This was not seen with normal marrow cells after culture with such conditioned media [318]. The implication from this work is that a human RNA leukemia virus is present in an overt form in the leukemic cells and in a cryptic form in the suppressed "normal" cells in these patients. When the "normal" remission cells are stimulated to proliferate by the conditioned medium, this viral infection becomes overtly expressed and identifiable. A similar phenomenon has been reported with cultures of leukemic cells stimulated by human embryo-conditioned media [319].

These observations are of extreme interest and are in urgent need of confirmation. If true, they provide very illuminating examples of the way in which a virus and regulatory factor might interact in the complex process leading to the emergence of a leukemic clone. It is also urgent to determine whether the active factor is GM-CSF or some other regulatory factor.

As to whether the above observation disproves the proposition that remission cells are normal is a more complex question. In the context of the present discussion, "normality" would be defined as a normal pattern of proliferative activity leading to apparently normal maturation of progeny to nondividing end cells whose functional activity was normal or near normal.

By this definition, the cells need not be free of an integrated RNA leukemia virus. An analogous situation exists in AKR mice where probably most lymphoid cells in the body contain the Gross leukemia virus, either in a smouldering replicative form or integrated into the genome. In early and middle life, such lymphocytes function as essentially normal cells, and if the thymus is removed, the animal will not develop lymphoid leukemia despite the persistent infection throughout life of the lymphoid cells.

In the human context, the reverse transcriptase observations have raised the bogey that it may be impossible ever to expect to cure a patient with acute leukemia if the normal cells are also infected. The answer obviously will have to await an analysis of the fate of persons presently alive with apparently complete long-term remissions. My prediction from the mouse models would be that a person with a long-term complete remission might well be at higher than normal risk of reinduction of a new leukemic clone but might well be able to remain in good health for life despite the presence of a persistent infection in the normal cells. The immediate concern is whether the cells differentiate to nondividing progeny and whether such cells are functionally adequate. By these criteria, remission populations appear to be clearly classifiable as normal.

In view of the complete contrast between the proliferative pattern of relapse and remission marrows, it could be predicted that if a culture analysis is made of marrows from patients with an incomplete remission, a very confusing set of data could be collected. This seems likely to be the explanation of a published account in which persisting abnormalities were found in the remission period [307].

A somewhat similar problem is encountered in analyzing marrows from patients with CML following therapy. Colony numbers may be reduced and the cell cycle status of the colony-forming cells may change but the colony cells remain Ph^1-positive, and it is very uncertain whether in CML a true remission occurs of the type seen in AML. Indeed, there is in most patients little evidence for the existence of a suppressed Ph^1-negative population. However, in a few patients after intensive aplasia induced by chemotherapy, a regenerating Ph^1 negative population has been described [303, 320], and this might be the origin of the mixed data indicating Ph^1-positive and negative colonies in cultures from treated CML patients reported b y CHERVENICK et al. [285].

The observations that no normal GM-CFCs are demonstrable in most pretreatment AML patients but that these cells reappear during remissions permit the deduction that normal ancestors of GM-CFCs must exist in the leukemic patient in a suppressed state. While these ancestral cells are, by definition, in the stem cell compartment, the present evidence has not proved that normal *multipotential* stem cells exist in such patients. While this is a reasonable extrapolation, it could be documented readily enough by culturing erythroid colonies using remission marrow cells from a patient with a karyotypic marker in the leukemic population. Such a study is well worth undertaking in view of the potential therapeutic use of remission bone marrows in autologous infusions if adequate proof of the presence of normal multipotential stem cells can be gathered.

G. GM-CSF and Inhibitor Levels in Leukemia

In mice with transplanted myelomonocytic leukemia, serum GM-CSF levels were found to be consistently elevated [16]. Furthermore, in such mice, as the disease progressed, serum inhibitor levels fell [238].

However, other observations in mice suggest that the elevated GM-CSF levels are not specifically related to myeloid or myelomonocytic leukemia. Elevated serum GM-CSF levels were also observed in conventional and germfree AKR mice with lymphoid leukemia [95, 214], in Swiss mice with Buffett virus-induced lymphoid leukemia [237], in BALB/c mice with Moloney virus-induced lymphoid leukemia [221], and in DBA/1 mice with Friend virus-induced erythroleukemia [221]. While there is an accentuated granulopoiesis in both AKR leukemia [190, 321] and Friend virus-induced leukemia [322], it is doubtful whether the elevated GM-CSF levels indicate much more than a general response of the mouse to the tumor-bearing state since elevated levels were also observed in mice with transplanted breast tumors and plasmacytomas [190]. There is also an obvious difficulty in eliminating the possibility that elevated GM-CSF levels are due to secondary infections or endotoxemia in mice that are becoming progressively sicker as tumors increase in size.

Somewhat similar problems exist in interpreting GM-CSF levels in humans with leukemia since infections are also common in acute leukemia, and the use of certain drugs, e.g., cytosine arabinoside, has been found to markedly influence serum or urine GM-CSF levels [223, 30, 299, 225].

A number of surveys have been made of the capacity of serum or urine from leukemic patients to stimulate GM-colony formation by mouse bone marrow cells. In a sequential study of 33 patients with AML or AMML, 30% of 251 serum samples showed elevated colony-stimulating activity (0.1 ml of serum stimulating more than 20 colonies), as did 53% of 1422 24-h urine specimens [223]. All patients at some stage in their illness showed periods

Table 14. Stimulation by dialyzed human sera of GM-colony formation by mouse bone marrow cells[a]

Disease	Number of sera assayed	% Sera with elevated colony-stimulating activity[b]	Mean GM-CSF levels[c]
Normal blood donors	65	6%	10.4 ± 5.3
Miscellaneous hemopoietic disorders	230	22%	14.7 ± 15.2
Lymphoma/reticulum cell sarcoma	19	32%	20.9 ± 20.9
CLL/lymphosarcoma	67	27%	17.5 ± 21.1
ALL	48	35%	18.7 ± 18.0
Hodgkin's disease	28	11%	12.2 ± 15.6
AMML	37	35%	21.9 ± 21.7
AML—untreated or relapse	133	37%	21.4 ± 21.8
AML remission	98	21%	13.0 ± 12.5
Subacute myeloid leukemia	18	28%	16.7 ± 18.9
CML	86	45%	24.6 ± 23.0
CML — acute transformation	75	65%	41.8 ± 36.3

[a] All assays performed in cultures of 75,000 C_{57}BL marrow cells containing 0.1 ml dialyzed serum.
[b] % sera stimulating more than 20 colonies.
[c] Mean colony counts ± SD.

during which serum and/or urine GM-CSF levels were elevated. In this initial study, it was observed that relapse patients tended to be unable to elevate serum CSF levels during infections. In confirmation of earlier studies, it was shown in this survey that approximately half of the sera from patients with acute leukemia exhibited subnormal or undetectable inhibitor levels for GM-colony formation by mouse marrow cells [242, 239, 223]. A correlation was observed between subnormal inhibitor levels and short survival.

In a subsequent more extensive study, serum GM-CSF levels were determined in a number of types of leukemic patients and in patients with other hemopoietic disorders (METCALF, D., unpublished data). All patients had had a sufficiently severe disturbance of hemopoiesis to warrant a diagnostic bone marrow biopsy. The results (Table 14) indicated that approximately 20–25% of the sera from all of the different categories of patients exhibited elevated colony-stimulating activity. Sometimes these patients had coincidental infections, but in other patients no obvious reason was apparent for the elevation, and as in the mouse, it may have been due to a variety of reasons including a systemic response to infiltration of hemopoietic tissue by tumor cells or to other abnormalities in the hemopoietic tissues.

In untreated or relapse patients with AML or AMML, a slightly higher proportion of sera was observed to have increased colony-stimulating activity. In this survey, a lower proportion of sera from remission patients exhibited elevated activity than was seen with sera from pretreatment or relapse patients although the difference was of only marginal statistical significance. The most clearly evident abnormality was in the sera from patients with CML. Such patients are not noted for their susceptibility to infections, but 45% of the sera exhibited increased colony-stimulating activity. An even more striking abnormality was observed in patients in the acute transformation stage of CML where 65% of the sera showed very high levels of colony-stimulating activity.

Table 15. Serum inhibitor levels in human sera for GM-colony formation by mouse bone marrow cells

Disease	No. of patients studied	No. of sera analyzed	No. (%) with subnormal inhibitor levels[a]
Normal donors	187	187	4 (2%)
Miscellaneous hemopoietic disorders	10	34	2 (6%)
Miscellaneous nonhemopoietic cancer	25	106	13 (12%)
CLL/lymphosarcoma	14	25	3 (12%)
ALL	30	58	13 (22%)
AML or AMML	35	323	172 (53%)
CML	13	18	4 (22%)
CML—acute transformation	3	13	12 (92%)

[a] Assays performed in cultures of 75,000 C_{57}BL marrow cells. Inhibitor levels assessed as subnormal if serum failed to reduce colony numbers stimulated by postendotoxin serum by more than 50%. (Data from METCALF and CHAN, 323).

Although the culture pattern in vitro of cells from AML and acute transformation patients is similar, it seems likely that these patients differ in the level of GM-CSF impinging on the leukemic populations.

In a study of serum inhibitor levels (Table 15), about half the sera from patients with AML exhibited subnormal or undetectable inhibitor levels when assayed against normal GM-colony formation by mouse bone marrow cells. Inhibitor levels in the serum from other types of patients were essentially normal, again with the notable exception of sera from patients with CML in acute transformation where most sera exhibited subnormal inhibitor levels [323]. As was discussed in Chapter 5, conflicting estimates of inhibitory activity in human sera have been made using different methods for measuring this activity, and the significance of the above observations is uncertain. Furthermore, in a limited series of tests using GM-colony formation by human marrow cells, examples of AML sera were encountered with no detectable inhibitory activity in mouse bone marrow cultures but with strong inhibitory activity for human cultures (METCALF, D. and RUSSELL, S., unpublished data).

While inhibitor levels appear to be abnormal in patients with AML and CML in acute transformation, the significance of these abnormalities for the control of granulopoiesis remains to be determined.

Several problems exist with respect to the increased colony stimulating activity observed in the sera from many leukemic patients:

1. As was discussed in Chapter 5, parallel assays of human sera on mouse and human marrows commonly do not agree in ranking the sera in order of colony-stimulating activity [181, 182]. At this stage, the mouse marrow system seems less complex and more likely to be able to measure GM-CSF levels since anti-GM-CSF sera completely inhibited colony formation with mouse but not human marrow cells [182], but the assays could be misleading since foreign species target cells are used.
2. It was reported that serum from patients with chronic lymphoid leukemia (CLL) were particularly active in stimulating colony formation by human marrow cells [324], but this was not observed in a similar study in this laboratory [182]. Indirect evidence was also produced that acute leukemic sera might contain an inhibitor for human GM-colonies [324], but other studies failed to detect such an inhibitor [325].

3. With the demonstration that chloroform-extractable material from serum has colony-stimulating activity for human but not mouse marrow cells (ROBINSON, W. A., personal communication), it will be necessary to carry out parallel assays for this factor in various leukemic sera.
4. If substantial local production of GM-CSF occurs in the marrow, it may be that serum GM-CSF levels give a quite inadequate estimate of GM-CSF concentrations in the marrow, the site of most target cells. This situation has already been documented in experimental animals [156].

These uncertainties indicate the need for caution in interpreting the data. Nonspecific rises in colony-stimulating activity appear to be common, as might be expected in patients who are severely ill and at risk of infections. It is also by no means clear whether the correct techniques have yet been used to assess colony-stimulating activity. Despite these limitations, the data do strongly suggest that regulator levels may be abnormal in patients with myeloid leukemia, particularly in patients with CML in acute transformation. Although chemotherapy has been shown to alter GM-CSF levels, from an analysis of the patients in Table 14, no difference was observed between pretreatment sera and sera from patients with AML in relapse and under intensive chemotherapy.

Although AML and CML leukemic cells have been shown to be responsive to GM-CSF, it could be questioned whether the levels of GM-CSF in sera are sufficiently high to stimulate these cells. This was investigated in a comparative analysis of titrations of monkey lung and human white cell-conditioned media on human marrow cells on one hand and an analysis of these conditioned media versus leukemic sera on mouse marrow target cells. Calculations from these comparative assays indicated that the levels of GM-CSF even in normal human sera were 2–3 times the concentration of GM-CSF in conditioned medium capable of delivering a plateau stimulation to human marrow cells [286]. As mentioned earlier, addition of such sera will stimulate GM-colony formation by human marrow cells even at the 1:10 dilution involved in adding 0.1 ml of serum to a 1 ml culture. However, in this latter case it has yet to be demonstrated that the GM-CSF in the added serum is actually what stimulates colony formation since, unlike in mouse marrow cultures, colony formation is only partially prevented by use of antihuman urine GM-CSF sera [182].

It would appear therefore that even normal serum levels of GM-CSF represent a significant proliferative stimulus for leukemic cells. Despite the reservations about the correct method for estimating human GM-CSF, the normal and elevated levels demonstrated so far in leukemic patients almost certainly represent a significant proliferative stimulus for the leukemic populations in these patients.

H. Can Leukemic Cells Produce GM-CSF?

One question of considerable interest is whether CML or AML populations can produce GM-CSF, and if so, since the leukemic cells are responsive to GM-CSF, whether this represents a self-priming system leading to progressive expansion of the leukemic population. Strictly speaking this question should be rephrased as two questions: (1) can leukemic colony-forming cells make GM-CSF, and (2) can the more mature progeny of leukemic colony-forming cells, e.g., polymorphs, monocytes, or macrophages make GM-CSF?

To recapitulate the evidence regarding normal populations, cell separation studies have shown that the colony-stimulating cells can be separated from colony-forming cells, and following such separation, colony-forming cells are unable to proliferate without exogenous GM-CSF. Furthermore, monocytes and macrophages were shown to be a rich source of GM-CSF while polymorphs were not and in fact could release material inhibiting the production of GM-CSF by other cells. At face value, this evidence implies the existence in normal populations of a system in which the ancestral cell is unable to stimulate itself but is under the influence of two feedback control systems from its progeny—a positive feedback from the monocytes and macrophages stimulating proliferation and a negative feedback from the polymorphs inhibiting proliferation.

This is a satisfactory model which is quite consistent with ideas on regulatory control systems, but on critical scrutiny, there are a number of weaknesses which have not been explored. Most cultures of semipurified GM-CFCs have of necessity dealt with relatively small numbers of such cells, and there are in fact no published data on the behaviour of such cells in crowded cultures containing up to 1×10^6 cells per ml—the concentration commonly used to test the capacity of cells as underlayers or to produce conditioned medium. Furthermore, since these GM-CFC populations were usually only enriched and not pure populations, the possible inhibitory activity of associated nonadherent or light density cells cannot be excluded. Furthermore, the data on GM-CSF synthesis by monocytes and macrophages is by no means convincing. These cells can actively ingest GM-CSF, and the release GM-CSF following stimulation is not blocked by inhibitors of protein synthesis. Because of this, it is rather doubtful whether these cells really synthesize all of the GM-CSF which numerous experiments have shown them able to release.

In the case of the cloned mouse myelomonocytic leukemias discussed earlier, the situation is also not entirely clear. Tests for GM-CSF production by the leukemic colony-forming cells have not been sufficiently stringent to document or eliminate this possibility. The more mature cells of leukemic populations clearly can synthesize GM-CSF in vitro [326, 16], and even cloned populations have been shown to be active, but the current uncertainty regarding GM-CSF production by normal monocytes and macrophages makes it difficult to determine whether this capacity of leukemic cells is abnormal or no greater than that shown by normal cells.

Turning to the question of CML populations, the evidence is similar to that existing for normal populations. Unfractionated CML populations are capable of autostimulation of colony formation and of producing conditioned media capable of stimulating colony formation by normal or leukemic cells. However, in this latter regard, CML cells appear to be less effective than normal cells, and the activity of peripheral blood cells from these patients improves after therapy [281, 327, 44]. Separated low density CML GM-CFCs are usually not capable of proliferation without added GM-CSF, but again these tests have not been performed under cell density conditions where moderate GM-CSF production could have been detected [44]. Finally, CML fractions with colony-stimulating activity are highly heterogeneous, and while the data again correlate activity with monocytes and macrophages [44], it cannot be guaranteed that all of these cells are necessarily members of the Ph^1 leukemic clone. Cells from CML patients in acute transformation appeared to be unable to produce GM-CSF [281].

The behavior of AML cells appears to be variable. Unfractionated cells from many AML patients lack the capacity when in underlayers to stimulate colony formation by normal cells or to produce conditioned media with colony-stimulating activity [295, 45, 294, 44, 328]. In a study by Robinson and Entringer [295], acute undifferentiated or monocytic leukemic cells were active in underlayers but not AML cells. This was confirmed in a study by Goldman et al. [327] who found that underlayers of peripheral blood from acute monocytic leukemic patients exhibited higher activity than normal cells. This agrees with the observation that plasma levels of GM-CSF were higher in patients with acute monocytic leukemia than in other patients with leukemia [298].

AML populations freed of colony-stimulating cells do not appear to be able to proliferate in vitro [44, 85], but the same reservations must be applied to this data as were discussed for normal and CML cells.

At the present state of our knowledge, the autostimulating hypothesis as the basis of the progressive expansion of the leukemic population cannot be regarded as established although available data are consistent with this possibility. In essence, this hypothesis could apply equally to normal populations and, if so, reasons must be found for the limited growth of normal populations versus the apparently unlimited growth capacity of leukemic populations. A number of possible explanations could be advanced: (1) unresponsiveness of leukemic cells to feedback inhibition by polymorph-derived inhibitors or inhibitors of other origins, (2) hyperresponsiveness of leukemic cells to GM-CSF, (3) production by leukemic cells of abnormal GM-CSFs uniquely stimulating leukemic populations, or (4) intrinsic abnormalities in leukemic cells influencing the pattern of differentiation of progeny cells following stimulation by GM-CSF.

Each of these possibilities will now be discussed in some detail as the progressive, unrestrained growth of leukemic populations is *the* essential problem in leukemia.

1. Available information regarding inhibitors of granulopoiesis is too incomplete or difficult to interpret to adequately discuss the first possibility. Low molecular weight inhibitors of granulopoiesis have been shown to be released by normal and leukemic granulocytic cells, but these appear to be equally inhibitory for normal and leukemic cells in vitro [254]. There is also doubt regarding their specificity although in some experimental systems some specificity for granulopoiesis has been documented [250]. Low molecular weight inhibitors have so far not been detected in vivo [254].

The high molecular weight lipoproteins in serum which can inhibit granulocytic colony formation in vitro exhibit no specificity of action (at least in partially purified form) and inhibit colony formation by other hemopoietic cells. These materials also appear to have the capacity to inhibit leukemic cells as effectively as normal cells [102]. In some assay systems, levels of these serum inhibitors have been reported to be abnormally low in about half of the patients with AML but to be normal in patients with CML [242, 239, 223, 323]. However, other studies have failed to document this difference [243], and much appears to depend on the type of FCS being used in the assays.

Polymorphs in high concentrations inhibit granulocytic colony formation by inhibiting the production of GM-CSF by colony-stimulating cells [46]. It is possible such a system could operate in vivo at a local level to restrict granulopoiesis. The relative absence of mature polymorphs in AML may give such populations a growth advantage, and in CML the polymorphs have been shown to be functionally inactive in suppressing granulopoiesis by normal cells [46]. It is not yet clear whether leukemic-derived colony-stimulating cells are more or less responsive than normal cells to this polymorph-derived suppressor.

2. There is so far no evidence to support the second possibility that leukemic cells are hyperresponsive to GM-CSF, and in one study CML cells were slightly hyporesponsive. The data for AML cells were difficult to interpret from the unusual dose-response curves, but it is improbable that they were unusually responsive [286].

3. The phrase "stimulated by GM-CSF" has been used repeatedly in this chapter when referring to the stimulation of leukemic cultures by white cell underlayers or conditioned media. Is there any real justification for assuming that the active factor is GM-CSF since underlayers and conditioned medium must contain a multiplicity of biologically active materials? If the answer is yes, or a provisional yes, it is still necessary to raise the question of

whether abnormal forms of GM-CSF may be made in leukemic patients.

In the case of the mouse myeloid and myelomonocytic leukemias, it has been shown that the purified GM-CSF molecule is active in stimulating colony formation [269, Fig. 26]. Since no form of GM-CSF with activity on human cells has yet been purified, strictly speaking it is an assumption to use the term "stimulated by GM-CSF." However, purification studies in this laboratory on the GM-CSF in human placental-conditioned medium have succeeded in obtaining a highly enriched preparation free of most of the original contaminating protein [57]. This semipurified GM-CSF is equally effective in stimulating normal and leukemic cells from AML or CML patients in vitro and will now be surprising if the situation will be found to differ when this material is finally in pure form.

Despite this mounting evidence that human leukemic cells are stimulated by normal GM-CSF, it is quite proper to consider the possibility that leukemic or other cells in a leukemic patient may produce abnormal forms of GM-CSF to which the leukemic cells may be uniquely or preferentially responsive. Analysis of human urine and serum GM-CSF by physicochemical methods [161, 165] and the use of specific antisera have failed to document the existence of abnormal forms of GM-CSF in AML or CML. Antisera prepared in rabbits against human urine GM-CSF was equally effective in inhibiting GM-colony formation in mouse marrow cultures stimulated by leukemic or nonleukemic human serum or urine [176, 182]. However, studies on GM-CSF in the membranes of normal and leukemic white cells and the GM-CSF released by the cells in culture have documented some interesting differences between GM-CSFs derived from normal and leukemic cells. Most of the GM-CSF extractable from normal or leukemic white cells was shown to be present in or associated with the cell membrane [178]. When such material was analyzed by gel filtration, three distinct peaks were eluted with colony-stimulating activity for normal human marrow cells. A similar pattern of active material was observed with membrane extracts from AML or CML cells, with again active material eluting with approximate mol wt 14,000 36,000, and 93,000. In medium conditioned by normal white cells, again three peaks of active material were identified [177]. However, in media conditioned by leukemic cells, only a single peak of active material was observed which corresponded with the middle peak (36,000 mol wt) in the normal conditioned medium. A survey of cells from leukemic patients indicated that this characteristic was a consistent finding with leukemic cells [177].

These findings could indicate some imbalance in synthesis or release of certain forms of GM-CSF from leukemic cells but do not by themselves offer any evidence for the production of a qualitatively abnormal GM-CSF. In another study, it was shown that phytohemagglutinin stimulated a subpopulation of cells from the blood of patients with AML to produce a factor capable of stimulating ^{3}HTdR uptake by leukemic cells. These conditioned media also stimulated GM-colony formation by normal marrow cells, but it is not clear whether the factor stimulating the incorporation of thymidine is separable from GM-CSF [55, 329]. Differences were reported in low molecular weight stimulating factors derived from leukemic and normal sources [180].

4. Finally, and perhaps most probable of all, is the likelihood that leukemic cells have serious intrinsic derangements in the genetic mechanisms controlling differentiation and the capacity for proliferation. This is likely from the abnormal karyotype of many AML leukemic populations although a heritable abnormality of this type would not need to be caused by, or be associated with, clearly visible chromosomal abnormalities. Despite the observation that some clones of mouse myeloid leukemic cells can differentiate normally, the overwhelming evidence from comparable studies on human AML cells has indicated that the human cells are unable to differentiate normally. This indicates major intrinsic and heritable abnormalities in these leukemic populations.

Since the essence of the progressive growth involves a relative or complete failure of a sufficiently high proportion of progeny cells to differentiate to nondividing cells, the presence of intrinsic defects in this mechanism could alone be sufficient to account for the progressive proliferation or growth advantage of a leukemic population.

The evidence indicates that, because of their multipotentiality, the stem cells of the leukemic population both in AML and CML are probably located in the stem cell compartment. If this is so, it is likely that these cells exhibit a significant capacity for self-generation.

Nothing is known of the mechanisms controlling self-generation in normal hemopoietic stem cells, but these are likely to be local microenvironmental regulators. Restriction in the distribution of microenvironmental cells in the adult presumably limits both the total mass of hemopoietic tissue and the location of hemopoiesis to the marrow and spleen. From the capacity of leukemic populations to proliferate progressively in abnormal sites, it can be deduced that the proliferation of leukemic stem cells is not as dependent on, or responsive to, these microenvironmental factors as is normal stem self-generation.

Uncontrollable proliferation in the leukemic stem cell compartment may be the crucial factor leading to the progressive enlargement of a leukemic population. This would explain the present rather paradoxical observations that the slightly more mature leukemic cells now being monitored in agar cultures appear to respond to and depend on regulatory factors and to generate populations of the same size as normal cells, yet the leukemic population size increases progressively in the patient.

I. Suppression of Normal Cells by Leukemic Cells

The most spectacular single finding emerging from the agar culture of marrow or blood cells from patients with AML has been the documentation that in pretreatment patients there is usually a complete absence of detectable normal colony-forming cells. This indicates a profound suppression of normal granulopoietic populations at least from the level of GM-CFCs onward. As was shown by the analysis of AML patients in remission, normal stem cells do survive in these patients and can reestablish normal hemopoiesis.

Several animal models have been developed that mimic at least some aspects of human AML and permit studies on possible mechanisms by which normal populations might be suppressed by leukemic populations. TANAKA et al. [330]) described a transplantable myelomonocytic leukemia in RF mice in which a progressive decrease in normal hemopoiesis occurred and a somewhat similar transplantable myelomonocytic leukemia was developed in rats [331]. VAN BEKKUM et al [332] studied a carcinogen-induced transplantable myeloid leukemia in BN rats. The leukemic cells grew relatively slowly in vivo permitting the development of a semichronic model. As with human AML cells, the leukemic cells failed to produce colonies in vitro, but as the transplanted leukemia grew in vivo, a progressive reduction to zero occurred in GM-CFC levels in the marrow.

Conflicting evidence has been produced on the question of whether leukemic cells added to the culture dish can suppress colony formation by normal GM-CFCs. In the BN myeloid leukemia model just described, no suppression was documented [332], and as mentioned earlier, WEHI-3 myelomonocytic leukemic cells strongly stimulate colony formation by normal marrow cells when cocultivated with them [16]. With other nongrowing mouse myeloid leukemias, no inhibition of normal colonies was observed in mixed cultures (METCALF, D., unpublished data).

In human marrow cultures, CHIYODA et al. [333] reported inhibition of GM-colony formation by 2×10^5 normal human cells by the addition of as few as 2×10^4 AML or ALL cells. In an extension of this work, it was reported [334] that extracts of a number of AML marrows were able to inhibit GM-colony formation in vitro by normal human cells. Extracts from normal marrow had no such activity. Medium conditioned by the leukemic cells also reduced normal GM-colony formation.

A somewhat similar finding was reported by MORRIS et al. [335] who found that coculture of normal human marrow cells with peripheral blood or bone marrow from seven of nine patients with AMML (even in a ratio as low as four normal cells to one leukemic cell) led to a marked reduction in GM-colony formation by the normal cells. Direct cultures of marrow cells from these nine patients failed to develop colonies. Marrow cells taken from one of these patients during a subsequent remission failed to reveal inhibitory activity.

Conflicting results have been obtained by a number of workers who failed to find any evidence of inhibition of colony formation in vitro by normal human cells following coculture with a variety of leukemic cells [292, 294, 299, 296).

In a possible explanation of these discrepancies, BULL et al. [336]) observed that when the percentage of blasts in the marrow from a patient with AML exceeded 30–40%, no normal GM-colonies developed. The effects of mixing normal and leukemic cells appeared to depend on the histocompatibility of the mixed cells. Mixture of two normal matched marrows led to an increase in colony formation over expected numbers. Mixtures of matched leukemic and normal cells did not lead to inhibition, but if the leukemia was mismatched with the normal cells either partially or completely, inhibition occurred. It was suggested that antigenic differences between leukemic and normal cells in the patient might cause the same effect.

It is quite likely, of course, that many other mechanisms may be involved in the competitive interaction between leukemic and normal populations, e.g., cell contact processes, cell crowding, damage to microenvironmental or factor-producing cells in the marrow or elsewhere. Few of these possibilities can be tested directly in semisolid cultures, but it should be possible at least to resolve the present conflicting evidence from human and mouse cultures as to whether normal colony formation can or cannot be suppressed by leukemic cells in mixed cultures in vitro. If this phenomenon does occur, the simplicity of the semisolid cultures should permit the mechanism involved to be characterized.

J. Clinical Uses of Agar Culture Techniques

At present, more clinical use is being made of semisolid cultures to analyze bone marrow and blood cells from leukemic patients than cells from patients with any other type of disease.

To be of most value, the cultures for clinical analysis should be as simple as possible. From experience in this laboratory, the following procedures are recommended for each specimen and should provide the maximum of information with the mimimum of effort (Fig. 32):

1. Centrifuge the specimen through BSA of density 1.062 g/cm^3 and culture the unfractionated specimen, the supernatant and pelleted cells at two cell concentrations, 10,000 and 100,000 cells per culture dish.
2. Score cultures at 7 days, counting colonies and clusters.
3. Calculate the frequency of light and heavy density colony-forming and cluster-forming cells and the cluster to colony ratio.

This data will allow a diagnosis of the type of leukemia, an assessment of prognosis, detect an impending clinical change in the patient, and analyze the relapse/ remission status.

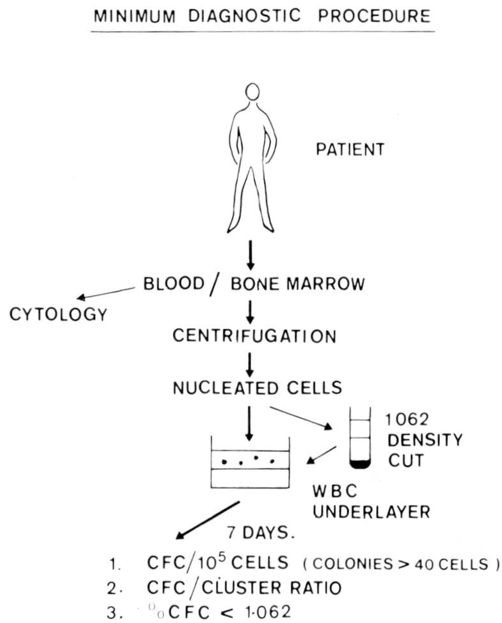

Fig. 32. Scheme of minimum culture procedures to apply in monitoring each blood or marrow specimen in patients with myeloid leukemia

The density centrifugation procedure is as follows: Cells are suspended in 5 ml of BSA (pH 5.1, osmolarity 269 mosmol) and of density 1.062 g/cm^3, layered over cell-free albumin of the same density and the interface mixed. The layer containing the cells is itself overlaid with BSA of lower density to prevent a cell-air interface from forming during centrifugation. The tube is centrifuged at 3500 g for 10 min. Cells of density equal to or lighter than 1.062 g/cm^3 remain in suspension and the denser cells form a pellet. Supernatant and pelleted cells are harvested separately, washed, viable cell counts performed, then cultured.

The clinical uses of agar culture techniques in the diagnosis and management of leukemia are as follows:

1. Diagnosis of AML. Occasional problem patients still occur, and the distinctive growth patterns of AML cells allow a virtually certain diagnosis. Conversely, we have seen several patients diagnosed as AML who had large numbers of colony-forming cells of normal density. Subsequent tests showed these patients to have had septicemia. The agar cultures will usually clearly discriminate between AML and ALL if this is difficult on morphological grounds.

2. Assessment of Likely Responses to Chemotherapy. From an analysis of cluster size, density of colony-forming cells, and cluster to colony ratios, it now seems possible to give a more sophisticated estimate of the probable response of AML patients to chemotherapy than was formerly possible using only the age of the patient, i.e., the poorer response of older patients. This may become of importance if major alternative forms of therapy are developed which could be substituted early in treatment for the usual therapeutic regimes.

3. Confirmation of Remission. The development of large numbers of colonies and the demonstration that these are generated by cells of normal density together with the development of a normal cluster to colony ratio are clear indications of the regrowth of a normal granulopoietic clone, i.e., of the development of the remission, regardless of the morphology of the marrow population. Chemotherapy should be modified accordingly.

4. Early Warning of Blast Transformation in CML. A progressive increase in morphological abnormalities in colony and cluster cells, a decrease in frequency of colony-forming cells, and a rising cluster to colony ratio all signal that clinically apparent acute transformation will develop within the next 2–6 months. It now needs to be established whether this early warning will allow improved results to be obtained with modified chemotherapy.

5. Transition of Myeloproliferative States to AML. To anticipate the discussion in Chapter 7, in patients with aplastic anemia, paroxysmal nocturnal hemoglobinuria, polycythemia vera, or refractory anemia in whom a higher than normal risk of leukemia development exists, monitoring the marrow and blood populations using agar cultures can again give early warning of the development of leukemia. While it again has yet to be shown whether the option of earlier therapy given by this information would improve ultimate results, the reassurance to patients and clinicians of the *nondevelopment* of acute leukemia is also an important factor.

6. Determination of Chemotherapy Appropriate for Individual Patients. It was an early hope that use of agar cultures would permit chemotherapy tests on the patient's own leukemic cells so that the most effective chemotherapy could be selected. Some initial studies in mouse cultures were published to document the type of dosages active in vitro [112], but so far no studies have been reported on cultures from patients, nor has an analysis been made of whether the substituted drugs chosen on the basis of in vitro tests would be in fact more effective than the usual treatment regimes. Although this potential use of agar cultures is still actively discussed, it seems improbable that it will ever be used with the present chemotherapeutic agents.

7. Assessment of Survival in Stored Bone Marrow. Agar cultures are ideal for monitoring the viability of marrow cells stored in liquid nitrogen for subsequent infusion to leukemic patients [337].

8. Analysis of the Nature of Human Leukemia. The discussion in this chapter has reemphasised a point which has always worried laboratory workers—that animal models may not exactly mimic the human disease and may on occasions be misleading. Thus, the M1 mouse model in which the leukemic cells are apparently able to revert to normal functional activity suggests strongly that remissions might be based on reversion of the functional activity of leukemic cells to normal. However, studies on AML patients indicate that the capacity to differentiate to anything resembling mature cells is uncommon. Conversely, in most patients, remissions involve the competitive rebound of a suppressed normal population. Use of the M1 leukemia as a model of human AML may therefore be potentially misleading. The primary clinical value of agar cultures may well be a long-term one, namely the ability to analyze the nature of *human* leukemia by direct studies on human hemopoietic populations.

K. Summary

In two mouse models, leukemic granulocytic and monocytic cells can proliferate and form colonies of cells in semisolid agar. Proliferation was found to be responsive to purified GM-CSF.

In humans, the proliferation of CML and AML cells in agar shows an even more striking responsiveness to, and dependency on, stimulation by the normal regulator GM-CSF, and no patients have been found in whom the leukemic cells were *not* dependent on GM-CSF.

CML cells form colonies and clusters in vitro with a near normal differentiation, the major abnormalities being the extremely high frequency of GM-CFCs, particularly in the blood, the abnormally light buoyant density of these cells, and the long cell cycle times of these cells (or the high proportion of noncycling cells).

Cultures from AML patients usually contain no colony-forming cells, and the AML cells usually form only clusters of varying sizes or fail to proliferate. In a minority of patients, the leukemic cells appear able to form colonies. AML cluster and colony-forming cells have intrinsic abnormalities and their progeny usually do not differentiate normally in vitro. Again these cells are of abnormally light buoyant density and have an abnormally long cycle time (or have a high proportion of noncycling cells).

A two-stage culture system using preliminary incubation with PHA in a liquid phase may offer a selective culture system for leukemic cells. In remission, in most patients with AML, a suppressed normal granulopoietic population repopulates the marrow.

Abnormalities in serum and urine GM-CSF and inhibitor levels have been demonstrated in CML and AML patients. Since the leukemic populations in CML and AML patients are responsive to GM-CSF, these abnormal regulator levels may in part be responsible for the emergence and progressive proliferation of the leukemic clones.

Chapter 7

GM-Colony Formation in Myeloproliferative Disorders

The so-called "myeloproliferative disorders" include a complex group of poorly understood diseases such as aplastic anemia, polycythemia vera, refractory anemia, sideroblastic anemia, paroxysmal nocturnal hemoglobinuria, and others. They are characterized by proliferative abnormalities in one or more families of hemopoietic cells usually associated with the production of abnormal levels of end cells, often with abnormalities in maturation.

It is reasonable to expect that a thorough analysis of these diseases using in vitro cloning methods will eventually establish the exact nature of these diseases and the manner in which they are related to one another. While some studies have already been made on these subjects, the primary purpose of the discussion in this chapter is rather more specialized and will simply consider these diseases from the point of view of potential preleukemic disorders.

Chapter 6 has outlined the nature of CML and AML as analyzed by in vitro cloning methods. To understand the origin of these abnormalities, it would be highly desirable to be able to analyze the situation in patients before leukemia actually developed. Unfortunately, no preleukemic states are known for CML or for most patients with AML. However, in approximately one-third of patients developing AML, the disease is preceded by a hemopoietic disorder of sufficient severity to bring the patient to a hospital. These antecedent disorders are one or other of the various myeloproliferative diseases. It must be emphasized, however, that only a *minority* of patients with these diseases will develop leukemia.

An intensive analysis of the situation in patients with various myeloproliferative diseases therefore has several objectives: (1) to determine whether abnormalities exist in GM-CFC or regulator levels before AML develops, (2) to determine whether a sequence of abnormalities is demonstrable, (3) to identify which patients with myeloproliferative disorders are going to develop AML, and (4) perhaps of even greater importance, to identify which patients are *not* going to develop AML.

To recapitulate the findings in AML patients, the following abnormalities were demonstrated:

1. Where GM-CFCs were present, these were of abnormally light buoyant density, exhibited a low frequency of cells in S phase, and generated progeny whose differentiation was usually abnormal. Cultures usually exhibited an abnormally high cluster to colony ratio.
2. Most AML cells formed only clusters, cluster-forming cells were equally frequent in blood and marrow, were of abnormally light buoyant density, and few were in the S phase of the cell cycle. Cluster cells usually exhibited abnormal differentiation.
3. GM-CSF levels often were elevated, and serum inhibitor levels were often undetectable or subnormal. AML cells were themselves often poor sources of GM-CSF.

Specific questions to be raised concerning data from patients with myeloproliferative disorders are whether any of these abnormalities alone or in combination are demonstrable in these various diseases.

A. Aplastic Anemia

In marrow cultures from patients with aplastic anemia, a number of workers have observed a depression in GM-CFC frequency [263, 294, 85, 338]. In one study, it was noted in at least one-third of the patients that the GM-CFCs were also of abnormally light buoyant density [317]. In another study on patients with aplastic anemia [294], it was noted that the colony-stimulating activity of peripheral blood cells from these patients was markedly reduced compared with the activity of white cells from normal donors. In a study in this laboratory, 50% of sera from patients with aplastic anemia had GM-CSF levels above the upper normal limits (Table 16) although the infection status of these patients was not determined.

In a group of 16 patients with aplastic anemia studied by DICKE and LOWENBERG [339], 12 were found to have subnormal GM-CFC levels and in four, levels were normal. The colony-stimulating activity of the peripheral blood cells from all of the latter four patients was normal, as was the activity from seven of 12 of the patients with subnormal GM-CFC levels. Thus, three groups of patients were categorized (Table 17). As shown in table 17, patients with normal GM-CFC and colony-stimulting activity levels did well clinically, whereas a high mortality was observed where both GM-CFC levels and colony-stimulating activities were low. Of particular interest in the present context of potentially preleukemic diseases were the seven patients with low GM-CFC levels but normal colony-stimulating activity of the peripheral blood cells. Three of these seven patients developed acute leukemia during the relatively short observation period of the study.

B. Refractory Anemia

In refractory anemia, defects can be apparently confined to the erythroid series with marked erythroid hyperplasia together with megaloblastosis and ring sideroblastosis but with normal

Table 16. Stimulation of GM-colony formation by mouse bone marrow cells using dialyzed sera from patients with myeloproliferative disorders

Disease	No. of sera analyzed	% Sera with elevated colony-stimulating activity[a]	Mean serum GM-CSF[b]
Normal blood donors	65	6%	10.4 ± 5.3
Polycythemia vera	16	56%	23.4 ± 16.5
Paroxysmal nocturnal hemoglobinuria	5	80%	27.6 ± 13.2
Aplastic anemia	16	50%	21.1 ± 14.4
Refractory anemia	21	33%	17.9 ± 15.3
Myelofibrosis	28	61%	49.0 ± 46.0
Preleukemia	7	57%	27.9 ± 30.1

All assays performed by adding 0.1 ml of serum to cultures of 75,000 $C_{57}BL$ marrow cells.
[a] % Sera stimulating more than 20 colonies, the upper limit of colony numbers stimulated by 0.1 ml of normal serum.
[b] Mean number of colonies stimulated by 0.1 ml of serum ± standard deviations.

Table 17. Correlation in patients with aplastic anemia between GM-CFC levels, colony-stimulating activity of peripheral blood cells and clinical course[a]

	No. of patients	GM-CFC levels	Peripheral blood colony-stimulating activity	Clinical course
Category I	5	Low	Low	Frequent need for transfusions 4/5 dead
Category II	7	Low	Normal/high	Frequent need for transfusions 3/7 acute leukemia
Category III	4	Normal/high	Normal/high	In hematological balance

[a] Data adapted from DICKE and LOWENBERG [339].

neutrophil and platelet production. These patients have been classified as refractory anemia type 1 by VILTER et al. [340]. In other patients, these defects in erythropoiesis are accompanied by neutropenia, pancytopenia, thrombocytopenia, or abnormalities in granulocyte maturation. These are classified as refractory anemia type 3 patients.

In a study of refractory anemia patients (excluding patients diagnosed as preleukemia or chronic Di Guglielmo's syndrome), MOORE and SPITZER [338] observed that patients of type 1 exhibited a normal frequency of GM-CFCs in the marrow and a normal ratio of colonies to clusters. GM-CFCs were not elevated in the peripheral blood. However, cells from all 15 patients with type 3 refractory anemia exhibited abnormal proliferative activity in vitro. Cells from ten of the 15 patients produced reduced numbers of colonies although the cluster to colony ratio and colony cell differentiation were normal. Cells from the other patients either produced low numbers of colonies with abnormal cluster to colony ratios and/or colonies and clusters with abnormal maturation (Table 18). In two of the three patients whose cells produced only clusters in culture, acute leukemia developed within 6 months. It was noted that GM-CFCs from all type 3 patients with refractory anemia had an abnormally light buoyant density with 20–100% of the GM-CFCs being of lighter density than 1.062 g/cm^3 [338, 317].

Table 18. GM-colony and cluster formation by cells from patients with refractory anemia[a]

Type of disease	No. of patients	Bone marrow Colonies/10^5 cells	Bone marrow Clusters/10^5 cells	Cluster/Colony Ratio	Blood Colonies/10^5 cells	Blood Clusters/10^5 cells
Refractory anemia type 1	6	47	262	6.2	0	0
Refractory anemia type 3	10	1.5	13	5.2	0	1
	1	3	48[b]	16	0	0
	1	110	3300[b]	30	—	—
	3	0	560[b]	>560	0	0
AML preceded by refractory anemia type 3	4	0	412[b]	>412	0	16

[a] Data modified from MOORE and SPITZER [338].
[b] Maturation defects in vitro.

Cells from four patients with AML who had had a previous history of refractory anemia type 3 produced clusters in culture typical of AML with no antecedent clinical disease.
A somewhat similar group of patients to type 3 refractory anemia subjects was studied by GREENBERG et al. [341] under the diagnosis of "preleukemia." Depressed colony numbers and an elevated proportion of light density GM-CFCs were observed. In a proportion of these patients, urine GM-CSF levels were elevated.

In a study on serum GM-CSF levels (METCALF, D., unpublished data, Table 16) one-third of sera from refractory anemia patients were found to have levels above the upper normal limit.

C. Myelofibrosis

Although the risk of acute leukemia development in myelofibrosis does not appear to be as high as in other myeloproliferative disorders, interesting abnormalities in GM-CFC levels have been observed. As might be anticipated, marrow GM-CFC levels are usually reduced. However, circulating levels of GM-CFCs are elevated, and although the colonies generated exhibit normal maturation, these GM-CFCs have been found to be of abnormally light buoyant density [338]. Cells from two of seven patients analyzed by MOORE and SPITZER [338] formed no granulocytic colonies and only generated clusters. In the latter patients, an elevated blood level of myeloblasts was observed, and the patients may have had early acute leukemia. Patients with myelofibrosis have been observed to have exceptionally high serum GM-CSF levels (METCALF, D., unpublished data), and in one study (Table 16), 17 of 28 sera had levels above the upper limit of normal with a mean level more than 4 times that seen in normal subjects.
In view of the known capacity of the bone marrow stromal cells to produce GM-CSF, one interesting possibility raised by the very high serum GM-CSF levels is that the so-called "fibrous" tissue occupying the marrow cavity in myelofibrosis may be a functional tumor of GM-CSF-producing cells.

D. Polycythemia Vera

In a study of 12 patients with polycythemia vera, in five patients with normal peripheral blood white cell levels, the frequency of GM-CFCs was normal in the marrow and peripheral blood, and the density of the colony-forming cells was also normal [338]. Similar results were obtained by GREENBERG et al. [341]. However, in patients with elevated white cell levels with immature cells in the peripheral blood, GM-CFC levels were increased in the peripheral blood, and there was an elevation in the proportion of light density cells [338, 317]. If myelofibrosis supervened, these changes became more marked (Table 19).
Cells from two patients with acute leukemia who had had polycythemia vera exhibited a growth pattern typical for AML cells—cluster formation by cells of abnormally light buoyant density with defective maturation in the cluster cells.
Serum GM-CSF levels were elevated above normal levels in nine of 16 patients analyzed with average levels almost twice those seen in normal subjects (Table 16).

Table 19. GM-CFC levels in polycythemia vera[a]

Type of disease	No. of patients	WBC × $10^3/mm^3$	Marrow		Blood		% GM-CFC < 1.062 g/cm^3
			Colonies/ 10^5 cells	Clusters/ 10^5 cells	Colonies/ 10^5 cells	Clusters/ 10^5 cells	
Polycythemia vera	5	11.6	141	800	1	8	4
Polycythemia vera with immature cells in blood	3	19.0	88	335	39	140	65
Polycythemia vera with immature cells in blood and myelofibrosis	2	14.0	—	—	212	870	81
AML with history of polycythemia vera	2	—	0	1540[b]	0	1810[b]	58

[a] Data from MOORE and SPITZER [338].
[b] Maturation defect in vitro.

E. Paroxysmal Nocturnal Hemoglobinuria

Few patients appear to have been analyzed in detail, but GM-colony-forming cells were reported to be of normal density [317]. In a study of serum GM-CSF levels, four of five sera tested had levels above the upper normal limit.

F. Preleukemia

The diagnosis "preleukemia" usually arouses scepticism and controversy amongst hematologists. This is not the place in which to discuss arguments for or against the proposition that a distinct clinical syndrome of preleukemia exists which can be identified on morphological or clinical grounds. Quite clearly, however, if sequential observations are being made on patients with myeloproliferative disorders who subsequently develop acute leukemia, at some stage in the observation period, the observations can validly be stated to have been on preleukemic patients. Indeed, it is very probable that in these particular patients the whole disease process is part of the preleukemic phase. Information has been gathered from a number of sequential studies on patients terminating in acute leukemia which permits some statements to be made on culture patterns in the interval immediately preceding leukemia development.

In one of the earliest studies, GREENBERG et al. [294] described seven patients with preleukemia. In six, GM-CFC levels were severely depressed and the colony-stimulating activity of the peripheral white cells from these patients was subnormal. In an extension of this study, GREENBERG et al. [341] observed depressed GM-CFC levels in 26 of 33 patients whose various diseases terminated in AML. In a mixed group of patients with CML, subacute myeloid leukemia, preleukemia, or essential thrombocytopenia, the GM-CFCs were of abnormally light buoyant density in 15 of 16 patients. Seven of eight of these patients where more than 35% of colony-forming cells were of abnormally light buoyant density subsequently developed acute leukemia. Elevated urine GM-CSF levels were observed in 17 of 31 patients and in ten of 12 who developed acute leukemia within 10 months of the study period. Six of seven patients who had both elevated urine GM-CSF levels and low GM-CFC levels developed acute transformation within 10 months.

This particular study suggests strongly that if a patient with a myeloproliferative disorder exhibits two or more abnormalities of the following: low GM-CFC levels, a high proportion of the light density GM-CFCs, high cluster to colony ratios, or elevated GM-CSF levels, the onset of acute leukemia within months is likely.

Other studies by MOORE and SPITZER [338] and MOORE [317] also documented the presence of multiple abnormalities in refractory anemia and polycythemia vera patients who subsequently progressed to acute leukemia within the subsequent 6 months. In at least several of these patients, the marrow contained no colony-forming cells but large numbers of cluster-forming cells of abnormally light buoyant density. This culture pattern is essentially similar to that of acute leukemia. However, the difference in these myeloproliferative patients was that no abnormal findings were obtained from culture of the peripheral blood. The development of clinically apparent leukemia coincided with the appearance of large numbers of cluster-forming cells in the peripheral blood, completing the characteristic findings of AML as seen in culture.

In some patients at least, a marrow population with highly abnormal in vitro proliferative characteristics can be present for many months before leukemia supervenes. SENN and PINKERTON [342] described three patients with markedly depressed GM-CFC levels for 5, 15, and 27 months before acute leukemia developed.

Using the PHA-primed culture system for detecting AML cells, SPITZER et al. [311] reported that in four of ten patients with probable preleukemia or early leukemia, marrow cells were able to grow without GM-CSF in PHA-primed cultures (the characteristic of AML cells), suggesting the early appearance of cells of the leukemic clone.

As discussed earlier, CML commonly terminates in an acute terminal phase which exhibits many of the features of AML. Indeed, some workers regard CML as merely a prolonged hyperplastic preleukemic disorder antedating the real disease—AML [343, 344]. As described earlier, the progressive changes in culture pattern observed prior to acute transformation (reduction in GM-CFC levels, rising cluster to colony ratios, abnormal maturation of colony and cluster cells, and high serum GM-CSF levels) are similar to the changes just described in myeloproliferative disease patients during leukemia development. The appearance of PHA-primed colony-forming cells in such patients is also consistent with these progressive changes [311].

G. Clonal Succession in AML Development

While the above culture observations are admittedly fragmentary as is inevitable in clinical studies, there is a strong implication of progression in the abnormalities detectable in culture as these patients with myeloproliferative disorders progress to acute leukemia. These initial findings are of sufficient interest to warrant more extensive studies deliberately designed to permit long-term longitudinal studies on these patients.

Current concepts of carcinogenesis suggest that neoplastic populations are often clonal and usually emerge as a consequence of a series of changes in which progressively more abnormal subpopulations emerge and outgrow or dominate preexisting normal or abnormal populations. In at least some of the myeloproliferative disorders, the abnormal hemopoietic populations have been shown to be clonal, e.g., in polycythemia vera [345].

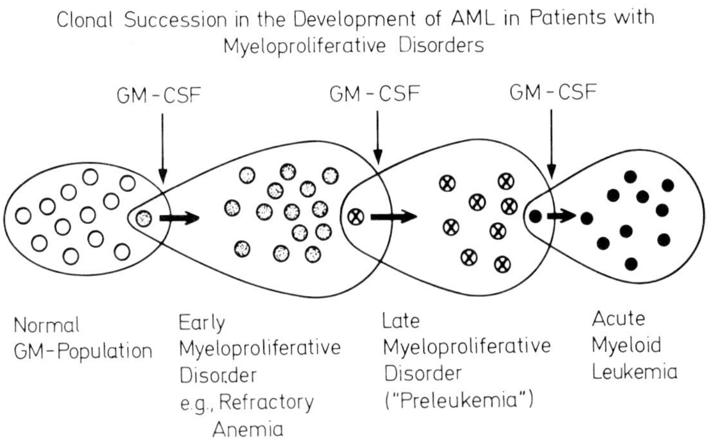

Fig. 33. Schematic representation of sequential events leading to myeloid leukemia development. An altered normal cell generates a dominant clone of hemopoietic cells (myeloproliferative disorder), and this event may be repeated a number of times during the evolution of the myeloproliferative disorder. Leukemia commences when a fully developed leukemic cell emerges and generates a dominant leukemic clone. Sequential events are dependent on continued stimulation by normal or abnormal levels of GM-CSF

The evidence just discussed implies that early in these diseases the granulopoietic populations often exhibit one or two abnormalities in culture whereas late in the disease immediately prior to leukemia development several abnormalities are demonstrable. This suggests the existence of at least three episodes of clonal succession in these patients as the disease develops (Fig. 33).

From the practical point of view, evidence of clonal progression as indicated by in vitro culture patterns in a patient with a myeloproliferative suggests the probable development of acute leukemia within the next 2–12 months. Conversely, failure to exhibit signs of progression can be regarded as a favorable sign, at least in terms of the unlikelihood of acute leukemia development.

From the biological point of view, experiments in both mice and cats have shown that various myeloproliferative disorders and acute leukemia can be initiated by probably the same RNA leukemia viruses [346, 347, 348]. While the evidence is still incomplete in humans, it is reasonable to postulate the existence of similar RNA viruses and the concept that these initiate the sequence of clonal succession of abnormal granulopoietic populations referred to above. If, as seems likely, infection by such viruses in man is transmitted vertically, the granulopoietic populations are already infected at birth, and it cannot be hoped to interrupt the sequence of changes leading to acute leukemia development simply by vaccination directed against the virus. There is, however, increasing evidence that viral infection, or transformation, of a hemopoietic population is not in itself sufficient to lead to the emergence of a leukemic clone [349]. Disturbances in regulator balance and the action of such regulators on viral-altered populations appear to be essential for the emergence of successively more and more abnormal hemopoietic clones. If this concept is correct, then regulatory factors are essential cofactors in the emergence and progressive proliferation of leukemic cells. On this basis, an alternative method for preventing or controlling acute leukemia becomes possible since the leukemic and preleukemic populations remain responsive to, and dependent on, GM-CSF, It may therefore become of some importance to devise methods for altering GM-CSF levels on a long-term basis.

The present type of studies on patients with myeloproliferative disorders have a number of potentially important applications: (1) they can document whether the above concept of clonal succession by progressively more abnormal granulopoietic populations accurately describes the situation during acute leukemia development, (2) it should be possible by parallel studies on the erythropoietic, eosinophilic and lymphoid populations to determine whether or not comparable sequential abnormalities occur in these related populations, and hence to determine to what degree the clonal abnormalities extend back into the stem cell compartment, and (3) the existence of abnormal regulator levels or abnormal regulators in myeloproliferative disorders can be sought for.

On the question of regulator abnormalities, negative correlations are of equal importance to positive findings. For example, if GM-CSF levels are rarely elevated in patients who do not progress to acute leukemia, indirect evidence is obtained that elevated GM-CSF levels may be of importance in forcing clonal progression in acute leukemia. Indeed, until convincing evidence is obtained that elevated GM-CSF levels are always present during the development of acute leukemia, there seems little justification for attempting therapeutic manipulations of regulator levels in such patients.

H. Summary

The complex and confusing group of interrelated myeloproliferative disorders have yet to be analyzed thoroughly in semisolid cultures. However, the data already available indicate that abnormalities in growth patterns are demonstrable in GM populations in such patients. These are commonly associated with elevations of serum and/or urine GM-CSF levels.

The abnormalities—depressed GM-CFC levels, abnormally light buoyant density of GM-CFCs, elevated cluster to colony ratios, abnormal cellular differentiation, and elevated GM-CSF levels—are qualitatively similar to the changes seen in AML.

As patients with myeloproliferative disorders progress to AML, GM populations exhibit more of the abnormalities seen in AML populations. This suggests a clonal succession of progressively more abnormal GM populations in these patients.

In general the culture data support the hypothesis that AML development is a multistage process occurring in the presence of, and probably dependent on, disturbance in regulator levels.

Chapter 8

Eosinophil Colony Formation

Eosinophil colony formation in vitro was first described by ISCOVE et al [53] and CHERVENICK and BOGGS [13] in cultures of human marrow and peripheral blood cells. These observations were confirmed and extended by several groups working with cultures of human marrow cells [86, 57, 75].

Formation of eosinophil colonies by mouse bone marrow cells had been observed in earlier work on mixed cultures of WEHI-3 myelomonocytic leukemic cells and mouse marrow cells [16], but at that time the cells comprising these curiously shaped colonies were not recognized as eosinophils. Subsequent studies by METCALF et al. [19] with highly active lymphocyte-conditioned media showed that these media had the capacity to stimulate the formation of eosinophil colonies in addition to neutrophil and macrophage colonies. As shall be discussed in Chapter 9, active conditioned media of this type usually also have the capacity to stimulate megakaryocyte colony formation.

A. Technical Aspects

The growth of human eosinophil colonies is stimulated by the same underlayers of human peripheral blood cells or medium conditioned by such cells as are active in stimulating GM-colony formation. More recently, human placental-conditioned medium has been shown to be effective in stimulating eosinophil colony formation [57]. Although the original description of eosinophil colonies was made in methylcellulose cultures, use of this suspending medium is not critical, and similar eosinophil colonies develop in agar cultures of human marrow cells.

Human eosinophil colony formation does, however, highlight one of the technical weaknesses in semisolid cultures—the difficulty in determining colony types solely on the basis of gross morphology. Human eosinophil colonies are small and tightly packed and cannot be distinguished in unstained cultures from myeloblast cultures which have a similar size and shape. To identify a colony as containing eosinophils, it is therefore necessary to pick it off and stain the smeared colony cells with Giemsa or other histochemical reagents. This can be done using methylcellulose cultures but is a slow and tedious process requiring care to ensure that a representative sample of colonies is examined. The sampling procedure does not really permit typing or enumeration of clusters or accurate estimates of the number of cells in individual colonies. The cumbersome nature of this typing procedure seems to have restricted studies on the frequency and nature of cells generating human eosinophil colonies since very few data have been published on the frequency of these cells in various disease states.

A method has now been developed for staining the entire culture dish with eosin (see Chapter 3). This procedure allows the enumeration of eosinophil colonies and clusters in the entire culture dish, and accurate cell counts can be perfomed on these. With somewhat more difficulty, neutrophil, monocyte, and macrophage colonies and clusters can also be enumerated. Again, the technique demands concentration and is slow, but it does allow a complete analysis of the culture dish free of any worry concerning sampling errors. This technique should now permit a wide range of investigations on eosinophil CFCs in various diseases.

For some curious reason the morphology of the one type of readily recognizable mouse eosinophil colony is almost the opposite of that of human eosinophil colonies. These mouse eosinophil colonies are characteristically large and loosely dispersed globular aggregates of cells which are relatively easy to identify and count in an unstained culture. While data on these mouse eosinophil colony-forming cells are therefore easier to gather than for corresponding human cells, some caution must be exercised in interpreting the data. Direct staining of mouse cultures is less satisfactory than for human cultures because of the less prominent granules in mouse eosinophils. Even so, these stained cultures have revealed the occurrence of small, tight colonies of eosinophils that cannot be distinguished from neutrophil colonies on the basis of their general shape. Therefore, the frequencies of eosinophil colony-forming cells in cultures of mouse cells established from counts on dispersed colonies are certain to be underestimates by a factor of at least two. The stained cultures also reveal the presence of eosinophil clusters in about the same ratio to colonies as is seen with neutrophil colonies and clusters. Future studies will need to document the frequency of the smaller eosinophil colonies and clusters. However, the present description will be based entirely on the large, loosely dispersed eosinophil colonies.

Cultures supporting the growth of mouse eosinophil colonies can be prepared using a single layer culture system and adding to the cultures 0.2 ml of medium conditioned by mouse spleen or lymph node cells. For the preparation of active conditioned media, $2-5 \times 10^6$ spleen or lymph node cells per ml are incubated in RPMI 1640 medium containing 5% heat inactivated human plasma for 7–14 days in the presence either of 0.05 ml of 1:15 dilution pokeweed mitogen per ml or 5×10^{-5}M 2-mercaptoethanol. The media are harvested, centrifuged free of cellular debris, and used without dialysis or heat inactivation. Such media will not maximally stimulate eosinophil colony formation, and for this purpose the media need to be concentrated by freeze-drying, ammonium sulphate precipitation, or dialysis against polyethylene glycol. It must be emphasized that this conditioned media also contains high concentrations of GM-CSF so the cultures develop large numbers of granulocytic and macrophage colonies which can make eosinophil colonies difficult to count if more than 75,000 bone marrow cells per ml are cultured. As shall be discussed in Chapter 9, this same media stimulates the formation of megakaryocyte colonies. Much also depends on the FCS used in the cultures, and not all sera supporting GM-colony formation necessarily support good eosinophil or megakaryocyte colony formation.

The enumeration of the large loose mouse eosinophil colonies depends on identifying their characteristic gross morphology. With a little experience, the loose eosinophil colonies are readily identifiable because of their large globular shape, uniformly dispersed cells, and the translucent appearance of the small cells making up the colonies.

B. Eosinophil Colony Formation in Cultures of Mouse Marrow

Although mouse eosinophil colonies vary in size as do all normal hemopoietic colonies, they are strikingly uniform in morphological appearance, being loose globular aggregates of remarkably uniformly dispersed cells with a pale translucence [19] (Fig. 34). Where cells abut

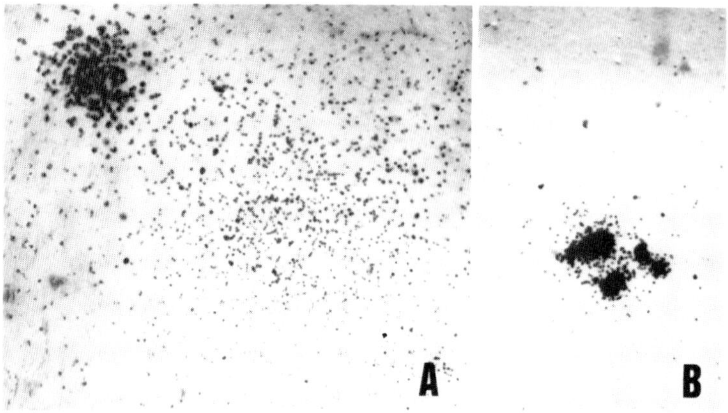

Fig. 34A and B. 7-day culture of mouse bone marrow cells stimulated by mouse lymphocyte-conditioned medium. Note in (A) a macrophage colony (upper left) and a large loose eosinophil colony, and in (B) a multicentric neutrophil colony. (From METCALF et al., [19]. Reproduced with permission from J. Cellular Physiology)

on the upper or lower surface of the agar, the cells disperse freely over this surface as a loose monolayer of unattached cells. The colony cells are intermediate in size between neutrophils and macrophages, and although appearing uniform, in fact vary considerably in size, most cells becoming smaller as differentiation proceeds.

Developing mouse eosinophil colonies first become identifiable with confidence at 4–5 days of incubation and increase in size progressively so that by 7 days the volume occupied is very large and scoring is quite easy. Eosinophil colonies frequently continue to enlarge progressively during the 2nd week of incubation and can develop into extremely large colonies of 5000 or more cells.

On cytological examination, all cells in the colony are found to contain the indistinct eosinophilic granules characteristic of mouse eosinophils [19], the nucleus either being ring-shaped or in a twisted figure eight (Fig. 35). As expected from the rapid growth of these colonies, mitotic activity is high and many cells in 7-day colonies are immature with basophilic cytoplasm. Examination of such cells from 7–11-day colonies in the electron-microscope has confirmed their identification as eosinophils. However, granule maturation appears to be incomplete, and the granules do not contain the characteristic central crystals seen in mature mouse eosinophils in vivo (METCALF, D. and MANDEL, T., unpublished data).

Analysis of mouse eosinophil colony cells has shown them to be nonphagocytic and nonadherent [74]. Indeed, these cells appear to be able to move relatively freely in the agar to produce the dispersed cloud of cells typical of an eosinophil colony. They are peculiarly easy to harvest since merely touching the surface of the agar over a colony causes the cells to gush upward through the disrupted gel, again suggesting that these cells are only loosely enmeshed in the agar gel and may even have liquified the surrounding gel.

Analysis of harvested mouse eosinophil colony cells has shown that most develop receptors for the Fc portion of IgG, but unlike colony neutrophils or macrophages, lack receptors for the C3 component of complement [74]. The cells also lack detectable membrane immunoglobulin (METCALF, D. and WARNER, N. L., unpublished data).

The complete absence of C3 receptors on colony eosinophils represents a useful functional assay confirming the morphological evidence that discrete eosinophil colonies never contain

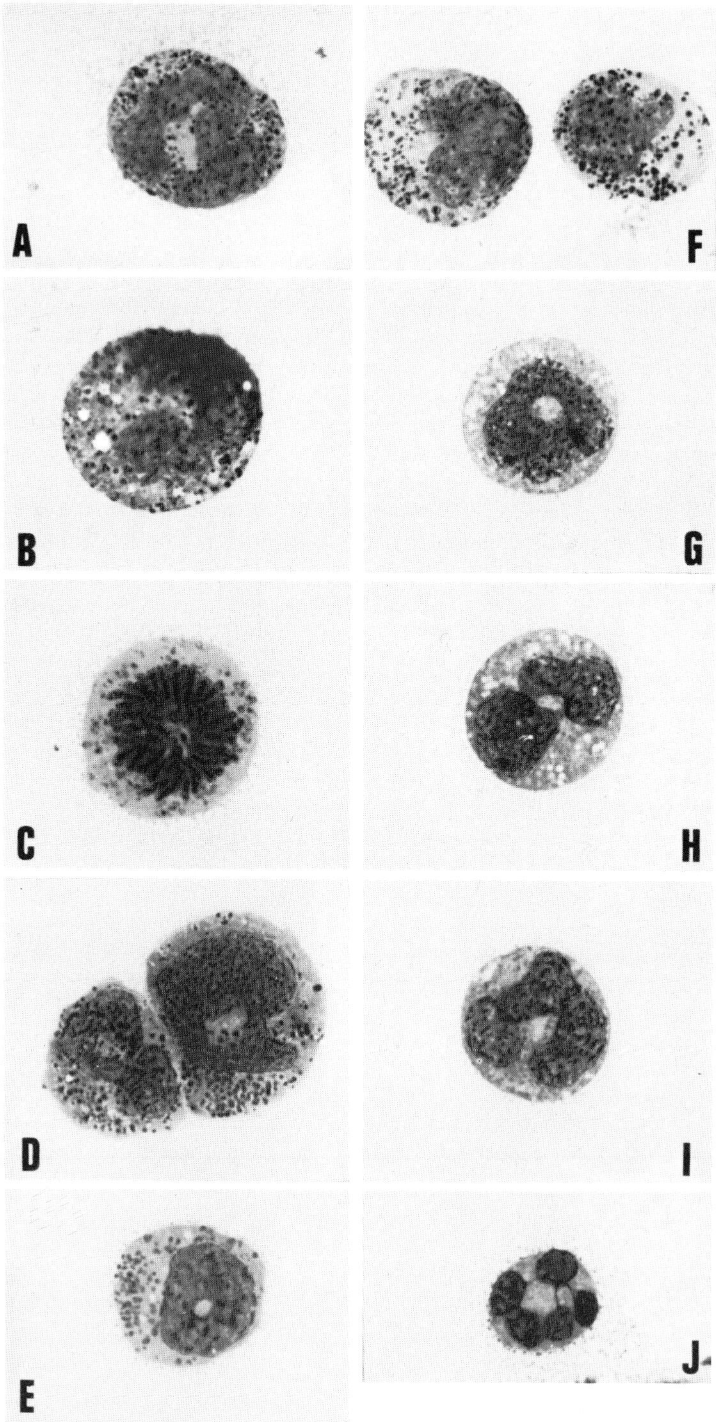

Fig. 35A–J. Giemsa-stained cells from eosinophil colonies grown from mouse bone marrow cells (A–F) and for comparison, comparable cells from neutrophil colonies (G–J). Note the eosinosinophil colony cells. (From METCALF et al., [19]. Reproduced with permission from J. Cellular Physiology)

second populations of neutrophils or macrophages. This is an important point that establishes eosinophil formation in the mouse as a clearly separate lineage distinct from either neutrophil or macrophage formation.

C. Eosinophil Colony Formation in Cultures of Human Marrow Cells

The proliferation of eosinophils in cultures of human marrow is significantly delayed in comparison with the growth of neutrophil and monocyte colonies. This appears to be a genuine delay rather than a uniformly slower growth rate since, once initiated, eosinophil colony growth rates appear to be similar to those of neutrophil and monocyte colonies. The reason for the initial delay can only be speculated upon at the present time.

As a consequence of this initial delay, if cultures are scored on day 7 of incubation, although eosinophil clusters are present, none of these is large enough to be scored as a colony. This situation changes radically at 10 to 14 days of incubation when the proportion of eosinophil colonies increases progressively to 20–30% of all colonies (DRESCH, C. and METCALF, D., unpublished data). A frequency of 50% of all colonies has been reported in cultures of human peripheral blood after 2–3 weeks of incubation [13].

Most eosinophil colonies remain compact aggregates of cells even though on the basis of granule size and density the cells are relatively mature. The ratio of eosinophil clusters to colonies at day 14 is approximately 5:1.

The most important point emerging from a careful analysis of marrow cultures from normal subjects and patients with various diseases is that eosinophils are *never* observed in neutrophil or monocyte colonies, and conversely, neutrophils and monocytes are never observed in eosinophil colonies. This is true even at the level of eosinophil clusters. The spectacular purity of eosinophil colonies is similar to that seen in mouse cultures and was confirmed in colony transfer studies by DAO (DAO, C., unpublished data). Early 2–3-day colonies were removed from cultures of human marrow cells by micromanipulation and transferred to fresh cultures containing conditioned medium or underlayers of peripheral blood cells but no other marrow cells. Such transferred colonies usually continued to increase in size and developed mature cells as incubation continued. No eosinophils were observed in transferred GM-colonies and vice versa.

These morphological data support the cell membrane marker studies on mouse eosinophil colonies and establish eosinophils as a lineage of hemopoietic cells quite separate from either neutrophils, monocytes, or macrophages.

The cells of human eosinophil colonies develop more prominent eosinophil granules than do mouse cells, but in the electronmicroscope, granule maturation appears to be incomplete, and the granules exhibit a low electron-dense core rather than the usual crystal [31, 86]. However, cytochemical analysis of human colony eosinophils using Luxol fast blue, eosin, and the Sakagauchi reaction for arginine has confirmed that the granules exhibit the typical properties of eosinophil granules [75].

D. Eosinophil Colony-Forming Cells (EO-CFC)

The relative frequency of EO-CFCs in the mouse marrow as assessed by dispersed colonies is distinctly lower than in the human, and EO-CFCs rarely total more than 10% of total colony-forming cells. However, as pointed out earlier, this frequency is artificially low, and the proportion of EO-CFCs relative to GM-CFCs could be as high as 20%, which would be comparable with the level in human marrow cultures.

EO-CFCs can be detected in the spleen and fetal liver, but the frequency is much lower than in the marrow [19]. EO-CFCs have also been demonstrated in spleen colonies from irradiated mice injected with hemopoietic stem cells, but again the frequency of such cells is low (METCALF, D. and JOHNSON, G. R., unpublished data). No studies have yet been reported on the frequency of these cells in conditions associated with eosinophilia, e.g., worm infestations.

In view of the report [350] that eosinophil formation in vivo is dependent on products released from activated lymphocytes, it is of interest that normal frequencies of EO-CFCs were observed in the marrow of nu/nu (congenitally athymic) mice, and the generation of EO-CFCs does not appear to be dependent on normal levels of T-lymphocytes [19]. No major age or strain-related variations were observed in EO-CFC levels in mice. Similarly, no changes in EO-CFC levels were observed following the injection of Freund's adjuvant, following whole body irradiation or in mice bearing a variety of transplanted tumors (19, METCALF, D., unpublished data).

In velocity sedimentation separation studies on C_{57}BL marrow cells, EO-CFCs segregated as a single peak (peak sedimentation velocity 4.0 mm/h), and the profile of EO-CFCs was significantly displaced to the more slowly sedimenting (smaller cells) fractions in comparison with GM-CFCs [19]. Although no information is available on the density of EO-CFCs, the data suggest that, on average, EO-CFCs may be slightly smaller in size than GM-CFCs.

Only limited studies have been performed on the frequency of EO-CFCs in human marrow suspensions. In cultures of marrow cells from patients with no significant hemopoietic disease, the mean frequency of EO-CFCs was approximately 20% of all colony-forming cells (i.e., at day 14, 8 ± 7 EO-CFCs/10^5 cells, DRESCH, C., unpublished data).

At day 14, eosinophil colonies and clusters formed about one-third of all colonies and clusters in cultures stimulated by human placental-conditioned medium. In six patients with untreated AML or AML in relapse, EO-CFCs were absent although eosinophil clusters were present. This is a potentially interesting situation. The suppression of EO-CFCs is similar to that seen with normal GM-CFCs. However, the presence of eosinophil clusters raises the possibility that eosinophils may be members of the leukemic clone in AML. In this context, eosinophil colonies and clusters have been observed in cultures of light density fractions from blood and bone marrow of patients with CML (METCALF, D. and DRESCH, C., unpublished data) suggesting that at least some of these cells are of abnormally light buoyant density and are possibly members of the abnormal light density leukemic clone.

In AML patients in remission, the relative frequency of EO-CFCs and cluster-forming cells was abnormally high in three of four patients analyzed. One other disease in which levels of EO-CFCs and cluster-forming cells were observed to be abnormally high was idiopathic thrombocytopenic purpura and this requires further investigation.

The report by CHERVENICK and BOGGS [13] of a 50% frequency of EO-CFCs in cultures of peripheral blood raises the possibility that these cells may be relatively more frequent in the blood than in the bone marrow, but this needs checking in parallel cultures of peripheral blood and marrow from individual subjects.

E. Eosinophil Colony-Stimulating Factor (EO-CSF)

Although the low frequency of eosinophil colonies has made quantitative studies on EO-CSF difficult, there is a clear reduction in colony numbers and size as progressively lower concentrations of lymphocyte-conditioned media are used to stimulate colony formation [19]. A similar effect has been seen in human marrow cultures stimulated by progressively lower concentrations of placental-conditioned medium.

As is true of granulocyte and macrophage colony formation, the special eosinophilic stimulating factor in lymphocyte-conditioned medium must be present continuously for eosinophil colony survival and progressive growth. Transfer of developing eosinophil colonies to cultures lacking any type of CSF or to cultures containing only GM-CSF leads to cessation of colony growth and death of all colony cells within 1–4 days [19]. These studies indicate that the special factor cannot be replaced by GM-CSF even when colony formation is well advanced. Since the type of lymphocyte-conditioned media used also contains high concentrations of GM-CSF, it can also be concluded that because eosinophil colonies remain pure populations, the colony cells must be incapable of differentiation into either the neutrophil or macrophage pathways, even when bathed in effective concentrations of GM-CSF.

Evidence of the separate nature of EO-CSF was obtained from electrophoretic separation of lymphocyte-conditioned medium. Unlike GM-CSF which has an α or α-postalbumin mobility, the active factor stimulating eosinophil colony formation remained localized close to the origin in starch gel electrophoresis [19]. EO-CSF has been shown to be heat labile and nondialyzable, with an apparent mol wt of approximately 50,000 on Sephadex G-200 filtration. However, this factor has yet to be obtained in highly purified form.

Further evidence of the difference between EO-CSF and GM-CSF was obtained from an analysis of the action of a rabbit antiserum prepared against mouse lung-conditioned medium GM-CSF on colony formation stimulated by crude lymphocyte-conditioned media. This antiserum caused a selective suppression of macrophage and granulocyte colony formation but had little effect on eosinophil colony formation [19]. Conversely, the factor in normal mouse or human serum that strongly potentiates granulocyte and macrophage colony formation by mouse marrow cells had no apparent potentiating effect on eosinophil colony formation although alterations in the morphology of eosinophil colonies might have occurred and made it impossible to identify the colonies [48].

The ability of lymphocytes stimulated by pokeweed mitogen or mercaptoethanol to release a factor stimulating eosinophil colony formation is of considerable interest in view of the demonstration that eosinophil production in vivo also appeared to be dependent on a factor released by activated lymphocytes [350].

Ruscetti et al. [211] observed that addition of *Trichinella* antigen to *Trichinella*-sensitized mouse lymphocytes increased the resulting level of GM-CSF in the conditioned medium. Although they were unable to identify eosinophilic colonies, such conditioned media stimulated an increased production of eosinophils in liquid cultures of mouse marrow cells. Similar results were obtained following the addition of PPD to cells from BCG-infected mice.

These experiments strongly suggest that the phenomenon observed in vitro is probably of physiological significance in vivo.

Although many mouse tissues contain GM-CSF and many such as bone, lung, heart, and kidney can produce high concentrations of GM-CSF in vitro, careful tests of such conditioned media have failed to detect any eosinophil colony-stimulating activity, even

Table 20. Capacity of various $C_{57}BL$ tissues to produce GM-CSF and the factors stimulating eosinophil and megakaryocyte colony formation[a]

Tissue used to condition medium[b]	Mean No. of colonies stimulated[c]		
	Neutrophil and/or macrophage	Eosinophil	Megakaryocyte
Spleen cells	48	12	3
	136	20	6
Spleen cells + irradiated DBA spleen cells	136	24	9
	96	20	8
Lymph node cells	44	6	0
	35	2	0
Lymph node cells + irradiated DBA spleen cells	300	20	8
	172	48	9
Thymus cells	0	0	0
	0	0	0
Thymus cells + irradiated DBA spleen cells	43	4	3
	96	16	5
Peritoneal cells	21	0	0
	18	0	0
Peritoneal cells + irradiated DBA spleen cells	82	0	0
	70	0	1
Pleural cells	11	0	0
Marrow cells	1	0	0
	1	0	0
Femur shaft cells	36	0	0
	52	0	0
Lung	124	0	0
	116	0	0
Heart	96	0	0
	176	0	0
Kidney	24	0	0
	12	0	0

[a] Data from METCALF et al. [20].
[b] All cultures contained 50μ M mercaptoethanol and were incubated for 7 days. Cells were cultured at concentrations of 5×10^6/4 ml of culture; minced tissues were 1 lung, 1 heart, 1 kidney, or 1 femur per 4 ml of culture medium.
[c] Calculated number of colonies stimulated by 0.2 ml of medium in cultures of 75,000 $C_{57}BL$ marrow cells.

following the addition of pokeweed mitogen or mercaptoethanol during the conditioning period [19, 20] (Table 20). The only exception to this has been the capacity of WEHI-3 myelomonocytic leukemic cells to produce low levels of EO-CSF [19].

While mouse spleen and lymph node cells are good sources of EO-CSF in cultures containing pokeweed mitogen or 2-mercaptoethanol, thymus cells do not produce the factor unless

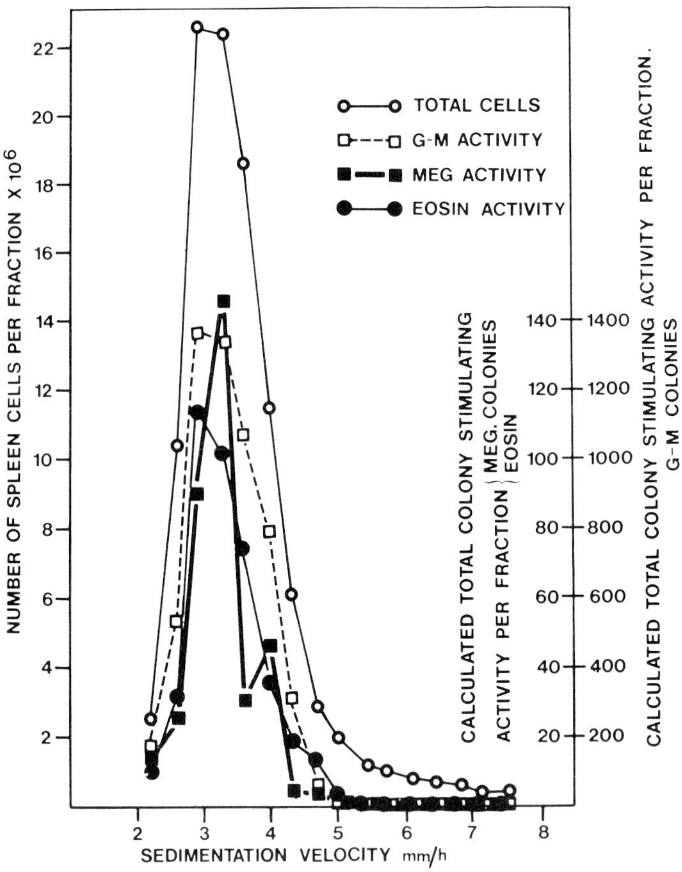

Fig. 36. Velocity sedimentation separation of mouse spleen cells showing distribution of cells which, on cocultivation with irradiated allogeneic cells, produced the factors stimulating neutrophil and macrophage (GM), eosinophil (EOSIN) and megakaryocyte (MEG) colony formation by C_{57}BL mouse marrow cells. Also shown is distribution of nucleated cells in original fractionation. Equal numbers of cells cultured from each fraction. Colony-stimulating activity calculated as total activity per fraction. (From METCALF et al., [20]. Reproduced with permission from Proc. Nat. Acad. Sci. U.S.A.)

subjected to the double mitogenic stimulus of mixed leucocyte cultures with irradiated allogeneic cells [19, 20]. Since preirradiation of the lymphocyte suspensions inhibits their capacity to produce EO-CSF it is probable that, as in the case of GM-CSF production, at least blast transformation is a prerequisite for factor production although actual cell proliferation may not be necessary [20]. It is of some interest that mouse lymphoid leukemic cells can often produce high concentrations of GM-CSF after culture with pokeweed mitogen but appear not to be able to produce EO-CSF [19], and this might be a useful functional marker to apply in studies on the nature of the intrinsic abnormalities in lymphoid leukemic cells.

Studies on spleen cells separated by velocity sedimentation have indicated that most EO-CSF is produced by small lymphocytes as is true also for GM-CSF production [20] (Fig. 36). The interesting problem raised by these observations is whether subpopulations of small lymphocytes exist with the specific capacity after appropriate stimulation to produce EO-CSF whereas other populations produce GM-CSF. Until more sophisticated methods are developed for separating subpopulations of lymphocytes, this intriguing question can only be speculated upon.

Unfractionated human placental-conditioned medium is capable of stimulating both GM and eosinophil colony formation by human marrow cells but only GM-colony formation by mouse bone marrow cells. Both GM and eosinophil colony-stimulating activities for human cells have remained associated after a series of sequential separative procedures, and both have an approximate mol wt of 30,000 (METCALF, D., BURGESS, A. W., DRESCH, C., unpublished data). It remains to be determined whether further separative procedures will be successful in separating these two biological activities or whether they reside in a single molecule.

Despite careful searching, EO-CSF has not been detected in postendotoxin mouse serum or the serum from other types of mice. However, this result needs to be accepted with some caution as the addition of many sera seem to inhibit eosinophil colony formation and the presence of EO-CSF may be being masked by inhibitors.

F. Comment

The eosinophil colony technique has not really been exploited to its full extent at the present time. Technically, work with human eosinophil colonies is difficult, and while work with mouse eosinophil colonies presents fewer problems, not all eosinophil colonies are able to be scored by direct counting.

EO-CSF appears to be separable from GM-CSF, and eosinophil colony formation provides dramatic proof both of the clonality of colonies and the genetic preprogramming that rigidly determines the pathway of differentiation followed by clones of hemopoietic cells. Production of GM-CSF, EO-CSF, and MEG-CSF by activated lymphocytes offers many exciting possibilities for analysis either by separation of subpopulations of lymphocytes or by selective activation of individual cells to produce one or more specific regulatory factors. At the present level of technology, it is difficult to explore this phenomenon more deeply, but the development of fluorescein and rhodamine-conjugated specific antisera to the various CSFs would make such studies technically feasible.

In general, the pattern of eosinophil formation as demonstrated by colony formation in vitro is remarkably similar to that shown by neutrophil and macrophage populations. The progenitor cells for both appear to be distinct, but future studies assisted by in vitro cloning should be able to determine what interrelationships exist between these populations in the stem cell to progenitor cell stage.

Chapter 9

Megakaryocyte Colony Formation

The literature on this subject is small, but the technique for obtaining megakaryocyte colony formation in vitro appears to offer exciting possibilities for future studies on the formation of normal and abnormal megakaryocytes. So far, only mouse megakaryocyte colonies have been successfully cultured in vitro, and the technique has yet to be adapted to the culture of human cells.

A. Culture Technique

In an early study, PORTER and GENGOZIAN [351] described the development of megakaryocyte-like cells in liquid cultures of marmoset cells. NAKEFF et al. [352] noted the development of megakaryocytes in cells mass-harvested from agar cultures of marrow cells from mice pretreated with vinblastine and cultured over underlayers of mouse embryo fibroblasts. In an addendum to this report, the occurrence of small colonies of megakaryocytes was described in such cultures. Although this study provided useful information on the nature of these cells, it is likely that the stimulating system used was not sufficiently strong to obtain good megakaryocyte colony formation.

METCALF et al. [20] reported the growth of megakaryocyte colonies in single layer agar cultures of normal mouse bone marrow cells. The medium used was the standard formula described in Chapter 3, and the stimulus for colony formation was provided by inclusion in the cultures of 0.2 ml of medium harvested from liquid suspension cultures of mouse spleen lymphocytes. Although many mitogens can provoke GM-CSF production in suspension cultures of mouse lymphocytes, only two agents—pokeweed mitogen or 2-mercaptoethanol—were found also to stimulate the formation of the special factors required for eosinophil and megakaryocyte formation.

As was true for the production of EO-CSF, the production of megakaryocyte CSF (MEG-CSF) is strongly dependent on the batch of serum used. In some studies, RPMI-1640 medium appeared to be superior to Dulbecco's modified Eagle's medium, but this was not a consistent finding. Suspensions of 2–5 $\times$ 10^6 spleen lymphocytes per ml are cultured in flasks or tubes in RPMI-1640 medium containing 5% heat inactivated human plasma. Mitogenic stimulation is supplied by the addition of 0.05 ml of freshly prepared 1:15 dilution pokeweed mitogen per ml (Difco) or sufficient 2-mercaptoethanol to produce a 5×10^{-5}M concentration. Colony-stimulating activity rises slowly in the medium harvested from such cultures and is maximal between 7–14 days of incubation. In most studies, untreated medium has been used without subsequent dialysis or heat inactivation. Even with a good batch of conditioned medium, megakaryocyte colony-stimulating activity is not sufficient to stimulate maximum levels of colony formation, and for this purpose the medium can be concentrated further by Amicon PM-10 filtration or freeze-drying with dialysis.

An outstanding association has been observed in such conditioned medium between the capacity to stimulate eosinophil and megakaryocyte colony formation [20]. All conditioned media capable of stimulating megakaryocyte formation also have the capacity to stimulate eosinophil colony formation, levels of the latter activity usually being relatively higher. The possible significance of this association will be discussed later.

Mixed leukocyte cultures of spleen lymphocytes from allogeneic mouse strains also have the capacity to produce EO-CSF and MEG-CSF but only in the presence of 2-mercaptoethanol, and levels of activity are usually not significantly higher than those achieved by the use of mercaptoethanol in syngeneic cultures [20].

The biggest practical problem encountered in working with megakaryocyte colonies has been the overcrowding of such cultures by other colonies due to the presence of GM-CSF and EO-CSF in the crude lymphocyte-conditioned medium. Scoring of such colonies is slow and tedious work, and not all observers appear to be capable of the concentration required to work for long periods analyzing such cultures. An alternative solution to this problem has recently been described [353]. Marrow cultures are prepared in 0.1 ml plasma gel cultures in microwell cultures. After culture, intact gels are stained for acetylcholinesterase, before scoring megakaryocytic clusters and colonies.

This appears to be an equally tedious method, and in the long term, the best solution to this problem is probably to attempt chemical fractionation of the conditioned medium to eliminate GM-CSF, and hopefully EO-CSF, thus producing a reagent with monospecific growth-stimulating activity.

B. Megakaryocyte Colonies in vitro

Two types of megakaryocyte colony have been observed to develop in cultures of mouse bone marrow cells: (1) small loose aggregates of up to 40 very large cells, all of which are identifiable as megakaryocytes, and (2) loose colonies of up to 120 large cells, often with a tight central region and containing in addition a mixed population of cells of varying sizes (Fig. 37). Only the largest of these cells are clearly identifiable as megakaryocytes, the smaller cells having round or indented nuclei and looking similar to early granulocytic cells. Pure aggregates outnumber mixed aggregates by 2:1 [20]. The smaller cells in these mixed colonies are commonly polyploid [20], and on the basis of their acetylcholinesterase content [353, 20], appear to be early megakaryocytes.

In strongly stimulated cultures, individual megakaryocytes are recognizable with some confidence in unstained cultures under the dissection microscope because of their very large size, characteristic smoothly undulating cytoplasmic edge, and the prominent bulge overlying the nucleus. Frequently, in agar cultures, these cells are surrounded by a faint halo of opaque material which may be platelets although this has not yet been documented by electron-microscopy. Platelet release by megakaryocytes grown in plasma gel cultures has been demonstrated by McLeod et al. [88] who grew megakaryocyte colonies from mouse marrow cells. In such cultures, platelets were clearly visible in the gel surrounding the megakaryocytes. The few megakaryocytes in the original cultured bone marrow population disintegrate in the first 1–2 days of culture and developing megakaryocyte colonies first become visible at 3–4 days of incubation [20, 353]. Cell size at this time is not as large as in fully developed colonies. Colony growth is progressive until 7 days, after which megakaryocytes usually disintegrate. Because of these growth characteristics, colony counts are performed routinely at 7 days of incubation, scoring all aggregates of three or more cells as colonies. Since such

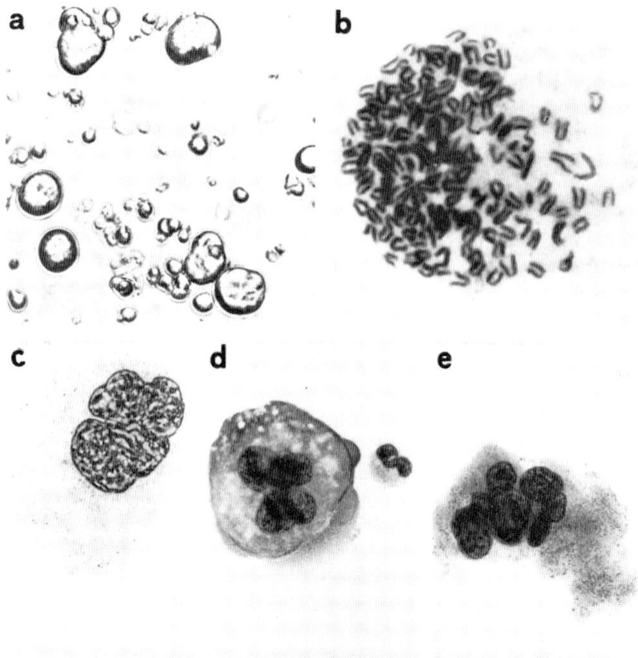

Fig. 37a–e. Cells from megakaryocyte colonies grown in agar from mouse bone marrow cells. (a) Portion of a mixed colony in situ containing megakaryocytes and smaller cells (phase contrast); (b) a polyploid mitosis (chromosome number approximately 160), (c), (d), (e) three different maturation stages of colony megakaryocytes. Note neutrophil in (d) for size comparison (Leishmann). (From METCALF et al., [20]. Reproduced with permission from Proc. Nat. Acad. Sci. U.S.A.)

colonies are almost invariably loosely dispersed, care needs to be taken in counting all colony cells.

In suboptimal cultures, cell size is often smaller, and because all preparations of lymphocyte-conditioned medium contain GM-CSF, the cultures contain many macrophage clusters which sometimes can be confused with small megakaryocyte colonies. It is necessary therefore in scoring these cultures to pick off all aggregates which might possibly be megakaryocyte colonies and perform the final definitive colony count on stained preparations of these, a tedious procedure limiting the number of cultures which can be processed.

In Giemsa-stained preparations, megakaryocyte colony cells are 60–80 microns in diameter with the large multilobulated nucleus characteristic of megakaryocytes (Fig. 37). The cytoplasm is often basophilic, and fully mature cells with the morphology of platelet-shedding megakaryocytes are rarely seen in agar cultures (354, METCALF, D., unpublished data).Better maturation of megakaryocytes can be obtained if heat inactivated human serum or plasma is substituted for the FCS in the culture medium (METCALF, D., unpublished data). The cells are not phagocytic and differ from large macrophages in being nonadherent when in contact with the bottom of the culture dish. The cytoplasm of the megakaryocytic colony cells is rich in acetylcholinesterase, a characteristic of megakaryocytes [20, 353]. While mitotic activity is uncommon after day 5 of incubation, an analysis of metaphase preparations has shown that dividing cells are polyploid (Fig. 37). Furthermore, analysis by microspectrophotometry [20]

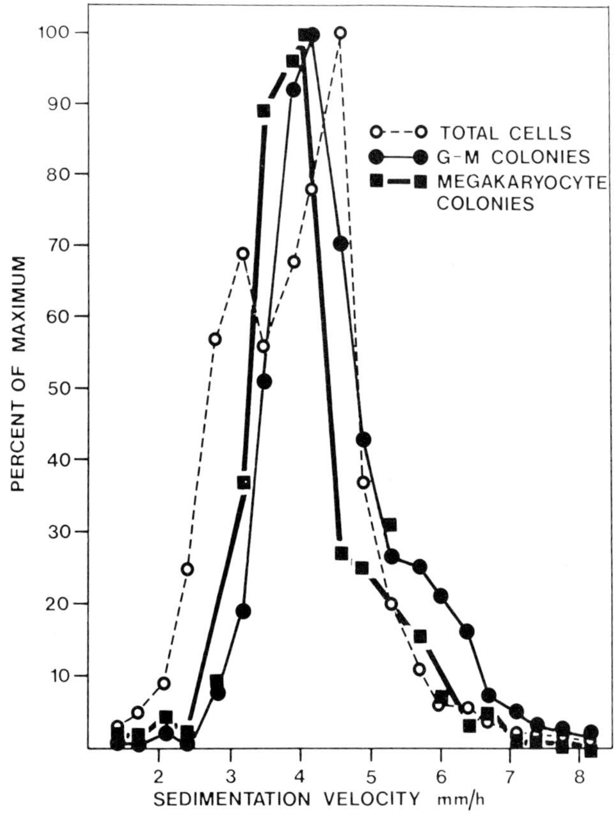

Fig. 38. Velocity sedimentation separation of C_{57}BL mouse marrow cells showing distribution of cells forming megakaryocyte and GM-colonies, and profile of total nucleated cells in various fractions. (From METCALF et al., [20]. Reproduced with permission from Proc. Nat. Acad. Sci. U.S.A.)

of individual Feulgen-stained colony cells from mixed and pure colonies showed that cellular DNA values varied from 4 N to 32 N, with a distribution similar to that observed in megakaryocytes in vivo.

The megakaryocytic nature of these cells has been confirmed by the use of fluorescein-conjugated antitelet antiplatelet with which the cytoplasm of the colony cells shows an intense fluorescence [352]. In the electronmicroscope, the cytoplasmic morphology of colony cells places them clearly in the megakaryocyte class although fully matured particle-containing intracytoplasmic platelets are rare in agar cultures of the above type (352, METCALF, D. and ODARTCHENKO, N., unpublished data). Subsequent studies by MCLEOD et al. [88] using plasma gel cultures and anemic sheep plasma (Stage III erythropoietin) showed that the megakaryocytes developing in these cultures exhibited full cytoplasmic maturation with extensive platelet formation. It has yet to be determined whether this more complete maturation is due to the plasma gel or some component in the crude erythropoietin preparation used.

Although maturation is reasonably uniform in the smaller pure colonies, maturation is markedly asynchronous in the mixed colonies. It is possible that in mixed colonies the full developmental sequence from the small megakaryocytic colony-forming cells (see later) to mature megakaryocytes is being observed. By analogy with granulocytic and macrophage colonies, the smaller and more frequent pure megakaryocytic colonies may be clusters formed by the progeny of megakaryocytic colony-forming cells. Being derived from relatively mature cells, such progeny would be likely to be relatively uniform.

Because work on megakaryocyte colony formation has been relatively recent, it is uncertain whether the present maximum size achieved (up to 120 cells) is the maximum possible size attainable by such colonies. However, even this colony size compares favorably with the quite small size of megakaryocytic colonies generated by stem cells in the spleens of irradiated mice, which suggests that the largest colonies grown in vitro may indeed be approaching the true clonal size limit for megakaryocytic proliferation.

There is some evidence that in crowded cultures colonies achieve a larger average size than in less crowded cultures, the mechanism of this autopotentiation being unknown [20].

With the demonstration that megakaryocyte colony formation can be stimulated by lymphocyte-conditioned medium and supported successfully by the culture medium being used, the invariable absence of these distinctive cells from various colonies permits certain deductions regarding the nature of the cells forming these latter colonies. Since megakaryocytes have never been observed in uncrowded cultures of adult mouse bone marrow in granulocytic, multiple granulocytic, macrophage, or eosinophilic colonies growing in the same culture dish in response to stimulation by the lymphocyte-conditioned medium, it can be concluded that the vast majority of the cells generating these colonies are probably not multipotential, i.e., are not stem cells.

C. Megakaryocyte Colony-Forming Cells (MEG-CFC)

Megakaryocyte colony formation shows an approximately linear relationship between the number of cells cultured and the number of colonies developing [20, 353]. Because only a few widely separated colonies develop in any one culture dish, it is a reasonable assumption that the colonies are clones derived from single colony-forming cells.

In the adult mouse marrow, the frequency of MEG-CFCs appears to be 10–$20/10^5$ cells [20, 353, 88], and in this laboratory, no major strain or age differences have been observed in the frequency of these cells. However, NAKEFF [355] has reported relatively high frequencies of MEG-CFCs in BALB/c and AKR mice. MEG-CFCs have also been detected in the spleen although the frequency is lower than in the marrow—1–$5/10^6$ cells. Exceptions are the spleen of SJL and NZB mice which on aging can develop MEG-CFC levels approaching those in the bone marrow. MEG-CFCs are not present in the lymph nodes, thymus, peritoneal, or pleural populations. As might be anticipated, MEG-CFCs are demonstrable in some spleen colonies generated by marrow CFUs in irradiated recipients and in the liver, spleen and marrow of fetal mice (METCALF, D. and JOHNSON, G., unpublished data).

The most informative technique applied to the analysis of MEG-CFCs has been velocity sedimentation separation. With this procedure, the large megakaryocytes in bone marrow sediment extremely rapidly and have been shown to be incapable themselves of colony formation [20]. MEG-CFCs were found to segregate as a single peak (peak sedimentation velocity 4.2 mm/h) and an average sedimentation rate slightly slower than that of GM-CFCs (Fig. 38). MEG-CFCs in discontinuous albumin gradients segregated as a single peak of density 1.075 g/cm^3 [355]. These data make it probable that the cells forming megakaryocytic

colonies are of relatively small size, similar to those forming neutrophilic, macrophage, and eosinophil colonies. This confirms the indirect data from labeling studies in vivo which indicated that megakaryocytic precursor cells are relatively small, inconspicuous cells (see review by EBBE, 356).
The injection of rabbit antimouse platelet serum to mice was reported to increase the frequency of MEG-CFCs in the bone marrow three to fourfold within 2 h, an effect which was no longer observable after 24 h [355].

D. Megakaryocyte Colony-Stimulating Factor (MEG-CSF)

From the above description, the reader familiar with experimental hematology will detect an apparent dichotomy between work performed in vitro and in vivo on the control of megakaryocyte and platelet formation.
There is an extensive literature on a serum factor, thrombopoietin, levels of which are elevated by prebleeding and which on injection in vivo stimulates megakaryocyte formation and the appearance in the blood of increased levels of platelets. Using other assay procedures, it is possible to demonstrate increased uptake of radioisotopic selenium into developing megakaryocytes [357, 358]. Some evidence has been produced that thrombopoietin is a polypeptide, but its site of production in the body is unknown.
Studies on the effects of human serum in mice have been less extensive, but there have been reports that the injection of serum from thrombocytopenic patients elevates platelet levels in mice. One implication from this work is that human thrombopoietin may be active on mouse target cells.
How can this background of in vivo data on thrombopoietin be fitted into what has so far been demonstrated regarding the control of megakaryocyte production in vitro? In an attempt to link the two areas, NAKEFF [355] explored the effects of thrombocytopenic mouse serum (produced by the injection of platelet antiserum) on megakaryocyte formation in vitro. Addition of such serum was found to double the number of megakaryocyte colonies developing whereas serum from mice injected with normal rabbit serum was inhibitory.
From studies in this laboratory, only mitogen-activated lymphocytes and unstimulated WEHI-3 myelomonocytic leukemic cells have the capacity to produce the specific factor MEG-CSF required to stimulate colony proliferation in vitro. Presumably, embryonic fibroblasts also have the capacity to produce low levels of MEG-CSF. Careful analysis of CSF-containing preparations extractable from all mouse organs have failed to detect the presence of MEG-CSF. Cultured marrow cells, bone shaft, heart, lung, kidney, fibroblasts, and salivary gland, while producing high levels of GM-CSF, appeared to produce no MEG-CSF [20].
Serum from normal mice of many different strains and ages and from mice following splenectomy, irradiation, bleeding, tumor transplantation, or the injection of cytotoxic drugs have all failed to stimulate megakaryocyte formation (METCALF, D., unpublished data). Since megakaryocyte formation normally occurs within the marrow and good evidence exists for a significant local production of GM-CSF within the marrow, the possible production of MEG-CSF by marrow stromal cells has been studied with particular emphasis. However, to date, no MEG-CSF has been detected in highly concentrated media harvested from cultured marrow or bone stromal cells [20].

Table 21. Potentiating activity of unheated human serum on colony formation stimulated by mouse lymphocyte-conditioned medium[a]

Serum used in medium	Mean No. of colonies[b]		
	Neutrophil/macrophage	Eosinophil	Megakaryocyte
FCS	20	2	2
Normal human serum 1	0	0	0
2	0	0	0
3	3	0	3
4	16	2	4
5	3	1	4
6	0	0	0
7	4	0	1
8	72	10	15
9	0	0	0
10	77	4	15
11	0	0	0
12	0	0	0
Histiocytic lymphoma	82	3	12
Lymphocytic lymphoma	0	0	0
Histiocytic lymphoma	34	1	11
Pancytopenia	4	0	6
Iron deficiency anemia	31	2	7
Iron deficiency anemia	1	0	0
Lymphocytic lymphoma	0	0	0
Histiocytic lymphoma	0	0	0
Hodgkin's disease	3	0	6
Aplastic anemia	55	6	11
AML	2	0	6
AML	0	0	0

[a] All cultures contained 20% serum (either FCS or unheated test human serum) and 75,000 $C_{57}BL$ marrow cells. Colony formation was stimulated by 0.2 ml of conditioned medium from $C_{57}BL$ spleen cells cultured with pokeweed mitogen.
[b] Mean number of colonies from duplicate cultures.

It has been reported [353] that small megakaryocyte colonies of up to 12 cells can be stimulated to develop in plasma gel cultures not only by medium conditioned by pokeweed mitogen-stimulated mouse spleen cells but also by PHA-stimulated lymphocyte-conditioned medium and L-cell-conditioned medium. These plasma gel cultures contained much higher cell concentrations (1×10^6 cells/ml) than used in agar cultures, and it is possible that in plasma gel cultures marrow cells may be able to produce a factor stimulating a low level of proliferative activity.

In view of the reports that human thrombopoietin is active on injection into mice, particular attention has also been paid to the effects of the addition of 0.1 ml of human serum or plasma to cultures of mouse marrow cells. To date, the effects on mouse marrow cultures of more than 4000 sera from patients with all major types of hemopoietic disturbance have been analyzed, but megakaryocyte colony formation has never been observed. Many of these sera can be presumed to have contained thrombopoietin detectable by the in vivo assays.

This negative data would imply that these human sera or plasmas contained no megakaryocyte-stimulating material detectable in agar cultures.

A quite different phenomenon has been encountered in observing the effects of substituting human serum for the FCS in cultures of mouse bone marrow cells that contain lymphocyte-conditioned medium. In the data from one such experiment shown in Table 21, it is clear that some human sera strongly potentiated megakaryocyte colony formation. On analysis, the following characteristics were observed: (1) the sera had no capacity to stimulate megakaryocytic colony formation in the absence of lymphocyte-conditioned medium, (2) colony size as well as colony numbers were increased, and colony megakaryocytes frequently exhibited an unusual degree of maturation, (3) no correlation existed between disease state and serum activity, many normal sera exhibiting high activity, (4) almost all sera developed potentiating activity after heating to 56°C for 30 min, and (5) potentiating activity for megakaryocyte colony formation correlated strongly with potentiating activity for neutrophil and macrophage colony formation in the same culture dishes but in parallel cultures did not correlate with the capacity to stimulate B-lymphocyte colony formation (Table 22).

The significance of this potentiation by human serum is obscure at present, but the phenomenon is a useful practical maneuver for obtaining good megakaryocyte colony formation.

Clearly, there are difficulties in linking thrombopoietin with MEG-CSF which will only be resolved by further work. To speculate at this early stage, one of a number of possibilities may account for the inconsistencies:

1. Megakaryocyte proliferation in the artificial conditions obtaining in vitro may depend on a factor (MEG-CSF) which is of no relevance in vivo and is therefore undetectable in vivo.

Table 22. Correlation in individual human sera between potentiating activity for megakaryocyte, GM, and B-lymphocyte colony formation by mouse cells

	No. of sera	
	Potentiating megakaryocyte colony formation	Not active on megakaryocyte colony formation
Sera potentiating GM-colony formation	29	5
Sera not active on GM-colony formation	43	106

$\chi^2 = 34.6$. Megakaryocyte potentiating activity strongly correlates with GM-potentiating activity ($P < 0.01$)

	No. of sera	
	Potentiating megakaryocyte colony formation	Not active on megakaryocyte colony formation
Sera potentiating B-lymphocyte colony formation	22	23
Sera not active on B-lymphocyte colony formation	39	57

$\chi^2 = 1.8$. No significant correlation between megakaryocyte potentiating activity and B-lymphocyte potentiating activity.

2. Megakaryocyte colony formation may be able to be stimulated by thrombopoietin, but the colony forming system may be very insensitive and not able to detect circulating levels of this regulator. (From what is known of the responsiveness of other colony types in vitro, this seems improbable.)
3. A likely possibility is that some other component in serum may interfere with the action in vitro of thrombopoietin and prevent its detection.
4. It may be that thrombopoietin is not a direct stimulus of megakaryocyte proliferation but either acts indirectly via some other cell population or may need to be metabolically modified before becoming an effective stimulus.

At the present time, little purpose is served by these speculations, and the only experimental approach open is to characterize the MEG-CSF which can be produced and detected in vitro. Spleen and lymph node cells appear to be equally effective in producing MEG-CSF. No activity was detectable in media harvested from thymic lymphocytes cultured with 2-mercaptoethanol but was produced if thymic cells were cocultivated with irradiated allogeneic spleen cells in the presence of mercaptoethanol (20). Irradiated spleen cells cultured with mercaptoethanol did not produce MEG-CSF. The results are in agreement with the fact that 2-mercaptoethanol acts as a T cell mitogen if T-lymphocytes are stimulated by allogeneic antigens [359] and implies that blast cell transformation and/or proliferation are essential steps preceding the production or release of MEG-CSF.

When spleen populations were fractionated by velocity sedimentation separation prior to culture with mercaptoethanol in the presence of allogeneic irradiated cells, the major portion of MEG-CSF obtained was produced by cells with the slow sedimentation velocity of small lymphocytes [20] (Fig. 36). These same cell fractions also produced most of the detectable EO-CSF and GM-CSF. These observations have raised two interesting alternatives:

1. Do all small lymphocytes have the capacity to make all three regulatory factors, and if so, do they produce these simultaneously? or
2. Are there subpopulations of small lymphocytes each of which is capable of producing only one factor, the various subpopulations all being activated by mercaptoethanol or pokeweed mitogen?

Little work has been performed to characterize the nature of MEG-CSF. Preliminary studies have shown that the active factor is nondialyzable and heat labile. In view of the constant association of EO-CSF with MEG-CSF, it is of considerable importance for future work to determine whether these two factors are separable or whether they are really a single factor which is capable of stimulating two different target cell populations.

E. Comment

The present cloning system, although tedious to score, does provide for the first time a method for analyzing the nature of megakaryocyte precursor populations and the factors controlling their proliferation.

Outstanding problems to be resolved are: (1) the nature of the unidentified cells in mixed megakaryocytic colonies, (2) the relationship of MEG-CSF to thrombopoietin, (3) the relationship of EO-CSF to MEG-CSF, (4) whether MEG-CSF exists in vivo, and (5) whether activated lymphocytes are a significant source of MEG-CSF in vivo. On this latter question, it may seem improbable that lymphocytes should function as significant regulators of megakaryocyte and platelet production. However, at least in the mouse, there are two situations in which these two populations behave in an abnormal fashion. In NZB mice with chronic autoimmune hemolytic anemia, and thus with a continuous stimulation of lymphocyte proliferation, megakaryocyte accumulation can be extreme in the spleen. Similarly, in mice bearing antigenic tumors, it is common to find megakaryocytic hyperplasia. It may be therefore that the two populations do have unsuspected functional interrelationships.

Finally, it is a matter of some urgency to adapt this culture technique to the culture of human megakaryocyte colonies. Until this is achieved, it is not possible to contemplate the direct analysis of such interesting abnormalities as megakaryocytic myelosis and the relation of this disease to the osteofibrosis-osteosclerosis syndrome.

Chapter 10

Erythroid Colony Formation

Short-term liquid cultures of marrow erythropoietic cells have been used extensively to monitor erythropoietin-dependent heme synthesis, but it is doubtful whether such cultures can support significant erythropoietic proliferation.

The first report of erythroid colony formation in semisolid medium was made by STEPHENSON et al. [8] who described the use of plasma gel cultures to obtain rapidly developing, small colonies of erythropoietic cells in cultures of mouse fetal liver cells. Subsequent work by this group using an improved culture system [9] showed that a more slowly developing multicentric ("burst") colony of erythropoietic cells could also be grown [360]. This sequence of observations has given rise to a curious terminology—CFU-E (colony-forming unit, erythroid) for the cells forming the small, rapidly developing colonies and BFU-E (burst forming unit, erythroid) for the cells forming the larger multicentric aggregates.

As will be seen from the description to follow, the cells forming the early colonies are probably more mature than the cells forming the multicentric burst colonies, the known properties of the latter being consistent with an interpretation that they are progenitor cells. Furthermore, the small size of the rapidly developing colonies makes them equivalent to clusters in the granulocyte-macrophage system. While the terminology introduced by the Canadian workers will be followed throughout this chapter, the probable relationship to other terminology and cell populations is indicated in Table 23.

A. Early Developing Erythroid Colonies

In the original technique described by STEPHENSON et al. [8], mouse fetal liver cells were grown in plasma gel cultures in the presence of erythropoietin and were found to produce within 48 h small colonies of up to 32 cells. Cytological examination of the cells in these colonies showed that they had the morphology of late-stage nucleated erythroid cells and were benzidine-positive.

Because of the compact nature of these colonies, the small number of cells per colony, and the small size of individual colonies, these 48-h "colonies" are in fact very small objects that cannot be seen satisfactorily using a dissection microscope. It is necessary for scoring not only to use an inverted microscope but probably also to prestain the preparations with benzidine, taking care not to count small clusters of granulocytes.

The original technique was improved to permit the growth of similar colonies from adult mouse marrow cells [9], and the harvesting of such colony cells was made possible by the substitution of methylcellulose for the plasma gel [63].

In cultures of mouse bone marrow cells, the erythroid colonies after 48 h are composed of orthochromic erythroblasts (normoblasts) with small numbers of nonnucleated erythroid cells. By 72 h, most colony cells are nonnucleated with extruded nuclei lying in the vicinity. The peak frequency of colonies (aggregates of more than eight cells are scored as colonies) is at 48 h, and colony numbers fall rapidly after this time due to lysis of colony cells.

Table 23. Mouse erythropoietic colony-forming cells

Canadian terminology	Probable equivalent in GM-system	Type of progeny	Properties of colony-forming cells
CFU-E	Cluster-forming cells	Small aggregates of up to 32 cells within 48 h	Sedimentation velocity 6.4 mm/h
BFU-E	Colony-forming (progenitor) cells (GM-CFC)	Multicentric aggregates totaling up to 1000 cells formed by 7–10 days	Sedimentation velocity 3.9 mm/h

Data from HEATH et al. [360].

In an analysis of colony size at 48 h, MCLEOD et al. [9] observed a size heterogeneity typical of all normal hemopoietic colonies, with the vast majority of colonies containing 32 or fewer cells. Modal values of four, eight, and 16 cells were observed suggesting that initially in colony development there was both symmetry and synchrony of cell divisions.

Proof of the clonality of early developing erythroid colonies has recently been obtained by AXELRAD and his co-workers (AXELRAD, A. A., personal communication). Time-lapse studies on monolayer cultures of mouse fetal liver cells showed that colonies arose from single cells. Furthermore, although division times were rather variable in colony cells, for daughters of any one cell the cycle times were very similar and essentially cell division occurred synchronously. This confirms the indication of synchrony and symmetry from the earlier data and is reminiscent of the synchrony and symmetry observed in early granulocytic colony formation [81].

In the absence of erythropoietin, a small amount of multiplication by mouse erythropoietic cells appears to be possible, and this leads to the formation of aggregates of 2–5 cells. However, erythropoietin is absolutely necessary for sustained erythropoietic proliferation to form colonies (greater than eight cells), and colony numbers and size rise with increasing erythropoietin concentrations. Maximum colony numbers were observed with 0.01–0.02 U/ml concentrations, but colony numbers fell if higher concentrations of Stage III material were used [9]. Subsequent studies by ISCOVE and SIEBER [62] showed that this fall with increasing erythropoietin concentrations was due to impurities in the preparations and did not occur if these were first removed by further purification.

In methylcellulose cultures, the frequency of colony-forming cells appears to be lower (1/600 marrow cells) than reported for the improved plasma gel system [9], and peak colony numbers were not achieved until an erythropoietin concentration of 0.4 U/ml was used [62]. In another study using methylcellulose cultures, maximum colony numbers were achieved with an erythropoietin concentration of 0.17 U/ml [361]. Addition of β-mercaptoethanol at an optimal concentration of 10^{-4} M or α-thioglycerol increased up to fivefold the number of colonies obtained [62].

For both marrow and spleen populations, a linear relationship was observed between the number of cells cultured and the number of colonies developing. Limiting dilutions indicated that colonies were probably produced by single cells [9]. The frequency of colony-forming cells in C3H marrow populations averaged three per 10^3 cells, and colony-forming cells were 10 times less frequent in the spleen (four per 10^4 cells). In mouse fetal liver, the average frequency of colony-forming cells was 25 per 10^3 cells.

Studies by COOPER et al. [361] using an antierythroid serum showed that all relatively mature nucleated erythroid cells could be destroyed in fetal liver populations by exposure of the population to this antiserum in the presence of complement. This pretreatment left a population which was greatly enriched (to 99%) for nonhemoglobinized precursor cells (proerythroblasts and basophilic erythroblasts). Up to 5% of these cells were able to form 48-h colonies. While this does not permit a positive identification of all of the colony-forming cells, the observations make it unlikely that more mature (hemoglobinized) nucleated red cells are able to form colonies and suggests that erythroblasts or more ancestral cells might be the cells forming early erythroid colonies.

The limited proliferative potential observed in 48-h colonies strongly suggests that the cells forming these colonies are analogous with cluster-forming cells in the granulocyte-macrophage culture system.

Another approach to characterizing the cells generating 48-h colonies was made by HEATH et al. [360] using velocity sedimentation separation. The results indicated that these cells had a relatively high peak sedimentation velocity of 6.4 mm/h, suggesting a moderately large cell volume.

Indirect evidence for the *relative* maturity of CFU-E (48-h colony-forming cells) was obtained by GREGORY et al. [362] who showed that the frequency of these cells in the bone marrow and spleen was lowered by hypertransfusion. This suggests that the precursors leading to the formation of these colony-forming cells must themselves by erythropoietin-dependent (that is, relatively late maturation stages). Furthermore, in individual spleen colonies generated by stem cells in irradiated recipients, a relationship was observed between CFU and GM-CFC content but not between CFU and CFU-E content, again suggesting that the latter two populations are more remote from one another than the stem cell-progenitor cell relationship shown between CFUs and GM-CFCs.

In view of the known effects of androgenic steroids in stimulating erythropoiesis, it is of interest that addition of synthetic derivatives of testosterone to cultures of rat bone marrow increased the number of early erythroid colonies developing in the presence of erythropoietin [365].

In further studies using rat marrow cells fractionated by velocity sedimentation separation, evidence was presented that the cells forming early erythroid colonies were heterogeneous, and populations responding to fluoxymesterone were able to be distinguished from populations responding to etiocholanolone [366].

B. Late Developing Multicentric (Burst) Erythroid Colonies

If cultures of the above type are prepared so as to contain high initial concentrations of erythropoietin and/or are refed with erythropoietin and maintained for 7–10 days of incubation, a second type of erythroid colony develops. These have been termed "burst" colonies since they are composed of a loose collection of aggregates, each of the component aggregates corresponding in size and cellular composition to a 48-h colony [363].

Burst colonies only begin to appear after 6 days of incubation and reach maximum numbers between days 7–9, after which colony numbers decline due to the same process responsible for the disappearance of early colonies—maturation of individual colony cells to nonnucleated cells, with rapid subsequent disintegration. In many burst colonies, however, many of the colony cells are less differentiated and contain no detectable hemoglobin [360]. It is important to reiterate the sequence of events in such cultures of mouse marrow cells. In the first 2 days, there is a rapid appearance of numerous small colonies which then quickly disappear. The cultures for a brief interval appear almost empty, then develop the multicentric or burst colonies, each segment of which is essentially similar to an early colony —a small aggregate of rapidly maturing erythroid cells.

The frequency of burst-forming cells was assessed as two per 50,000 mouse marrow cells by AXELRAD et al. [363]. It is of interest that the relation between the number of cells cultured and the number of bursts developing is nonlinear [360]. Few bursts developed at cell concentrations less than 10^5/0.5 ml culture. Conversely, cell separation studies showed that cells were present in the rapidly sedimenting fractions which could inhibit burst formation.

Unlike early erythroid colony-forming cells whose numbers are sharply affected by hypertransfusion or erythropoietin injections [363, 362], the frequency of BFU-E was not decreased by hypertransfusion. Analysis of the sedimentation velocity of BFU-E indicated a peak sedimentation velocity of 3.9 mm/h [360], suggesting a size even smaller than GM-CFCs and possibly intermediate between that of progenitor and stem cells.

In parallel studies on late developing erythroid colony cells grown from mouse marrow cells, ISCOVE and SIEBER [62] found that individual colonies grew better in methylcellulose than in plasma and could contain up to 10,000 cells. Colonies were often single aggregates but still contained the typical component aggregates similar to early colonies. They obtained a frequency of 25 BFU-E per 10^5 marrow cells, considerably higher than the original estimate of AXELRAD et al. [363] and in the frequency range of colony-forming (progenitor) cells in other hemopoietic populations. As was the case with early erythroid colonies, the number of late erythroid colonies was increased by the addition of mercaptoethanol or α-thioglycerol.

The proliferation of burst colonies requires the use of erythropoietin concentrations tenfold higher than for early colony cells, and maximum colony numbers were only obtained with a concentration of 3 U/ml. Thus, if the erythropoietin preparation being used contains contaminating inhibitory material, the necessity to use such high concentrations seems to result in an inevitable reduction in the observed number of colonies.

For both early and late erythroid colony formation, there is a departure from linearity between the number of cells cultured and the number of colonies developing if low cell numbers are cultured. For some curious reason, addition of 1% deionized BSA restores linearity for early colony formation [9, 62].

C. Comment

At the present stage, a fairly satisfying sequence seems to have been documented by the combined in vitro and in vivo studies. This sequence is CFU—BFU-E—CFU-E, with BFU-E formation being erythropoietin-independent but the transition of BFU-E to CFU-E both in vitro and in vivo being erythropoietin-dependent (Fig. 39).

An intriguing similarity exists between the low responsiveness to erythropoietin of the BFU-E that form multicentric burst colonies (tenfold higher erythropoietin concentrations required than for CFU-E) and the low responsiveness of the GM-CFCs that form multiple granulocytic colonies (requiring 10–20-fold higher GM-CSF concentrations than other GM-CFCs). Although multicentric GM-colonies can reach a large size and each portion equal a granulocytic colony in size, it is doubtful whether the analogy with the erythroid colony system can be seriously sustained. Multiple granulocytic colonies never transform to macrophage colonies, and if the cells forming multiple granulocytic colonies were in fact the

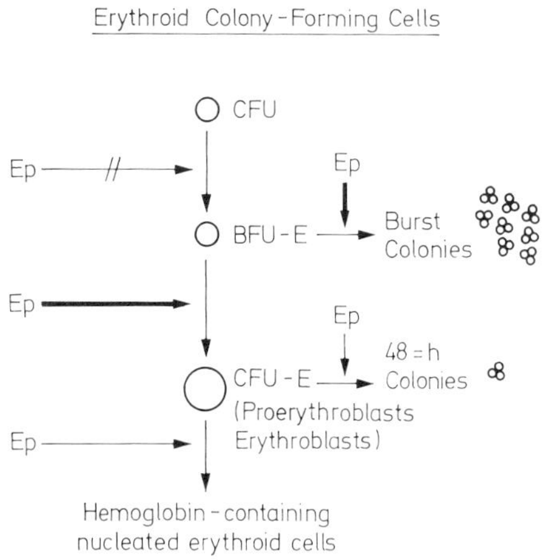

Fig. 39. Schematic representation of the interrelationships between types of erythroid colony-forming cells and CFUs in the mouse

immediate ancestors of other GM-CFCs, it would be expected that most of the subcolonies within a multiple colony would transform to macrophages. Nevertheless, the similarities are intriguing and are worthy of further exploration.

While the in vitro analysis of erythropoietic populations has suggested a fairly simple and logical hierarchy of cells, several comments need to be made:

1. As pointed out by ISCOVE and SIEBER [62], current estimates give the following frequencies in the mouse marrow: BFU-E 25 per 10^5; CFU-E 325 per 10^5; earliest recognizable precursors (proerythroblasts) 1000–2000 per 10^5. From such figures and the fact that there are approximately 10^4 nucleated erythroid cells per 10^5 marrow cells, it is obvious that, as is the case with other hemopoietic populations, colony-forming cells are only a small minority of cells compared with the size of the morphologically recognizable compartment.
2. Logically, all nonhemoglobinized or hemoglobinized identifiable erythropoietic precursors that are capable of some proliferation in vivo should also be capable of proliferation in vitro. From the above figures, it seems either that the morphologically recognizable cells are unable to proliferate in vitro, or more likely, the one or two divisions that they can undergo are difficult to detect in the cultures.
3. Apart from the differing requirements for erythropoietin between BFU-E and CFU-E, there has so far been only one report of heterogeneity in either subpopulation [366]. The proliferation of erythroid cells does seem to be more uniform than corresponding granulopoietic populations. It is likely, however, that at least some heterogeneity in proliferative capacity and/or responsiveness to erythropoietin exists within both subpopulations, and this question requires further analysis.
4. ISCOVE et al. [63] have presented convincing evidence that the factor stimulating erythroid colony formation in vitro is in fact erythropoietin as assayed in vivo. Again, in comparison with the multiplicity of GM-CSFs, erythropoietic regulation appears to be markedly simpler with only one described form of erythropoietin with a mol wt of approximately 45,000. It must be emphasized, however, that the studies characterizing erythropoietin have so far only been concerned with two source materials—anemic sheep

plasma and anemic human urine. If GM-CSF studies had been limited to two source materials, a similar satisfying uniformity might have emerged. Until attempts are made to search for and characterize erythropoietin in various tissues or conditioned media, the question of heterogeneity of erythropoietin and the associated possibility of heterogeneity in colony-forming target cells cannot be seriously discussed or dismissed. A similar comment can be made regarding the longstanding controversy on the renal or extrarenal origin of erythropoietin. It is pointless continuing this controversy from entrenched positions. The in vitro cultures offer a sensitive new system for screening the capacity of cells and tissues to produce small amounts of erythropoietin-like material. Rather than continue to assay such material in vivo [364], experience with semisolid cultures indicates that use of rapid in vitro screening systems will revolutionize such studies.

5. The phenomenon of burst erythroid colony formation is intriguing in that colony formation appears to be delayed 6–7 days after initiation of the cultures. Since proliferation occurs relatively synchronously in the multiple fragments of each burst colony, it is obvious that some proliferation of the original colony-forming cells must have occurred during this 6–7-day interval to generate the cells (presumably CFU-E) that each generate a small subcolony. The formation of these loosely dispersed cells presumably cannot be detected against the background of surviving single cells in these cultures. What is of interest, however, is the nature of the mechanism delaying the formation of hemoglobin-containing progeny by these cells. It may be possible by manipulating culture conditions to modify the time of onset of burst formation and thus to characterize some of the cellular events involved.

D. Neoplastic Mouse Erythroid Colonies

Erythroleukemia can be induced in many strains of mice using the Friend or Rauscher leukemia viruses. The erythroleukemias are difficult to transplant because the virus in the transplanted cell suspension reinduces new leukemias in recipient mice. Studies have shown that the development of Rauscher erythroleukemia is suppressed by hypertransfusion of the animals before virus infection [367]. This implies strongly that the target cells for the virus are the progeny of erythropoietin-responsive cells.

The situation with the Friend virus is more complex. Different variants of the Friend virus exist, some capable of inducing anemia, others polycythemia. No exhaustive analysis has been performed of the effects of erythropoietin suppression on the induction of erythroleukemia by all variants of the Friend virus. In the case of the polycythemic strains of Friend virus, evidence has been produced that the target cells affected by the virus normally respond to erythropoietin by the formation of erythroid cells [368, 369]. When transformed by the Friend virus, the erythroleukemic cells are altered in that erythropoietin is no longer required for their continued erythroid differentiation [370, 371].

In an interesting series of studies, Liao and Axelrad [10] found that marrow cells from C3H mice infected with the polycythemic strain of Friend leukemia virus were able to form 48-h erythroid colonies in the absence of added erythropoietin. Furthermore, addition of antierythropoietin antibodies did not suppress colony formation, suggesting that the cells were not hypersensitive to erythropoietin and responding to the small concentrations of erythropoietin in the FCS. Studies with anti-Friend sera showed that the cells generating these colonies had been infected by the Friend virus and were exhibiting Friend virus-induced antigens. Maturation of leukemic colony cells occurred with exclusion of nuclei and the formation of nonnucleated erythrocytes. Colonies also developed in which cells showed less differentiation, and these were more common than in control cultures of normal marrow cells. Colony size in cultures of cells from Friend virus-infected mice was similar to that of control colonies (maximum size 32 cells), but the addition of erythropoietin (0.2 U per ml) did not increase colony size.

Colony-forming cells (CFU-E) were 5 times as frequent as in normal marrow, but colony numbers were only very slightly increased by addition of erythropoietin. In confirmation of previous studies with whole animals, prior hypertransfusion suppressed the development of erythropoietin-independent erythroid colonies following Friend virus infection, while bleeding had the reverse effect.

Subsequent experiments [11] showed that infection of normal C3H marrow cells in vitro with Friend virus followed within 1 h by culture in plasma gel cultures led to a fivefold increase in the number of erythropoietin-independent colonies developing. No erythropoietin-independent burst erythroid colonies were observed. The implication is strong that the erythropoietin-independent colonies developing in this experiment represent the progeny of cells transformed in vitro by the Friend virus.

Reduction in the concentration of FCS used in the cultures reduced the level of background erythroid colonies occurring in control normal mouse marrow cultures but did not significantly reduce the number of colonies developing following Friend virus infection. While this effect may have been due to reduction in the background levels of erythropoietin, it might also suggest that virally transformed erythroid cells have a lower serum requirement in culture than normal cells.

These observations are a dramatic demonstration that infection of hemopoietic cells by a neoplasia-inducing virus can alter the responsiveness or dependency of the cells on a normal growth regulator. In the case of the Friend virus, it would seem that information conveyed by the Friend virus genome is capable of substituting for the message generated by contact of erythropoietin with the cell. Although the neoplastic cells exhibited some loss of capacity to differentiate, differentiation was possible by at least some of the progeny of the virus-infected cells.

It is possible tht Friend virus infection causes a selective amplification of the very small numbers of apparently erythropoietin-independent cells in normal animals. However, the in vitro transformation data almost require the alternative explanation that direct viral transformation of cells is associated with the acquisition of erythropoietin independence. As maturation of erythroid cells proceeds normally enough in most colonies generated by virus-infected cells, the major abnormality in Friend virus-infected mice appears to be a marked hyperplasia of the CFU-E compartment.

The situation is superficially similar to that in CML with its extreme hyperplasia of the GM-CFC compartment. However, the two diseases differ fundamentally since in CML the cells retain full dependency on the normal regulator GM-CSF, whereas the affected CFU-E population in Friend virus-induced leukemia exhibits erythropoietin independence. Since BFU-Es appear to be the ancestors of CFU-Es, the behavior of these cells in mice infected by Friend virus is obviously in need of clarification.

In a parallel series of studies, Nooter and Ghio [372] analyzed erythroid colony formation in methylcellulose cultures of marrow cells from BALB/c mice infected with the Rauscher erythroleukemia virus. A 5–25-fold rise was noted in the frequency of marrow cells forming early erythroid colonies in the absence of added erythropoietin. Addition of erythropoietin did not increase the number of colonies developing, and use of irradiated bone marrow cells from virus-infected mice as feeder layers did not enhance erythroid colony formation. It was suggested from the latter experiment that virus-infected bone marrow cells do not produce erythropoietin, but this question needs further exploration as the number of cells tested (2×10^5/ml) was extremely low.

As was observed for Friend virus-infected cells, erythroid colony formation by Rauscher leukemia virus-infected cells was less serum-dependent than colony formation by normal erythroid cells. This has some similarity with the well-known ability of transformed fibroblasts to grow in low serum concentrations [1].

One interesting property noted for erythroid colony formation by Rauscher leukemia virus-infected cells was that the erythropoietin-independent colonies persisted for more than 2 weeks whereas normal erythropoietin-dependent colonies differentiated and disintegrated after 4 days. This capacity for sustained growth of transformed cells in vitro is, of course, the basis for all in vitro established continuous cell lines, e.g., EB-transformed human B-lymphocyte cell lines, and appears also to be true of mouse B-lymphocytes transformed in vitro by the Abelson virus. It could be postulated that, in the establishment of continuous cell lines in vitro from transformed cells, it is only a rare mutant cell that is responsible for the initiation of the cell line. However, the interesting information provided by the cloning experiments of Nooter and Ghio is the strong suggestion that an extended capacity for in vitro proliferation is probably shared by all or many of the viral-altered cells.

Circulating erythropoietin levels are somewhat elevated in mice infected with the Rauscher virus [373], and one possibility explored by Nooter and Ghio was that continuous high levels of erythropoietin might themselves lead to the emergence of erythropoietin-independent CFU-Es. This was tested in mice made anemic by phenylhydrazine treatment, but no rise in erythropoietin-independent CFU-Es was noted.

Friend leukemic cells exhibit little capacity for differentiation but after culture with dimenthylsulfoxide (DMSO) can be induced to respond to erythropoietin by hemoglobin synthesis [375]. Whereas Friend leukemic cells formed colonies of relatively undifferentiated cells in agar or plasma gel cultures [376, 377], preincubation for 1–2 days in the presence of DMSO altered the cells so that they formed colonies in which obvious erythroid differentiation occurred [377].

E. Erythroid Colony Formation by Human Cells

The technique for the culture of erythroid colonies was adapted for the culture of human cells by Tepperman et al. [374] and by Iscove et al. [63]. In an analysis of marrow cells from a variety of patients, a range of colony-forming cell frequencies from $30–500/10^5$ marrow cells was observed (aggregates of eight or more cells were scored as colonies).

The time of development of erythroid colonies differed from that in the mouse. Colonies were first detected at 3 days and reach maximum size at 7–9 days [374]. Linear relationships were noted between the number of cells cultured and the number of colonies developing.

Unlike the situation with mouse cultures where some background formation of erythroid colonies occurs in cultures containing no added erythropoietin, in human cultures background colony formation is extremely low (the opposite of the species differences for granulocytic colony formation).

On the addition of increasing concentrations of erythropoietin (either anemic sheep plasma, Connaught Laboratories Step III, or human urine erythropoietin), a graded increase was observed in the number and size of erythropoietic colonies developing. However, according to ISCOVE et al. [63], human cells are less responsive to erythropoietin than mouse cells and require a concentration of more than 1 U per ml to be stimulated. Similar data was provided by TEPPERMAN et al. [374] who found that the development of plateau numbers of colonies required erythropoietin concentrations of 2–5 U per ml.

Human colonies exhibited a wide size range at 7–9 days. When marrow cells were fractionated by velocity sedimentation prior to culture, cells forming small (less than 32 cells) clusters sedimented at a peak sedimentation velocity of approximately 5.5 mm/h, while cells forming colonies larger than 32 cells sedimented with a peak sedimentation velocity of approximately 3.5 mm/h. This is very similar to the data of HEATH et al. [360] on mouse marrow cells (sedimentation values for CFU-E 6.4 mm/h, BFU-E 3.9 mm/h) and suggests that the human cells forming large colonies may be analogous to BFU-E and the cells forming smaller colonies to CFU-E. In this context, the human cells forming large colonies were only maximally stimulated by 10 U of erythropoietin per ml, again similar to the requirement of BFU-E for higher erythropoietin concentrations. In these fractionation experiments, no correspondence was found between the distribution of colony-forming cells and erythroblasts, and this latter cell seems unlikely to be the cell generating the erythroid colonies formed by human marrow cells. The in vitro radiation sensitivity of human erythroid colony-forming cells was established as D_0 113 rads.

To date, no detailed description has been made of the morphology of the cells in human erythroid colonies at various stages in the development of the colonies.

F. Culture of Cells from Patients with Polycythemia Vera

Polycythemia vera is a myeloproliferative disorder involving abnormalities in more than one hemopoietic population. However, it is characterized by an excessive production of red cells in the presence of abnormally low erythropoietin levels. Patients are able to elevate erythropoietin levels in response to bleeding. Analyses using patients who were heterozygous for the enzyme G6PD have shown that the abnormal erythropoietic cells are a monoclonal population presumably derived from a single cell [345].

It has been reported by PRCHAL and AXELRAD [378] that marrow cells from patients with polycythemia vera are able to generate substantial numbers of erythroid colonies in cultures containing no added erythropoietin. This interesting situation implies either that the abnormal clone is erythropoietin-independent or that the cells are hyperresponsive to the minute amounts of erythropoietin present in the FCS used in the medium. Addition of erythropoietin does increase the number of colonies developing, however, with an abnormally flat titration curve. Conversely, addition of some batches of antierythropoietin sera completely suppress colony formation while other preparations only partially suppress colony formation (AXELRAD, A. A., personal communication). It is too early to be able to give a precise interpretation of the data, but clearly the disease is of considerable interest and has intriguing similarities to the in vitro behavior of Friend virus and Rauscher leukemia virus-infected cells. The clonal nature of polycythemia vera and the abnormal response to erythropoietin (whether these be independence or hyperresponsiveness) strongly suggest that polycythemia vera is in fact an erythroleukemia, albeit of a benign nature.

G. Comment

At this stage, the evidence emerging from the growth of cells from mice from viral-induced erythroleukemia and from humans with polycythemia vera suggest strongly that in both situations the abnormal erythropoietic population is erythropoietin-independent.

It is still not clear whether corresponding cells exist in the normal marrow or whether, particularly in cultures of normal mouse cells, some erythropoiesis is being stimulated by background levels of erythropoietin in the FCS. If such erythropoietin-independent cells exist, then these may be selectively involved in the above disease situations. However, this seems improbable as suppression of erythroleukemia by hypertransfusion tends to prevent viral-induced erythroleukemia, implying as a minimum requirement that the target cells for the virus are generated by erythropoietin-dependent cells.

A simpler hypothesis is to propose that following infection by the erythroleukemia virus, the altered cells are able to proliferate without erythropoietin stimulation either (1) because the viral genome activates the cell processes normally requiring activation by erythropoietin (a substitution hypothesis), or (2) because the virus-infected cell is so deranged that even though hemoglobin synthesis and some maturation to morphologically recognizable red cells can occur, this process is no longer an erythropoietin-dependent sequence (a derangement hypothesis).

The situation with both the Friend and Rauscher leukemia viruses is the more intriguing because of the vast amount of effort which has been put into fractionating both viruses and determining what genetic information is carried in their RNA. While a derangement hypothesis is a priori more likely, a substitution of viral genetic information for hormone-generated information has yet to be excluded, and if part of the viral-coded information is in fact the erythropoietin message, a wonderful opportunity exists to collect information of importance both to tumor virologists and reglator biologists. For those who distrust models and prefer to work directly with patients, the similarities emerging between polycythemia vera and viral-induced erythroleukemia are both reassuring and intriguing.

Possibly the most striking aspect of the erythroleukemia story is the difference from the apparent situation in AML or CML, where all granulocytic proliferation remains regulator-dependent. However, there is still need for some caution. It does not yet seem to have been convincingly excluded that erythropoietin may be generated within cultures of Friend virus or Rauscher virus-infected cells or polycythemia vera cells. Cloning studies using single cells are needed to document the absolute autonomy of cell proliferation and ideally erythropoietin levels in the serum used in the medium need to be effectively suppressed. Since AML and CML cells can be sources of GM-CSF, are erythroleukemia cells a source of erythropoietin? Can endogenously produced erythropoietin in an erythroleukemic cell remain entirely intracytoplasmic and there stimulate proliferation and differentiation of the cell itself? Possibly, experiments based on these questions will prove to be negative, but they are technically feasible using the in vitro cloning system and should at least be attempted to clarify what appears to be a very intriguing situation.

Chapter 11

Normal Mouse and Human Lymphocyte Colonies

If normal mouse thymus or lymph node cells are cultured in the agar medium normally used for growing bone marrow colonies, death of the cells occurs very rapidly. Most cells reharvested after 2–3 h are stainable by eosin and by 24 h, the only surviving cells are occasional macrophages. From 1966 onward, many attempts were made to obtain survival and proliferation of T- or B-lymphocytes in agar cultures, but these were unsuccessful, despite the use of a variety of conditioned media or underlayers.

Two observations were made during this period which are of some general interest. ROBINSON et al. [379] attempted cultures of mouse spleen cells in agar containing sheep red cells. They reported the development of plaques of lysed red cells in the center of which were often small clusters of presumably antibody-forming lymphoid cells. In retrospect, this cluster formation is of interest in view of the current use of red cells to potentiate the growth of colonies of antibody-forming B-lymphocytes (see below), and the small clusters were probably B-lymphocyte colonies attempting to grow under suboptimal conditions. In the other study, METCALF [66] showed that the addition of lymph node or thymus cells to cultures of mouse bone marrow cells increased the number and growth rate of granulocytic and macrophage colonies if the culture conditions were suboptimal. The phenomenon did not depend on the use of syngeneic lymphoid cells and was seen also with allogeneic cells and even with cells from mice preimmunized against the strain of origin of the cultured marrow cells. In these cultures, it was also clear that the added lymphoid cells survived for only a very short period, and in fact equally good potentiation could be obtained with lymphoid suspensions killed by freeze-thawing or heating. Studies with ^{3}HTdR-labeled lymphoid cells showed that the dividing marrow colony cells actively reutilized nuclear material from the lymphoid cells. The phenomenon was not unique to lymphoid populations and could be duplicated by the addition of bone marrow cells or even by colony crowding without the addition of any extra cells. Subsequent experiments have shown that interactions of this type between cultured cells and colonies, leading to potentiated colony growth, are also a very obvious feature of B-lymphocyte colony formation.

At the present time, the successful culture of lymphocyte colonies in semisolid medium has been achieved by one or other of two methods: (1) use of 2-mercaptoethanol in the culture medium, or (2) preliminary activation of lymphocytes by mitogenic stimulation in liquid culture before subsequent culture in agar. Lymphocytes show to an extreme degree the principle which seems to emerge from culturing many types of cells in agar—that cultured cells either proliferate or die rapidly in such cultures. Very few cells (macrophages are exceptions) appear to be able to survive in this type of culture medium unless they are actually proliferating or have been activated to proliferate.

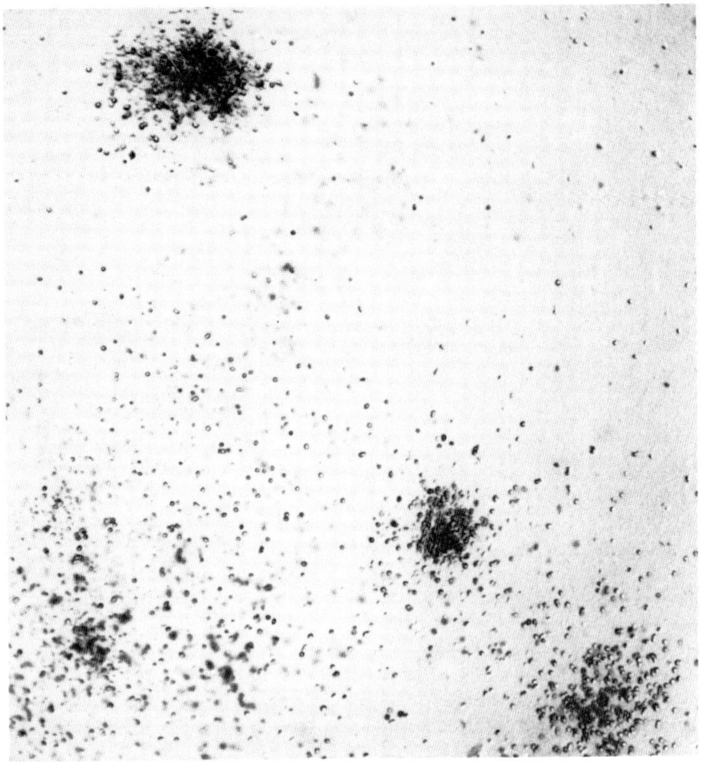

Fig. 40. A 7-day culture of $C_{57}BL$ lymph node cells showing four B-lymphocyte colonies

A. Mouse B-Lymphocyte Colonies

This work arose from attempts to culture, in agar, cells harvested from mixed leukocyte cultures of mouse spleen cells. The large macrophage-like cells in such mixed leukocyte cultures were able to form clusters in agar (METCALF, D., unpublished data), but occasional cultures also developed colonies of mononuclear cells. In these experiments, because of the high frequency of the cluster-forming cells, only 20,000 cells per dish were cultured, and subsequent studies have shown that the variable colony formation observed was due to this use of very low numbers of cultured cells.

The culture system included 2-mercaptoethanol in the agar medium because 2-mercaptoethanol had also been present in the liquid mixed leukocyte cultures. Use of 2-mercaptoethanol to increase the overall proliferative activity of lymphoid cells in vitro was introduced by CLICK et al. [24] and BROOME and JENG [25] who showed that addition of a variety of thiols or disulfides increased the proliferation of lymphocytes and antibody-forming cells in liquid cultures. Based on this work, METCALF [26] showed that 2-mercaptoethanol also strongly potentiated colony formation in agar by some murine plasmacytomas and CEROTTINI et al. [359] demonstrated that 2-mercaptoethanol permitted sustained T cell proliferation in mixed leukocyte cultures.

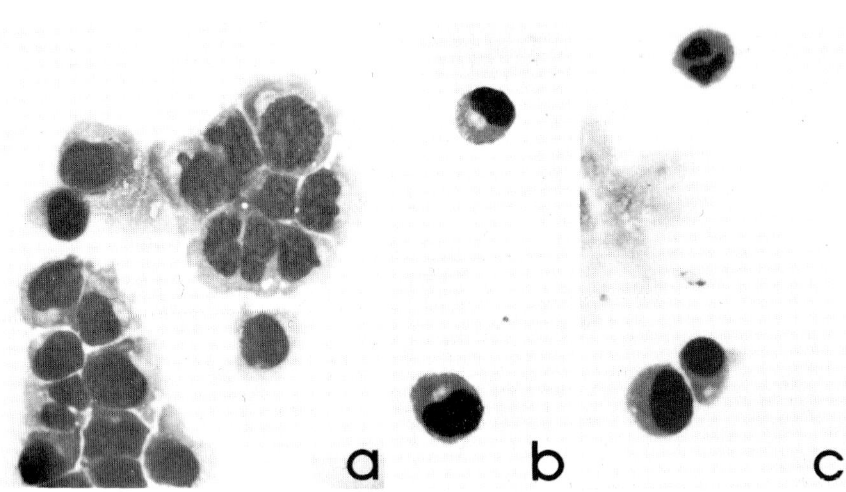

Fig. 41a–c. B-lymphocyte colony cells grown from $C_{57}BL$ lymph node cells. (a) large undifferentiated mononuclear blast cells in 4-day colonies; (b), (c) more differentiated cells resembling immature plasma cells in 7-day colonies. Note in (c) a degenerating cell with a clover leaf nucleus (May-Grunwald-Giemsa). (From METCALF et al., [28]. Reproduced with permission from J. Exp. Med.)

A systematic analysis by METCALF et al. [28] of the behaviour of mouse spleen and lymph node cells in agar cultures containing 2-mercaptoethanol showed that colony formation was readily obtained provided that the concentration of 2-mercaptoethanol was close to 5×10^{-5}M and that sufficiently large numbers of cells (more than 100,000/ml) were cultured. The general appearance of the colonies was similar to that of granulocytic or macrophage colonies (Fig. 40), and there was the same asynchrony of onset of proliferation and the same variation in colony size and shape previously described for granulocytic and macrophage colonies. As is true for all other types of hemopoietic cultures, more numerous smaller aggregates of cells (clusters) also developed in these cultures, and in fact clusters outnumbered colonies by about 5:1.

Early in colony development, the colony cells were uniform populations of large mononuclear blast cells rather similar to PHA-transformed lymphocytes (Fig. 41). By 7 days of incubation, although many colony cells remained as undifferentiated blast cells, others had matured to smaller cells with an excentric nucleus, basophilic cytoplasm, and a prominent perinuclear halo (Golgi region). These latter cells resembled relatively mature plasma cells, and examination in the elctronmicroscope confirmed this maturation towards plasma cells with the cytoplasm showing numerous flattened cisternae of rough endoplasmic reticulum, some polyribosomes, and a large Golgi apparatus (Fig. 42). Less commonly, some colony cells matured to cells resembling small and medium lymphocytes.

Although obvious maturation of colony cells occurs in these cultures, the process does not proceed to completion. Most of the colonies disintegrate between 7–10 days of incubation, and even immmediately before death, most cells retain their basophilic cytoplasm and fail to develop the morphology of typical mature eosinophilic plasma cells or small lymphocytes. In this failure to develop full maturation, the cells of lymphocyte colonies resemble those in most neutrophil, eosinophil, and megakaryocyte colonies grown in vitro.

Definitive identification of these colonies of mononuclear cells as B-lymphocyte colonies was

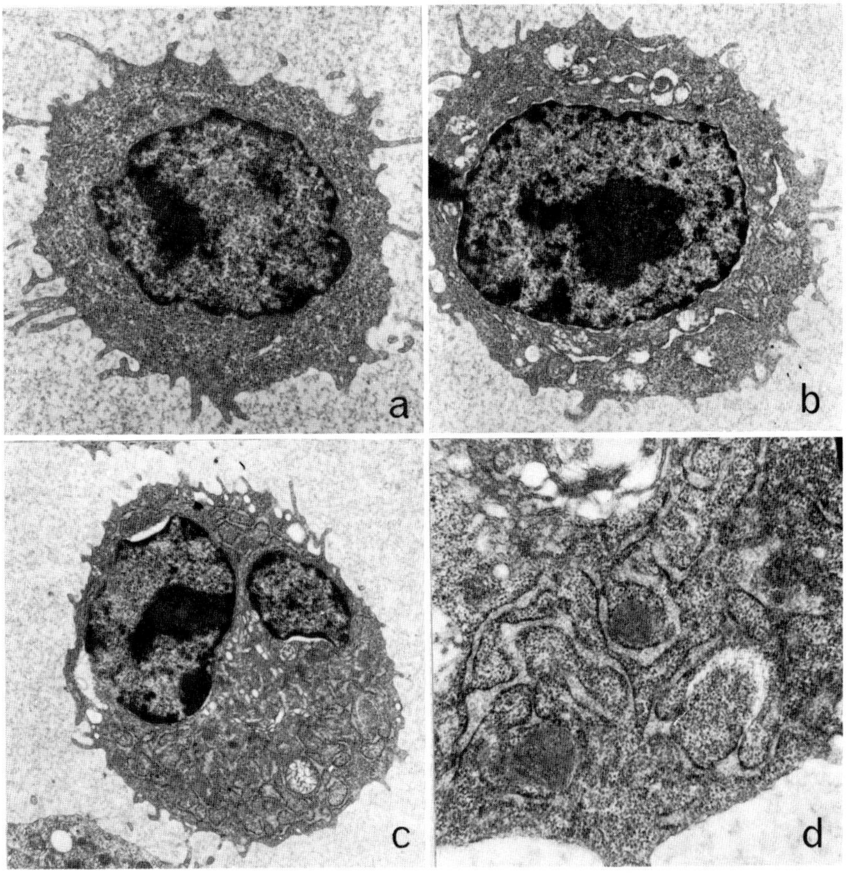

Fig. 42a–d. Electronmicroscopic morphology of 5-day B-lymphocyte colony cells grown from $C_{57}BL$ spleen cells. (a) a typical blast-like lymphoid cell, (b) early plasmablast, (c) a relatively well differentiated plasma cell, (d) a detail of the cytoplasm of a plasma cell similar in its differentiation to that in (c). (From METCALF et al., [28]. Reproduced with permission from J. Exp. Med.)

made by examining the membrane markers of harvested colony cells and determining the capacity of these cells to exhibit and secrete immunoglobulin.

As might be anticipated, there are some technical difficulties in washing colony cells harvested from agar. Mass-harvested cells are difficult to wash free of surrounding agar and sometimes react negatively in various tests. The highest and most consistent activity was observed with cells obtained from colonies by micromanipulation and individually washed in micro droplets. The results from a combination of these methods are listed in Table 24. It can be seen that virtually all colony cells exhibit membrane immunoglobulin, most exhibiting IgM and some 5–10% also exhibiting IgG_{2a}. There are some reservations about the significance of membrane IgG_{2a} as in other systems this has often been shown to be cytophilic immunoglobulin absorbed onto cells and not actively secreted by them. Proof that colony cells could synthesize immunoglobulin was obtained by culturing harvested colony cells in medium containing ^3H-leucine and demonstrating the synthesis of labeled immu-

Table 24. Membrane properties of pooled 7-day B-lymphocyte colony cells

Membrane marker		% Positive colony cells
Fc receptors (^{125}I-FGG, anti-FGG)		94%
C3 receptors (EAC rosettes)		1%
Membrane	IgM	92%
	IgA	<2%
	IgG_1	<1%
	IgG_2	5–10%
	IgD	<2%
Antisera against	Ly 1.2	<2%
	Ly 3.2	<2%
	Thy 1.2	<2%
	Ly 4.1	80%
	Ly 7.2	90%
	I-ABJEC	>90%
	I-ABJ	>90%
	I-J	<2%
	I-JEC	>90%

Data from METCALF et al. [28] and METCALF, D. and WARNER, N. L., (unpublished data).

noglobulin containing μ and L-chains [28]. The proportion of cells bearing IgG_{2a} did not differ markedly between colony cells grown from mice of different strains including nu/nu (congenitally athymic mice). No progression from IgM-bearing cells to IgG-bearing cells was observed as colony populations increased in size and matured. In colonies grown from Peyer's patch cells, no unusual frequency of IgA-bearing cells was observed. It should also be noted that colony cells were uniformly negative for IgD.

The majority (more than 90%) of colony cells exhibited Fc receptors, best demonstrated by the radioiodinated immune complex method (fowl gammaglobulin, rabbit antifowl gammaglobulin). Harvested colony cells were Ia-positive but lacked receptors for C3 as detected by rosette formation.

These observations characterized these colonies as being composed of B-lymphocytes. Evidence that each colony was a clone derived from a single cell was obtained by an analysis (1) of membrane immunoglobulin, and (2) antigen-binding characteristics [28]. An analysis of cells obtained from individual colonies by micromanipulation showed that all colony cells reacted with fluorescein-labeled anti-μ sera. If the cells also reacted with anti-γ_2 sera, then all cells in the colony exhibited this reactivity. There was also a notable intracolony homogeneity in the intensity of staining with these antisera.

Antigen-binding capacity was examined by growing colonies from CBA spleen cells enriched for NIP or DNP-binding cells by preliminary incubation of the cells on gelatin to which the hapten was coupled [28]. With spleen cells harvested from NIP-gelatin slabs, approximately 25% of the cultured cells were capable of binding the hapten, NIP. Analysis of mass-harvested colony cells grown from such cells showed again that approximately 25% of the colony cells bound NIP—the frequency of binding cells being unaffected by the presence of hapten in the culture dish during the incubation period. Analysis of individual colonies showed that about one colony in five was composed wholly of NIP-binding cells, and no NIP-binding cells were observed in other colonies [28]. Further analysis of such colonies showed that a proportion of NIP-binding cells was capable of producing hemolytic plaques when incubated with NIP-coated sheep red cells (METCALF, D. and PIKE, B., unpublished data) although the frequency of plaque-forming cells in relation to antigen-binding cells was lower than in liquid cultures of spleen cells enriched for NIP-binding cells.

This evidence strongly suggests that B-lymphocyte colonies are clones derived from single colony-forming cells and that the cells of individual colonies exhibit a remarkable degree of homogeneity.

B. Growth Requirements of Mouse B-Lymphocyte Colonies

Analysis of B-lymphocyte colony formation by mouse spleen or lymph node cells showed that the relationship between the number of cells cultured and the number of colonies developing was markedly nonlinear. When less than 100,000 cells per ml were cultured, few colonies developed, and these reached only a small size before dying prematurely [28].

Linearity of colony formation was achieved by adding to the cultures either (1) a suspension of sheep, human, or mouse red cells (optimal dose 0.1 ml of 10% cells) (Fig. 43), or (2) 10–20μg endotoxin to each culture dish. With both methods, linearity was maintained even in cultures containing fewer than 500 cells, and colonies achieved approximately the same size as in more crowded cultures [28, 61].

Both methods have disadvantages. The addition of sheep red cells makes the medium opaque. While this does not interfere with colony counting, which routinely is performed after first lysing the red cells with 0.5 ml of 3% acetic acid, it does make difficult any study requiring the identification of individual living colonies. As a compromise, useful potentiation can be achieved with as little as 0.1 ml of 0.5% red cells which allows many living colonies to be visualized. The use of endotoxin to potentiate colony growth is usually less effective than sheep red cells in terms of colony numbers and growth rates, but the potentiation can sometimes be strong (Fig. 44) and the colony cells are clearly visible. A major practical problem, however, is the fact that only some batches of FCS (three of 15 tested in one series) allow the endotoxin potentiation to be expressed, and care has to be taken to select a suitable batch before preparation of the cultures [61].

With different batches of FCS, the optimal serum concentration for colony formation varies from 5–15%, and as is true of all other colony formation, not all FCS batches are capable of supporting B-lymphocyte colony formation.

Addition of 2-mercaptoethanol to the cultures is mandatory for B-lymphocyte colony formation, and only a narrow concentration range is effective in stimulating colony formation (approximately 5×10^{-5}M). Analysis of the growth of transferred colonies indicated that 2-mercaptoethanol must be present throughout the incubation period for survival and proliferation of colony cells [61]. In part, the action of 2-mercaptoethanol is direct on the colony cells, but evidence was obtained that in the presence of 2-mercaptoethanol, spleen cells can release or produce a factor potentiating colony formation [61]. This suggests that in part the action of mercaptoethanol is indirect via some other cell type in the culture dish, a conclusion explaining the marked influence of cell crowding on colony formation.

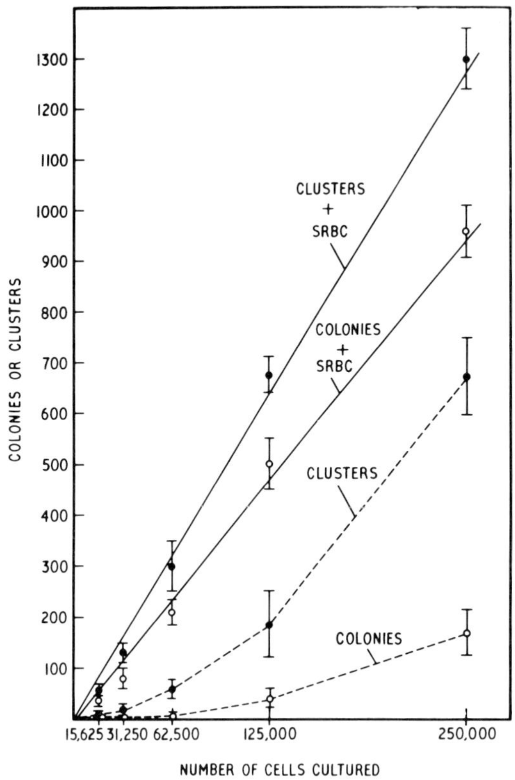

Fig. 43. Improvement in linearity and increase in colony and cluster numbers in B-lymphocyte cultures of $C_{57}BL$ lymph node cells following the addition of 0.1 ml of 5% sheep red cells (SRBC). (From METCALF et al., [28]. Reproduced with permission from J. Exp. Med.)

A parallel analysis of the action of endotoxin showed that in the absence of mercaptoethanol, endotoxin could not support cell survival or stimulate proliferation. In the presence of mercaptoethanol, at least part of the effect of endotoxin was a direct one on the actual colony cells [61].

The active factor in red cells responsible for the marked potentiation of B-lymphocyte colony growth has not been characterized, and it is not known whether it is the same factor as the red cell factor potentiating granulocyte and macrophage colony growth [65]. Use of fresh red cells was essential, and cells tended to lose their activity if stored beyond 1 week. Since red cells in underlayers can still potentiate colony growth, direct cell contact seems unnecessary. However, in cultures where red cells lysed prematurely, no potentiation of colony growth occurred, and lysis of red cells by osmotic shock or freeze-thawing destroyed their capacity to potentiate colony formation.

Superficially, B-lymphocyte colony formation differs from all other types of hemopoietic colony formation in not requiring a specific humoral factor for cell proliferation, the 2-mercaptoethanol appearing to substitute completely for such a factor. It is possible, however, that this difference is more apparent than real. Several lines of evidence suggest the existence of factors, possibly with a high degree of specificity, which could be operating in the culture dish:

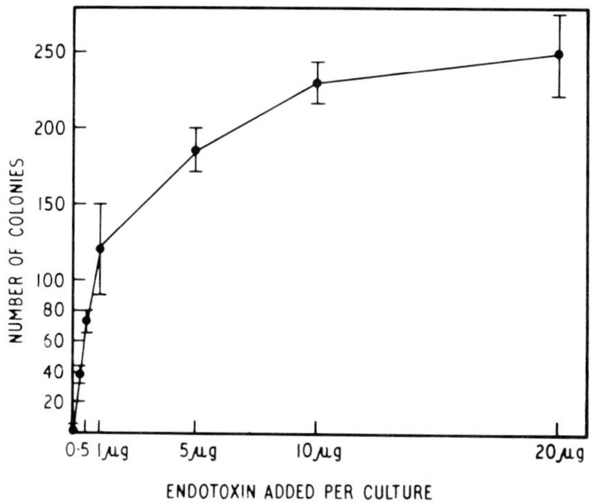

Fig. 44. Potentiating effects of endotoxin on B-lymphocyte colony formation in 1 ml cultures of 25,000 C_{57}BL spleen cells. (From METCALF, [61]. Reproduced with permission from J. Immunol.)

1. It has been shown by KINCADE et al. [380] that agar contains an extractable factor capable of stimulating B-lymphocyte colony formation in the presence of 2-mercaptoethanol, the factor possibly being polysaccharide in nature. B-lymphocyte colony formation in the presence of 2-mercaptoethanol did not occur in agarose but became possible when material extracted from agar was added.
2. As mentioned above, spleen and lymph node populations in the presence of 2-mercaptoethanol release or secrete a factor potentiating B-lymphocyte colony formation [61].
3. Addition of small numbers of macrophages from the spleen or peritoneal populations had a strong potentiating effect on colony growth [381].
4. Some potentiating activity was also observed following the addition of large numbers of thymic or irradiated spleen or lymph node cells [28].

As a minimal hypothesis, it might be speculated that a specific stimulating factor for B-lymphocyte colony formation is produced by macrophages in the presence of 2-mercaptoethanol and that this specific factor (equivalent to GM-CSF) is actively produced within the culture dish during colony formation.

Evidence for a B-lymphocyte growth factor of possibly another type has been obtained by METCALF and KOLBER [382] in a survey of the effects of different human sera on B-lymphocyte colony formation by mouse spleen cells. The vast majority of undiluted sera from normal blood donors or patients with nonneoplastic hemopoietic diseases or diseases of other organ systems either partially or completely inhibited colony formation (Table 25). This inhibitory effect may be due to the light density lipoproteins in serum since these light density fractions from mouse serum were found to be equally capable of inhibiting granulocytic and macrophage colony formation or B-lymphocyte colony formation [102].

In contrast, undiluted sera from 43–53% of patients with histiocytic lymphoma, Hodgkin's disease, or lymphocytic lymphoma stimulated B-lymphocyte colony formation. The degree of activity shown by the sera paralleled the clinical stage of the disease, being low in early Stage I and II patients, high in Stage III and IV patients and low again in remission patients.

Colony-stimulating activity was low or undetectable in three other diseases involving B-

Table 25. Potentiating effect of human sera on B-lymphocyte colony formation by mouse spleen cells

Disease state	No. of active sera/No. tested[a]	% Active sera
Normal blood donors	12/119	10%
Miscellaneous hemopoietic disorders[b]	2/47	4%
Histiocytic lymphoma	19/36	53%
Hodgkin's disease	25/54	46%
Lymphocytic lymphoma	40/92	43%
Multiple myeloma	6/19	28%
CLL	4/20	20%
ALL	7/15	47%
AML	30/57	53%
CML	4/14	29%
Myeloproliferative disorders	2/7	29%
Cancer (nonhemopoietic)	1/19	5%
Chronic renal disease	6/71	8%
Cardiovascular disease	0/20	0%
Autoimmune disease	1/31	3%
Gastrointestinal disease	1/9	11%
Miscellaneous other diseases	3/35	9%

[a] Sera were classified as active if more than 10 colonies developed in cultures of 25,000 $C_{57}BL$ spleen cells containing 0.1 ml of undiluted serum.
[b] Patients with iron deficiency anemia, macrocytic or hemolytic anemia, or polycythemia vera.
Data from METCALF and KOLBER [382].

lymphocytes—multiple myeloma, CLL, and autoimmune diseases. Of some interest was the fact that about half the sera from patients with ALL and AML showed moderate colony-stimulating activity but only after chemotherapy had been commenced.

Endotoxin and red cells were excluded as possible causes of the observed stimulating effect, and no correlation was observed between stimulating activity and donor blood group, serum hemoglobin, serum mouse red cell hemagglutinin titers, or serum GM-CSF levels.

The specificity and significance of this serum B-lymphocyte stimulating factor need to be explored in further studies, but potentially it is a candidate regulatory factor comparable with GM-CSF. The source of the factor is unknown, but it might conceivably be derived from neoplastic lymphoid cells or from normal host lymphoid or macrophage populations reacting to such cells. Such a factor might be released following cell damage induced by cytotoxic drugs in acute leukemia treatment although colony-stimulating activity in the serum was not observed to be elevated in patients with cancer or autoimmune diseases who were undergoing chemotherapy.

While B-lymphocyte colony formation remains a little unusual in its apparent growth requirements, the above fragmentary pieces of evidence are sufficient to make it possible that a specific B-lymphocyte growth-stimulating factor might be necessary for B-lymphocyte colony formation and might occur in vivo. Such a factor might be similar to the growth-stimulating blastogenic factor (or lymphokine) which numerous authors have reported to develop in liquid cultures of antigen or mitogen-stimulated lymphocytes [383, 384].

C. B-Lymphocyte Colony-Forming Cells (BL-CFC)

In young adult $C_{57}BL$ mice, the frequency of cells giving rise to B-lymphocyte colonies was determined in cultures supplemented by 0.1 ml of 10% sheep red cells to obtain maximal incidence figures. The data (Table 26) indicated that approximately one cell in 100–200 lymph node, spleen, thoracic duct, or peripheral blood cells formed a colony while cluster-forming cells, as mentioned above, were 5 times more frequent. Colony-forming cells were also common in pleural and peritoneal cavity populations. Bone marrow cells formed typical B-lymphocyte colonies, but the frequency of colony-forming cells was only about one-quarter to one-tenth that in lymph nodes or spleen. The most striking finding in this survey was that colony-forming cells were essentially absent from the thymus.

The data shown in Table 26 were obtained from a simultaneous series of cultures and give a valid estimate of the relative frequency of colony-forming cells in different tissues. However, subsequent experiments have shown that with optimal culture conditions, the frequency of colony-forming cells in spleen populations is at least one colony-forming cell per 30 cells. This, together with the higher frequency of cluster-forming cells, means that approximately 10–20% of all spleen cells are capable of proliferating in these agar cultures.

Comparative studies on the spleen in $C_{57}BL$, CBA, BALB/c, SJL, NZB, and nu/nu mice indicated that the frequency of colony-forming cells in the spleen was very similar in these strains with, if anything, a higher frequency in nu/nu (congenitally athymic) mice [381].

The SJL thymus has been shown to be abnormal in that, with increasing age, it accumulates a progressively increasing percentage of B-lymphocytes [385]. An analysis of the SJL thymus has shown an age-related rise in the content of BL-CFCs, and reciprocal thymus grafts between old and young animals showed that this was due to the development in old animals of a thymus-seeking population of BL-CFCs or cells capable of generating BL-CFCs [386].

Analysis of CBA and (CBA × $C_{57}BL)F_1$ embryos failed to detect BL-CFCs in the yolk sac at any stage of development. BL-CFCs first became detectable in the fetal liver at 17 days of gestation, and on the following day, these were detectable in the peripheral blood, spleen, and bone marrow. Levels in these latter tissues rose rapidly and reached adult values by 2

Table 26. Frequency of B-lymphocyte colony-forming cells in various tissues in young adult $C_{57}BL$ mice[a]

Tissue	Colony-forming cells per 10^6 cells
Spleen	8290 ± 4530
Subcutaneous lymph nodes	5500 ± 2800
Mesenteric lymph nodes	5400 + 2640
Peyer's patches	11,560 ± 3740
Peripheral blood	3760 ± 3090
Thoracic duct	4700 ± 3800
Thymus	9 ± 9
Bone marrow	1110 ± 420
Peritoneal cells	2670 ± 1360
Pleural cells	5540 ± 3370

[a] Data from METCALF et al. [28].

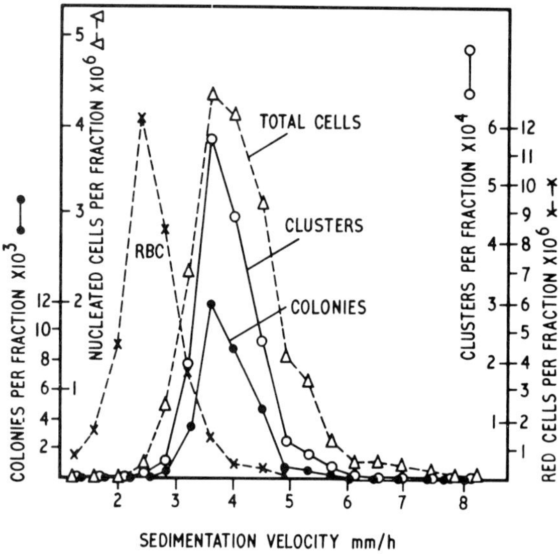

Fig. 45. Velocity sedimentation separation of $C_{57}BL$ spleen cells showing the distribution of red cells, total nucleated cells, and the cells forming clusters and colonies of B-lymphocytes. Note coincidence of colony-forming cell peak with that of spleen small lymphocytes. (From METCALF et al., [381]. Reproduced with permission from J. Cell. Physiol.)

days after birth [387]. Organ culture experiments in which intact 15-day fetal livers or spleens were cultured on millipore membranes for 5 days showed that in both organs BL-CFCs were able to develop independently from cell populations not detectable with the culture system used.

In another study [395], it was shown that BL-CFCs appear early in spleen colonies generated by CFUs in irradiated recipients. Using either adult marrow or 12-day fetal liver CFUs, 50–80% of colonies contained BL-CFCs by day 8 (Table 27) even though the primary

Table 27. Presence of B-lymphocyte colony-forming cells in spleen colonies formed by stem cells from adult marrow or 12-day fetal liver cells

Age of colonies in days	No. of colonies containing BL-CFCs/No. tested CBA BM→CBA	CBA FL→CBA	$C_{57}BL$ BM→$C_{57}BL$
7	—	—	1/15
8	16/20	9/17	6/15
9	9/20	15/20	4/36
10	19/40	—	9/16
11	4/10	—	1/8
12	—	7/13	69/100
13	—	4/14	—

BM = 3-month bone marrow cells FL = 12-day fetal liver cells.
Data from METCALF and JOHNSON [395].

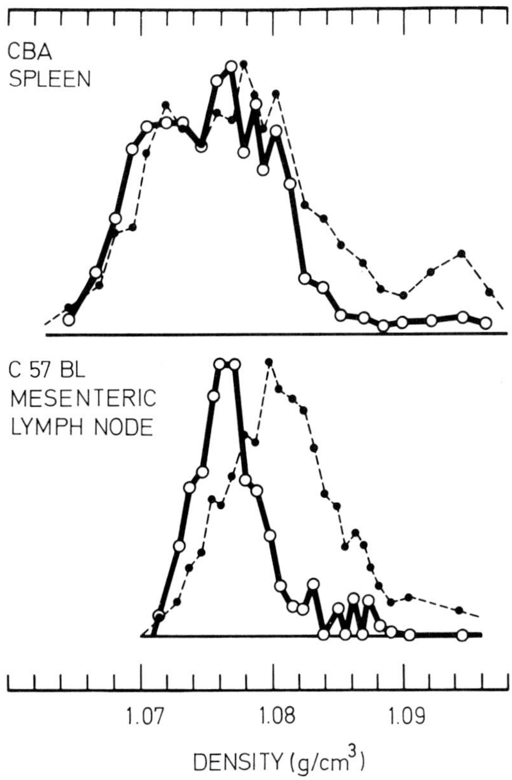

Fig. 46. Buoyant density separation of B-lymphocyte colony-forming cells in CBA spleen and C_{57}BL lymph node using continuous gradients of BSA. Data plotted as percent of numbers in fraction containing highest number of nucleated cells (broken line) or colony-forming cells (solid line). Note organ and strain variation but tendency of BL-CFC to be of relatively light buoyant density. (From METCALF et al., [381]. Reproduced with permission from J. Cell. Physiol.)

morphology of these colonies was either erythroid or granulocytic. A considerable animal to animal variation was observed in the levels of BL-CFCs in spleen colonies which may indicate that antigenic stimulation can influence the rate of appearance of these cells in colonies or that these cells may not be true members of the colony clone but have seeded out in the colonies from the circulation. This intriguing possibility is in need of further investigation, but the data so far obtained suggest that B-lymphocytes may not be as separate a population from other hemopoietic cells as was previously believed.

These data indicated (1) that BL-CFCs are cells which appear relatively late in embryonic development, (2) BL-CFCs and cluster-forming cells comprise 10–20% of the population in spleen and lymph nodes and are common in bone marrow, peripheral blood, and thoracic duct lymph, (3) the frequency of BL-CFCs is normal or higher than normal in nu/nu (T-lymphocyte deficient mice), and (4) BL-CFCs are almost certainly recirculating cells. Taken together, the data suggest strongly that BL-CFCs are in fact B-lymphocytes of a relatively mature type since virgin B-lymphocytes are believed not to recirculate.

Direct studies on the nature of BL-CFCs have supported these conclusions [381]. BL-CFCs were not destroyed by anti-θ (anti-Thy-1) sera in the presence of complement, but more than

90% formed Fc rosettes with antibody-coated sheep red cells. Most BL-CFCs were nonadherent to glass bead columns or Petri dishes, but, as mentioned earlier, addition of cells from the adherent population greatly potentiated colony formation by the BL-CFCs in the nonadherent fractions. In both fetal liver and adult spleen and lymph nodes, BL-CFCs sedimented as a single peak with a peak sedimentation velocity of 3.5 mm per h (that of small lymphocytes) (Fig. 45) although some BL-CFCs were present in all fractions indicating that some were of larger size. The buoyant density of BL-CFCs in spleen or lymph node populations was heterogeneous although most were slightly lighter in density than average (Fig. 46)—behavior typical of B-lymphocytes in these populations. Since BL-CFCs with NIP-binding capacity could be selectively enriched on NIP-gelatin slabs, it can be deduced that BL-CFCs must themselves exhibit immunoglobulin on their cell surface. Colony-forming cells were shown to be sensitive to cortisone and to whole body irradiation ($D_0$60 rads) [381].

The conclusion from these observations is that BL-CFCs are cells which themselves exhibit the properties of B-lymphocytes. Since 10–20% of spleen and lymph node populations proliferate and these populations contain less than 50% B-lymphocytes, one of two conclusions can be made: (1) the agar cultures are capable of growing all B-lymphocytes with an overall plating efficiency of 20–40%, or (2) the agar cultures may be capable of growing one or more major subpopulations of B-lymphocytes with a very high plating efficiency.

Until more is known about the properties of such B-lymphocyte populations as pre-B cells, virgin or naive B-lymphocytes, memory B-lymphocytes, etc., a functional identification of BL-CFCs cannot be made. However, from their late embryonic development, their ability to recirculate and their size, membrane immunoglobulin and Ia content, it is likely that BL-CFCs are not pre-B cells. The definition of pre-B cells is a little vague but corresponds roughly to progenitor cells in other hemopoietic classes. If the above interpretations are correct, B-lymphocyte colony formation differs sharply from the other types of hemopoietic colony formation in that the colony-forming cells are not progenitor cells but more numerous and more differentiated members of the B-lymphocyte class. To this difference may eventually be added an independence of specific regulators but this question has certainly not been settled at present.

D. Alternative B-Lymphocyte Culture Systems

ROZENSZAJN et al. [388] have reported an alternative method for obtaining B-lymphocyte colonies in vitro. This involves a two-stage culture system which will be described in full in connection with T-lymphocyte colony formation. In brief, mouse spleen or lymph node cells are incubated overnight in liquid cultures with endotoxin. After 15 h of incubation, the cells are cultured in agar medium over underlayers containing endotoxin. The system does not require the addition of 2-mercaptoethanol.

The reported frequency of colony-forming cells is approximately one per 1000 cells in spleen and lymph node populations and none in the thymus. The frequency of colonies was normal in nu/nu (congenitally athymic) mice. The colonies have yet to be thoroughly characterized as being composed of B-lymphocytes, but 90% of colony cells were reported to have detectable membrane immunoglobulin.

The relation of these colonies to those described earlier remains to be determined. The frequency of the colony-forming cells is at least tenfold lower than in the mercaptoethanol single-step culture system. This may simply reflect a less efficient culture system in the absence of mercaptoethanol or may indicate that a particular subpopulation of B-lymphocyte colony-forming cells is being cultured.

A similar system was reported by FIBACH et al. [389] in which human peripheral blood cells were incubated for 24 h with pokeweed mitogen, then cultured in agar over underlayers containing pokeweed mitogen. The frequency of colonies was 170 $\pm$ 33 per 5 $\times$ 10^5 cultured cells and the colonies contained up to 200 cells by day 7. Mass-harvested cells exhibited properties of both T and B cells—60% of the cells formed E rosettes (T cell marker), 25% formed EA and EAC rosettes (B cell markers), and 10% were stained with an anti-immunoglobulin (B cell marker). No report was made of an analysis on individual colonies, and the most likely explanation of the above observations is that a mixture of T and B colonies was present (or that T colonies were present together with surviving B-lymphocytes in the surrounding agar).

E. Comments

The capacity to grow clones of B-lymphocytes which are capable of specific immunoglobulin synthesis should represent an extremely useful ancillary technique for cellular immunologists despite the disadvantage of agar for harvesting cultured cells.

The culture system could be used to monitor B-lymphocyte responses to infections or tumors (particularly B-lymphoid tumors) and might well be able to be adapted to simultaneously detect colonies producing a specific antibody, e.g., by plaque formation around individual colonies.

Little evidence has been obtained so far that addition of antigen modifies the number or growth rate of B-lymphocyte colonies from preimmunized or unimmunized animals. It may be that mercaptoethanol and the agar mitogen are such a powerful polyclonal stimuli that they override or obscure the weaker mitogenic stimulus of specific antigens. Alternatively, it might be that MOLLER and COUTINHO [390] are correct in asserting that there is no such thing as specific antigen-immunoglobulin signaling for B-lymphocyte proliferation, simply a single nonspecific trigger stimulus—which in the present cultures is provided by the mercaptoethanol in conjunction with the agar factor.

F. Human T-Lymphocyte Colonies

The growth of colonies in agar cultures of mouse thymic lymphocytes was claimed in a brief report by BUJADOUX et al. [391]. In the apparent absence of any mitogen and in serum-free medium, colonies of small lymphocytes were reported to develop. The frequency of colony-forming cells was approximately one per 10^3 cells, and the number and growth rate of such colonies were increased by the addition of syngeneic red cells. No studies on surface characteristics of the colony cells were reported.

In subsequent studies, a two-stage method was developed by ROZENSZAJN et al. [29] in which human lymphocytes are first cultured in liquid with PHA, then, after an interval, the cells are washed and cultured in agar either on underlayers containing PHA or in a single layer culture system containing PHA.

In the technique, peripheral blood lymphocytes are separated from other white cells on glass columns [392], then cultured in Eagle's medium containing 20% autologous plasma and 1% bacto phytohemagglutinin M (Difco). After 15–18 h, the cells are washed and 10^6 cells cultured in 60 mm Petri dishes as a 1.7 ml layer containing approximately 0.3% agar in Eagle's medium with 18% FCS on a 5 ml underlayer containing 0.5% agar in Eagle's medium containing 20% FCS and 0.0625 ml of PHA.
The number of colonies developing depended on the length of the preliminary liquid culture phase, and for optimal colony formation, a minimum period of 12 h was necessary.
Although colony formation was maximal when PHA was included in the underlayer, some colony formation was possible when PHA was present in the lymphocyte-containing layer.
At high cell concentrations, a linear relationship was reported between the number of cells cultured and the number of colonies developing, and the frequency of colony-forming cells in the peripheral blood was one per 2000–3000 lymphocytes. In the spleen, the frequency of colonies per 10^6 cells was 60–150 and in the bone marrow 60–100. Colony size was maximal by 7–8 days of incubation, and colonies contained up to 500 large mononuclear blast cells. Karyotypic analysis of the dividing colony cells indicated a normal chromosome number. The morphology of the colony cells resembled that of PHA-transformed cells in liquid culture, and in the electronmicroscope the cells contained prominent nuclei, abundant ribosomes, and short filaments of endoplasmic reticulum. The cells were positive for esterase but negative for peroxidase, PAS, Luxol green, or toluidine blue. About 50–75% of colony cells formed rosettes with sheep red cells, and no membrane immunoglobulin was detectable by immunofluorescence.
In a subsequent study, FIBACH et al. [389] confirmed these observations using normal human lymphocytes isolated from peripheral blood on Ficoll-hypaque gradients. The frequency of colonies was 491 per 5×10^5 cells, and colony formation was shown to be nonlinear, falling to zero with cell concentrations below 10^5 cells per ml. Colonies also developed if pokeweed mitogen was substituted for PHA although the frequency of colonies obtained was only one-third of that with PHA. Mercaptoethanol was stated not to increase colony formation.
PHA or pokeweed mitogen were required continuously in both phases of the culture system, and a dependency of colony formation on the particular batch of FCS or human serum used is apparent from the conflicting published descriptions.
In mass-harvested colonies from pokeweed-stimulated cultures, about 10% of cells reacted with a fluorescent anti-Ig serum, and 25% of cells formed EA and EAC rosettes, suggesting that some colonies may have been composed of B-lymphocytes.
WILSON and DALTON [393] analyzed the potential value of the two-stage PHA-stimulated human T-lymphocyte colonies as an index of immunological reactivity in cancer patients. In normal subjects, 1000–2500 colonies formed per 10^6 peripheral blood lymphocytes, and 65% of the colony cells formed rosettes with AET-treated sheep red cells. The frequency of colony-forming cells was lower in the blood of cancer patients (350–1000 colonies per 10^6 lymphocytes). The depression of T-lymphocyte colony-forming cells was seen in all of 17 cancer patients analyzed and was a more consistent finding than depressed responsiveness as assessed by skin tests with five recall antigens or depressed thymidine incorporation by PHA-stimulated liquid cultures of the same peripheral blood lymphocytes.
CLAESSON et al. [394] developed an improved method for culturing T-lymphocyte colonies from human peripheral blood. Addition of sheep red cells to the culture medium (see Chapter 3) increased the frequency of colonies and even permitted the use of a single-step culture system, provided the polymorphs were first removed. The frequency of colonies in the one-step method was lower than in the two-step method, but agglutination problems were

avoided. Preliminary evidence has been obtained that if adherent mononuclear cells are added as an underlayer in these one-stage cultures, a colony frequency equal to that in the two-stage method is obtained (CLAESSON, M. H., unpublished data).

The maximum frequency of colony-forming cells observed with the improved two-stage method was one per 100 peripheral blood mononuclear cells and approximately 5% of all cells proliferated to form smaller aggregates. Up to 80% of colony cells exhibited rosette formation with sheep red cells, and no immunoglobulin-bearing cells were detected. Colony-forming cells were shown to have the sedimentation velocity of human small lymphocytes (4.0 mm/h), 90% had a density between 1.069–1.077 g/cm^3, most were found not to be in cell cycle, and most were able to be removed prior to culture by rosetting with sheep red cells [394].

The data suggest strongly that most of the cells forming T-lymphocyte colonies are small lymphocytes with properties identifying them as T-lymphocytes.

G. Mouse T-Lymphocyte Colonies

The general technique for growing human T-lymphocyte colonies was adapted by SREDNI et al. [89] for the growth of mouse T-lymphocyte colonies. Lymph node or spleen cells were cultured in liquid for 49 h with either PHA-M (Difco 0.0125 ml/ml) or Concanavalin A (Difco 30μg/ml) in Eagle's medium with 5% heat inactivated human serum. The cells were then washed and cultured in a double layer system, the upper layer containing the lymphoid cells and the lower layer containing the appropriate mitogen. Colonies reached up to 1000 cells by day 7–8 before degenerating. The maximum observed frequency of colony-forming cells in lymph nodes was only one per 10^4 cells, and no colonies were observed in cultures of nu/nu (congenitally athymic) mice. Harvested colony cells reacted positively with fluorescein-conjugated anti-θ (Thy-1) sera.

H. Comment

It seems clear from the above observations that it is possible to grow colonies of T-lymphocytes from human or mouse cells as a two-stage procedure using one or other of the known T cell mitogens—PHA, pokeweed mitogen, or Concanavalin A. There has been no formal proof that the colonies are clones, and as the precultured cells in the two-stage culture system are agglutinated and difficult to redisperse before reculture in agar, attention needs to be paid to this problem by the use of a number of antigenic markers available for T-lymphocyte subpopulations.

The nature of the cells forming the T-lymphocyte colonies is also in need of clarification. For both human and mouse peripheral blood or lymphoid populations the frequency of colony-forming cells as assessed by the two-stage system is very low, one per 2000–10,000 cells. These observations suggest very strongly that the cells forming T-lymphocyte colonies may not be typical T-lymphocytes and might well be a very small subpopulation of T-lymphocyte progenitor cells. The alternative is that two-stage cultures have an extremely low plating efficiency.

Using a modified one-stage or two-stage system including sheep red cells with or without added macrophages, a frequency of TL-CFCs of one per 100 peripheral blood mononuclear cells was obtained, and 5% of the cells exhibited some degree of proliferation [394]. The situation with human T-lymphocyte colonies is now approaching that with mouse B-lymhpocyte colonies. Either *all* peripheral blood T-lymphocytes are capable of proliferation (with a current plating efficiency of 5%) or the proliferating cells are a major subpopulation of peripheral T-lymphocytes, and hence presumably relatively mature cells.

Published accounts have been silent about the capacity or otherwise of *thymic* lymphocytes to proliferate and imply by default that only peripheral T-lymphocytes are able to proliferate. There is an urgent need to develop a reliable method for growing mouse T-lymphocyte colonies so that available selective antisera can be applied to determine which of the known subpopulations of T-lymphocytes can be grown in the agar culture system, e.g., cytotoxic cells, helper cells, suppressor cells, etc. and to determine at what stage of maturation these cells are.

The reported nonlinearity of the T colony-forming system at low cell concentrations suggests the operation of a growth factor produced in the culture dish, and in this respect, the T colony-forming system may again share features in common with the B-lymphocyte colony-forming system.

The general application of B and T-lymphocyte cloning systems should allow many aspects of the control of lymphoid populations to be clarified. Although the general disadvantage of the agar is apparent, it has not precluded studies on harvested colony cells, and the speed and simplicity of colony counting not only offers an exact method for assessing overall proliferation but offers the unique opportunity for analyzing the progeny of large numbers of individual cells.

Chapter 12

Neoplastic Lymphoid and Plasmacytoma Colonies

A. Lymphoid Leukemic Cells

Historically, lymphoid leukemic cells were the first hemopoietic cells to be cloned in agar. Despite this, it must be said that relatively little use has been made so far of the capacity of some transplantable mouse lymphoid tumors to form colonies in semisolid medium.

Many unsuccessful attempts have been made to culture spontaneous or primary lymphoid leukemias induced in mice by leukemia viruses or whole body irradiation. It was the consistent failure to grow AKR lymphoid leukemias in agar that originally led to the trial of feeder layer cultures and the accidental discovery that normal granulocytic and macrophage colonies developed in these feeder layers [4].

The situation is different with a number of long transplanted lymphoid leukemias in mice, particularly where the transplanted leukemias have been adapted to growth in liquid culture. Such leukemic cells can often proliferate in agar and generate large numbers of colonies of uniform size which sometimes tend to disintegrate early (after 5–7 days of incubation). The growth rate and frequency of colonies was not influenced by addition of high concentrations of GM-CSF (METCALF, D., unpublished data), but the influence of mitogens and mercaptoethanol has not been studied systematically. Recent studies on the growth in agar of cells from two transplanted murine B leukemias have shown them to be dependent on the addition of 2-mercaptoethanol for successful colony formation (HARRIS, A., personal communication).

The lipoproteins in mouse serum that inhibit GM-colony formation are also capable of inhibiting colony formation in agar by lymphoid leukemic and plasmacytoma cells (Fig. 47). As in the case of inhibition of GM-colony formation, it is quite uncertain whether this phenomenon represents anything more than an in vitro artifact.

By choice of a transplanted lymphoid tumor with a high cloning efficiency in agar and capable of forming tight, distinctive colonies of uniform size, experiments can be performed that are not yet possible with the myeloid leukemias. Thus, in cultures of cells from mouse spleen or lymph nodes being infiltrated by the leukemic cells, it is possible in the same culture dish to enumerate leukemic cells and also B-lymphocyte colony-forming cells (Fig. 48). Similar experiments can be performed using transplanted plasmacytomas. It has been reported that antibody-forming populations are selectively suppressed in mice bearing plasmacytomas [396], perhaps by some control system responding to total B cell numbers. However, in a study to test this proposition in mice bearing transplanted T leukemias, B leukemias, or plasmacytomas, all capable of colony formation in vitro, no selective suppression of normal BL-CFCs was observed in mice carrying either plasmacytomas or B leukemias (CLAESSON, M. H., unpublished data). Although the frequency of BL-CFCs in spleen and draining lymph nodes fell as the organs became progressively enlarged by the proliferation of tumor cells, calculations showed that total BL-CFC numbers were, if anything, higher than normal.

Lymphoid leukemic cells from patients with CLL or ALL do not proliferate in the standard

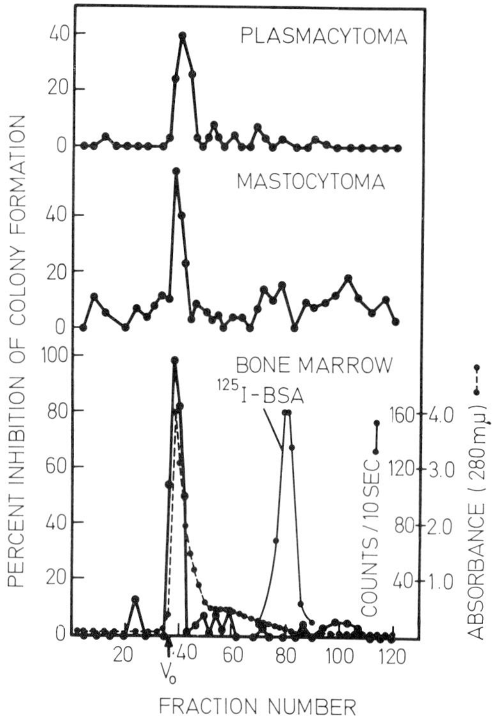

Fig. 47. Fractionation of light density lipoproteins from BALB/c serum on Sepharose 6B. Fractions assayed for inhibitory activity on GM-colonies produced by $C_{57}BL$ marrow cells, P815 mastocytoma cells, and a BALB/c plasmacytoma. (From METCALF and RUSSELL, [102]. Reproduced with permission from Exp. Hematol.)

agar culture system used for obtaining granulocytic and macrophage colonies, and no system has yet been reported which permits their clonal proliferation.

Various human lymphocytic cell lines which have been adapted to growth in vitro can produce colonies in agar. Studies have shown that the ability of such cells to adapt to continuous growth in liquid cultures depends on infection of the cells by the Epstein-Barr virus [397, 398]. The cell lines in most cases have been shown to be B-lymphocytes, and these transformed cells may well exhibit properties like leukemic cells or intermediate between those of normal and leukemic cells. The colonies produced in agar are regular in size and do not require the addition of mitogens or mercaptoethanol. They have been used in a number of studies on immunoglobulin production by cloned populations [399, 2].

In an interesting study, YAMAMOTO and HINUMA [400] demonstrated that exposure of human umbilical cord leukocytes in vitro to Epstein-Barr virus for 1 h permitted these cells to form progressively growing colonies in agar. These represented transformed cells since normal umbilical cord cells were unable to form colonies under the conditions used. A one-hit response relationship was observed between the number of colonies and the virus dose used. Colony cells were demonstrated by immunological methods to carry EBV-associated nuclear antigen, and viral transformation was prevented by the use of human sera containing EBV antibodies.

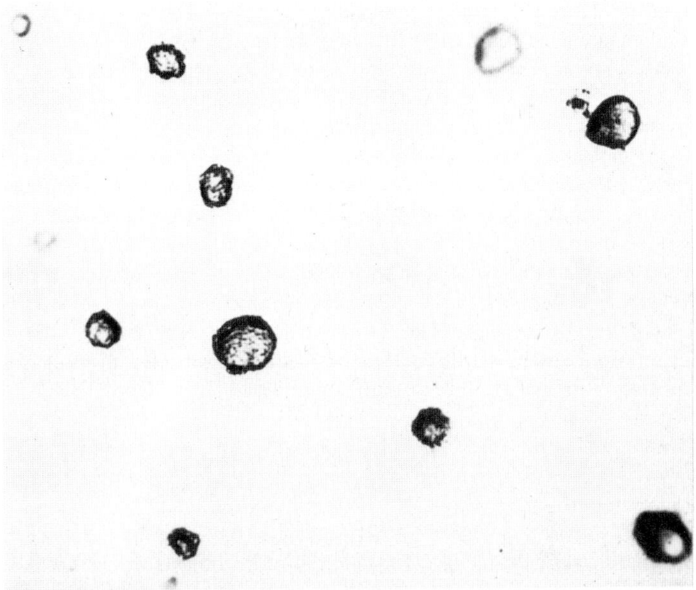

Fig. 48. Colonies of mouse B-leukemic cells (ABE-8) growing in agar. Note characteristic compact nature of the ABE-8 colonies compared with loose normal B-lymphocyte colonies as seen in Figure 40

B. Plasmacytoma Cells

As is true of most mouse lymphoid leukemias, most transplantable mouse plasmacytomas also fail to proliferate when cultured in agar medium. Exceptions are a few plasmacytomas which have been adapted to growth in liquid culture and these produce uniform colonies with high plating efficiency. Although plasmacytomas that have been adapted to continuous culture are uncommon and the tumor cells could be questioned as no longer being representative of the original tumor population, these plasmacytomas have proved of considerable value in analyzing the biosynthesis of immunoglobulins. SCHARFF and his coworkers [401] have cloned such plasmacytomas in agar and identified immunoglobulin-secreting clones by the addition of specific antisera to the cultures. Colonies producing immunoglobulin of a particular type are identified by the halo of antigen-antibody precipitate around the colony. Because every colony can be assumed to be a clone, culture of plasmacytomas in semisolid agar is a very useful screening procedure for rapidly examining many clones for possible mutants with an abnormal pathway of immunoglobulin synthesis.

Despite their value for studies in molecular biology, it is doubtful whether such plasmacytomas can offer much information of value for the analysis of factors regulating the growth and differentiation of this type of hemopoietic cell. The selection processes involved in obtaining successful adaptation to tissue culture are obviously severe, and cells adapting to in vitro conditions are likely to have undergone mutations or to represent a highly selected population derived from similar mutational episodes in vivo.

Plasmacytomas are unusual tumors in that, on continued transplantation, progressive changes, e.g., in cellular biosynthetic activity or chromosomal complement, are slow to occur relative to many other transplantable tumors. Such plasmacytoma cell lines can be transplanted for years and still continue to secrete a unique species of immunoglobulin—a relative stability which is not often seen in transplantable tumors.

Because of their relative stability it is possible that *recently* established transplantable plasmacytomas might still be useful populations to analyze in terms of their responsiveness to, or dependence on, various regulatory factors. Cells from most such plasmacytomas fail to form colonies in standard agar cultures. However, it was demonstrated by PARK et al. [402] that serially transplantable plasmacytomas would grow in agar if freshly prepared medium was used. Investigation showed that these cells had a specific requirement for ascorbic acid to proliferate in vitro and could form colonies if the medium was supplemented by the addition of ascorbic acid. In a modification of this technique, PARK et al. [403] also included underlayers of kidney tubules. Other studies by COFFINO et al. [404] showed that feeder layers of mouse, human, or rabbit cells or media conditioned by such cells could enhance colony formation in agar by three plasmacytomas which had previously been adapted to growth in vitro.

These studies raised the possibility of culturing plasmacytomas in agar by adding various growth factors although the studies were restricted to tumors that had already been adapted to in vitro growth.

In the course of a study by METCALF on the stromal tissue of transplantable tumors, a technique was used for growing colonies of fibroblasts from fibroblast progenitor cells [21]. In this technique, standard agar medium is supplemented by whole blood of which the plasma appears to be the important component for fibroblast colony formation. Some of the tumors were transplantable plasmacytomas, and it was observed that, when suspensions of tumor cells were cultured in medium containing whole blood, the plasmacytoma cells were capable of colony formation [23]. The colonies were characteristically compact and of relatively uniform size (Fig. 49) and colony cells had the morphology of plasmacytoma cells. Based on this phenomenon, a survey of other transplantable plasmacytomas showed that 19 of 25 could be cloned in agar if the medium was supplemented by whole mouse blood or washed red cells. The cloning efficiency for such tumors varied widely from 0.01% to 20%. In agreement with the observation of COFFINO et al. [404], some potentiation of colony formation was also

Fig. 49. Low power view of 7-day plasmacytoma colonies growing in medium containing sheep red cells

observed if thymic, spleen, or marrow cells were added to the cultures. The potentiation of plasmacytoma colony formation by whole red cells is very similar to the phenomenon in which colony formation by normal B-lymphocytes is potentiated by red cells [28]. It is reasonable to assume that the two phenomena are based on the same mechanism although this is as yet uncharacterized. As was true for normal B-lymphocyte colony formation, hemolyzed cells were not able to potentiate colony formation, and allogeneic or xenogeneic red cells were as effective as syngeneic cells in promoting plasmacytoma colony formation. Intimate contact was not required between the red cells and plasmacytoma cells for potentiation, and the red cells were as effective if used in an underlayer.

The potentiating effects of red cells on plasmacytoma colony formation appeared to be specific since no similar potentiation was observed with a series of myelomoncytic leukemias, fibrosarcomas, reticulum cell sarcomas, or T-lymphomas which were able to form colonies in agar.

In further studies with these plasmacytomas. it was shown that serum from mice injected with endotoxin also had the capacity to stimulate colony formation by some but not all plasmacytomas [23, 26]. Serum colony-stimulating activity arose sharply to a peak 2–3 h after endotoxin injection and had essentially returned to preinjection (inactive) levels by 6 h after

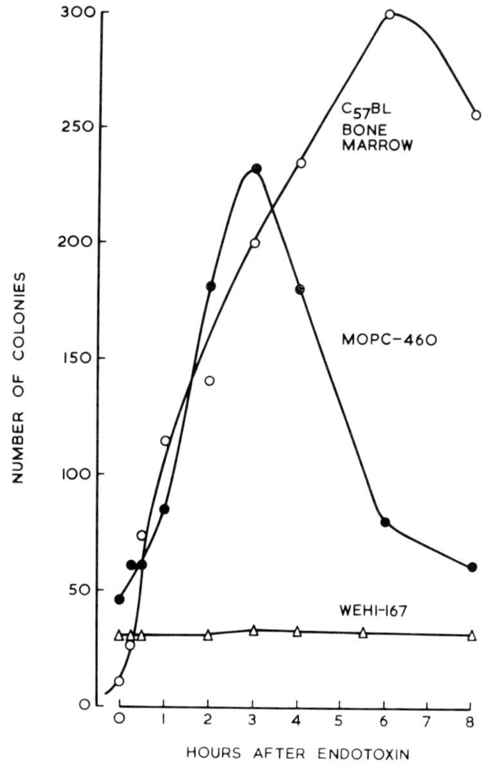

Fig. 50. Capacity of serum from $C_{57}BL$ mice injected with 5 μg endotoxin to stimulate GM-colony formation by $C_{57}BL$ marrow cells and colony formation by the plasmacytoma MOPC-460. Note that sera are inactive in cultures of the fibrosarcoma WEHI-167 and that there is no temporal correspondence between the peak GM-CSF content and peak activity in stimulating plasmacytoma colony formation. (From METCALF, [23]. Reproduced with permission from J. Cell. Physiol.)

injection (Fig. 50). This serum colony-stimulating activity again seemed to be specific for plasmacytoma cells, and the sera did not stimulate colony formation by other types of tumor cells. Direct addition of endotoxin to the culture dish did not stimulate colony formation. However, these experiments were performed before the critical importance of the type of FCS being used was recognized, and in the studies on plasmacytoma colony potentiation, only one batch of FCS was used. The negative effects with added endotoxin can therefore only be considered as a provisional observation.

Plasmacytoma colony formation was not stimulated by a variety of GM-CSF preparations, and the factor in post endotoxin serum stimulating plasmacytoma growth could be separated as a single peak in the β-region, separate from the GM-CSF in such serum (Fig. 51) [26]. Endotoxin was able to induce the appearance of plasmacytoma colony-stimulating activity in the sera of a number of mouse strains including the nu/nu (congenitally athymic) mouse, implying that production of the factor was not dependent on T-lymphocytes. Production of the active factor was also radioresistant. The onset of colony formation in unstimulated cultures was asynchronous, and in cultures containing added postendotoxin serum, the asynchrony persisted, but the number and rate of initiation of colonies were sharply increased.

A similar rise in serum colony-stimulating activity for plasmacytoma cells was able to be induced by the injection of the bacterial antigen, polymerized flagellin, and it was shown that preimmunization with this antigen prevented the development of serum colony-stimulating

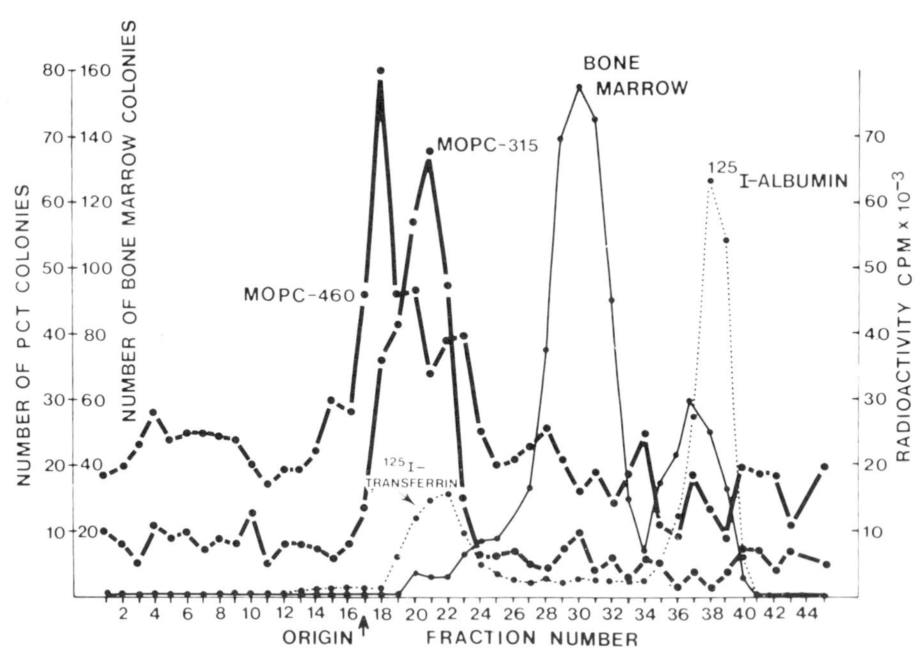

Fig. 51. Starch block electrophoretic separation of serum from $C_{57}BL$ mice injected 2 h previously with 5 μg endotoxin and assayed for GM-colony-stimulating activity on $C_{57}BL$ marrow cells or for colony-stimulating activity for two plasmacytomas, MOPC-315 and MOPC-460. Note peak of plasmacytoma-stimulating activity in the β-region, well separated from the GM-CSF. (From METCALF, [26]. Reproduced with permission from J. Immunol.)

activity following a challenge antigen injection [23]. A number of other bacterial antigens were also shown to be able to induce colony-stimulating activity [26]. It was also observed that the addition of 2-mercaptoethanol in molar concentrations of 10^{-4}–10^{-5} had a strong potentiating effect on colony formation by a number of plasmacytomas [26].

A high frequency of plasmacytomas can be induced in BALB/c and NZB mice by the injection of mineral oil, and the first generation transplantation of such tumors is also greatly facilitated by the preinjection of recipients with mineral oil [405]. In view of these observations, it was of some interest that the injection of mineral oil increased the capacity of serum to stimulate the plasmacytoma colony formation in vitro [26]. Injection of mineral oil also increased the capacity of peritoneal cells to stimulate plasmacytoma colony formation in mixed cultures of plasmacytoma and peritoneal cells. Essentially similar observations have been made by NAMBA and HANAOKA [406] on the growth requirements of a plasmacytoma (MOPC-104) in liquid cultures. Growth was stimulated by medium conditioned by macrophages or the serum of mice injected with Freund's adjuvant.

C. Comments

A number of comments can be made about the above observations on plasmacytoma colony formation:

1. Use of supplemental red cells permits most mouse plasmacytomas to be cloned in agar, and this should greatly expand the potential value of clonal studies on tumor variation and immunoglobulin synthesis.
2. There is a remarkable similarity between the growth requirements of normal B-lymphocytes and plasmacytoma cells in vitro even if the morphology of the colonies differs sharply. Both types of colony formation are greatly potentiated by red cells, both respond to the addition of mercaptoethanol, and both respond to added hemopoietic cells, particularly peritoneal cells. The implication is strong that plasmacytomas retain many of the growth requirements or responsiveness of normal B-lymphocyte populations.
3. The induction of plasmacytomas in mice requires the injection of mineral oil (see review by POTTER, 407) and appears to require a normal microbial flora since the induction regime does not induce plasmacytoma development in germfree mice [408]. The in vitro observations have provided a possible explanation of this observation by showing that both mineral oil and bacterial antigens induce the appearance of a circulating factor with the capacity to stimulate plasmacytoma cell proliferation. It is not impossible that such a factor might serve in vivo as a chronic proliferative stimulus impinging on B-lymphocyte populations, ultimately forcing one cell in the stimulated population to become fully neoplastic and generate a plasmacytoma. The continued responsiveness of the established plasmacytomas to the serum factor seems to be essentially similar to the continued dependency of myeloid leukemic cells on GM-CSF.
4. It should be possible to combine the present cloning techniques for normal B-lymphocytes with the technique used to transform mouse cells in liquid cultures using the rapidly acting Abelson leukemia virus [409, 410, 411]. The resulting pattern of colony formation might reveal whether or not transformation had occurred in vitro and might permit studies analogous to the elegant work with the Rous and Moloney sarcoma viruses on fibroblast transformation in vitro. Indeed, SCHER (SCHER, C. D., personal communication) has mixed normal lymphoid cells in vitro with Abelson virus and on subsequent agar culture,

has obtained small numbers of progressively growing colonies which may represent clones of transformed lymphocytes. If this observation can be confirmed, it might prove feasible to induce antibody-forming B-lymphoid tumors where the specificity of the antibody is known by first enriching lymphoid populations for cells binding with a known hapten [412], then infecting them with Abelson virus before cloning in agar. With present techniques, if transformation occurred, approximately one tumor in four might be secreting antibody against the hapten used.

As mentioned above a similar in vitro transformation of human blood cells (presumably B-lymphocytes) by the Epstein-Barr virus has been reported [400], but no study has yet been made of the nature or functional activity of the transformed cells.

Chapter 13

Hemopoietic Stromal Colonies

As mentioned in Chapter 2, there is a considerable body of experimental evidence derived mainly from in vivo experiments in irradiated mice to suggest that the production of progenitor cells from multipotential hemopoietic stem cells is regulated by microenvironmental cells in the various hemopoietic tissues, particularly the bone marrow and spleen (see review, 30).

Opinion is divided as to whether this microenvironmental influence is mediated by cell contact processes (the hemopoietic microenvironmental hypothesis) or by short-range humoral factors (the managerial cell hypothesis). Until tissue culture technology devises methods for creating three-dimensional matrices in which stromal cells enclose hemopoietic populations, it may be impossible to attempt to duplicate these regulatory events in vitro. There are, however, several promising leads which are worthy of discussion.

Studies by DEXTER and colleagues [413, 414, 415] have shown that, if marrow cells are cocultured in liquid with underlayers of either thymic or marrow-derived stromal cells, there can be an exceptional degree of self-maintenance of stem cells involving extensive self-duplication. It is not impossible that such a system could be adapted to a practicable system for mass production of animal or human hemopoietic stem cells although it has yet to be demonstrated that the eventual yield of stem cells is greater than could be achieved by the injection in vivo of the original number of stem cells.

It is of considerable interest that such cultures also generate large numbers of GM-CFCs and MEG-CFCs [413, 414, WILLIAMS, N., personal communication). The mechanisms involved have yet to be characterized but clearly involve some type of feeder layer action of stromal cells derived from the thymus or marrow. The feeder layer cells are obviously able to activate or support CFU proliferation and, to some degree at least, the formation of progenitor cells by CFUs.

While these experiments are potentially exciting, they are not yet capable of critical analysis because of the highly heterogeneous nature of the feeder cells involved. As is true for hemopoietic populations, an analysis of population interactions is only possible if the individual cells can be cloned and examined for functional activity as pure populations.

It has yet to be demonstrated whether semisolid cultures have anything to offer in this particular problem nor is it known what cell types function as microenvironmental or stromal cells. There is, however, fragmentary evidence both for the fact that fibroblast-like cells might function as stromal cells and that such cells could be cloned in semisolid cultures.

FRIEDENSTEIN and co-workers [416, 22] demonstrated that in liquid cultures of guinea pig or rabbit blood, bone marrow, spleen, and other hemopoietic populations, colonies of adherent fibroblast-like cells developed. The frequency of such cells in cultures of mouse bone marrow was approximately two per 10^5 marrow cells, and such colonies achieved a size of 50–1000 cells.

As shown in Table 28, the highest frequency of fibroblast colony-forming cells was in pleural cavity populations, although some colony-forming cells were demonstrable in lymphoid organs.

It was found that prior bleeding increased the frequency of colony-forming cells in the

Table 28. Relative frequency of fibroblast colony-forming cells in different organs in the adult guinea pig and mouse

Organ	Colony-forming cells per 10^5 cells	
	Guinea pig (liquid/Friedenstein)[a]	Mouse (Agar/Metcalf)[b]
Bone marrow	1.8	0.1
Spleen	1.0	0.1
Thymus	0.3	0.05
Lymph nodes	0.05	0
Peritoneal cavity	8.4	0.03
Pleural cavity	27.5	4.8

[a] Data from FRIEDENSTEIN et al. [22].
[b] Data from METCALF [21].

marrow two to threefold, and injection of diphtheria toxoid into the foot pad increased the frequency of colony-forming cells in the draining lymph nodes sixfold by 7 days after injection [22]. The fibroblast colony-forming cells were radiosensitive with a D_0 of 178 R [417].

What makes these colonies of unusual interest was the demonstration [417] that when marrow-derived colonies were harvested and grafted under the kidney capsule, bone trabeculae developed, enclosing foci of proliferating hemopoietic cells. Conversely, when fibroblast colony cells from spleen cultures were grafted under the kidney capsule, aggregates of lymphoid cells were found in the graft region. The implication from these experiments is that the "fibroblast" colonies were in fact hemopoietic stromal colonies and that, despite a similar morphology, these cells differed functionally in the type of hemopoietic cell proliferation they could support.

These observations are in urgent need of confirmation, particularly using reimplanted individual fibroblast-like colonies. If the experiments can be confirmed and extended, it may be possible that individual fibroblast colonies might be able to support the proliferation of hemopoietic cells of only one particular subclass.

Such glass-adherent colonies can be grown to a relatively large size and could be theoretically recloned and grown as large monolayer populations. The cells are, however, difficult to detach intact from glass surfaces, and for some experiments, it might be preferable to use colonies grown in semisolid medium and already growing in a three-dimensional shape, albeit in only a rudimentary matrix configuration.

In the original work on fibroblasts grown in agar cultures, it was apparently demonstrated to the satisfaction of tumor virologists that normal fibroblasts were unable to proliferate in agar (1) whereas viral-transformed cells could generate characteristic transformed colonies. It now seems extremely improbable that this distinction between normal and transformed cells is as sharp as was originally believed.

It was observed in this laboratory that if whole blood was incorporated in agar medium, normal mouse pleural cavity cells were able to generate large numbers of colonies of fibroblast-like cells [21] (Fig. 52). The frequency of colony-forming cells was 200 per 10^5 cells in the pleural cavity of neonatal mice and fell to approximately five per 10^5 cells in adult mice. Similar colonies could be generated by cells of the peritoneal cavity or cells from the

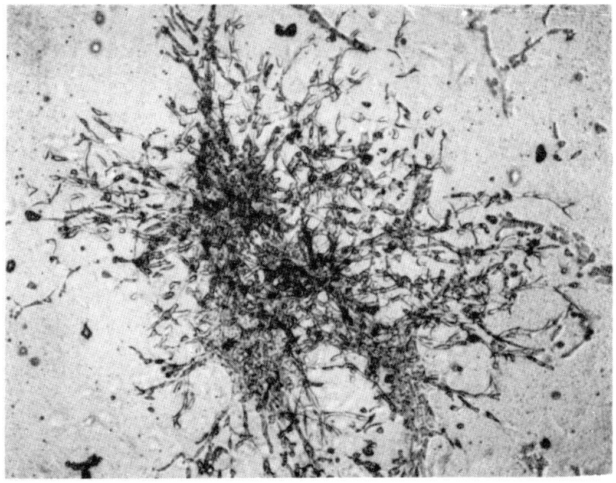

Fig. 52. Large stellate colony of fibroblast-like cells in a 7-day culture of $C_{57}BL$ pleural cavity cells in agar containing whole blood. (From METCALF, [21]. Reproduced with permission from J. Cell. Physiol.)

subcutaneous tissues although the frequency of colony-forming cells was markedly lower than in the pleural cavity.

It should be noted from Table 28 that the relative frequency of fibroblast colony-forming cells is similar using liquid or agar cultures, and the two techniques are probably detecting the same cells.

While few agar colony-forming cells were present in the normal adult peritoneal cavity, the injection of complete Freund's adjuvant caused a 1000-fold rise in the frequency of these cells within 3 days (Fig. 53). Injection of other irritants, e.g., scilica, had a similar though quantitatively smaller effect (METCALF, D., unpublished data).

The agar colony-forming cells from adult mice were not responsive to stimulation by GM-CSF. A factor required for their proliferation was present in mouse plasma but not in serum or washed red or white cells [21].

A linear relationship was noted between the number of pleural cavity cells cultured and the number of fibroblast colonies developing, and no inhibitory cells were noted in mixing experiments of pleural cavity cells with other cells [21]. Colony-forming cells were small round cells with a D_0 of 280 rads, indicating a significantly higher radioresistance than for CFUs or GM-CFCs. From experiments in which pleural cells were incubated in vitro with high concentrations of ^{3}HTdR, the colony-forming cells appeared not to be in cell cycle in adult mice. Levels of colony-forming cells in the pleural cavity were as high in germfree as in conventional mice. However, a considerable strain variation in frequency was observed with CBA and 129J mice having much lower levels than $C_{57}BL$ or BALB/c mice [21].

The biological function of these fibroblast colony-forming cells is quite unknown. Furthermore, morphological differences exist between the colonies grown from different locations, and it is possible that quite different cell types are being counted together. Thus, the colony-forming cells in the subcutaneous tissues may be the equivalent of pericytes believed to initiate focal proliferation of fibroblasts at wound edges, and the high frequency of colony-forming cells in the pleural cavity may explain the tendency for excessive fibroblast overgrowth following infections or injury in this cavity.

On the other hand, the fibroblast-like colonies grown from marrow or spleen populations might be quite different cells whose real function is to regulate various aspects of hemopoiesis.

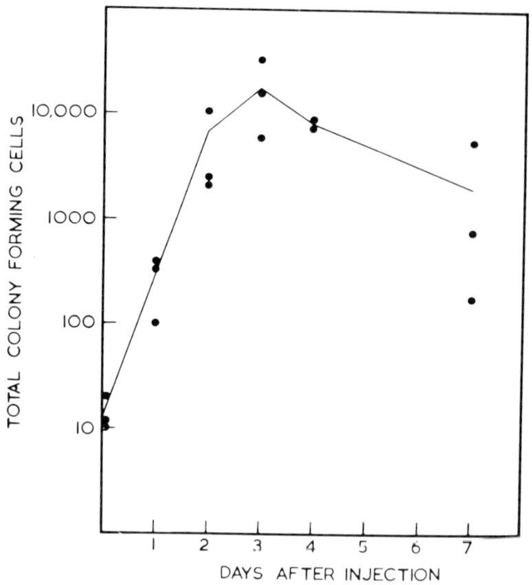

Fig. 53. Rise in total number of fibroblast colony-forming cells in the peritoneal cavity of $C_{57}BL$ mice following the injection of complete Freund's adjuvant. Each point represents data from a pool of three mice. (METCALF, D., unpublished data)

In this context, it is of interest that fibroblast colonies grown from mouse marrow populations have been reported to produce GM-CSF by WILSON et al. [418]. Fibroblast colonies (plaques) were observed attached to the bottom of the culture dish in methylcellulose cultures of mouse or dog bone marrow cells (5–50 per 10^6 cells). Because of the high concentration of cells cultured, it is not clear whether the cells forming the fibroblast plaques (termed PFU-C by the authors) required stimulation by GM-CSF for proliferation. The PFU-C were relatively radioresistant with a D_0 of 200–300 rads. When the original marrow suspension in methylcellulose was removed from the fibroblast plaques and a fresh layer of bone marrow cells in methylcellulose was added, GM-colony formation was stimulated. Although adherent macrophages were also present on the culture dishes and could have served as a source of GM-CSF, the authors concluded that the GM-CSF was actually produced by the fibroblast plaques, a conclusion supported by the more rapid growth rates of GM-colonies immediately adjacent to fibroblast colonies [418].

Removal by curettage of the marrow stromal elements reduced PFU-C levels but interestingly caused a fourfold rise in the frequency of these cells in the opposite intact femur [418].

These 'fibroblast' plaques are promising candidates for colonies of hemopoietic stromal cells, and the further analysis of these cells, particularly using mass cultures grown from individual plaques, is a project of some urgency.

It would be well worthwhile including in these studies a careful analysis of plaques cultured from Sl/Sl mutant mice known to have defective microenvironmental cells regulating the formation of progenitor cells from stem cells [30].

Less likely candidates for hemopoietic microenvironmental cells are the colonies of macrophage-like cells grown by LIN and STEWART from peritoneal cell populations from mice preinjected with thioglycollate medium [103]. These cells require stimulation by GM-CSF for their proliferation, and the colony-forming cells may be relatively mature members of the monocyte-macrophage arm of the GM-hemopoietic family [419]. The cells are of considerable intrinsic interest in that they demonstrate a greater capacity of such cells for proliferation than was formerly suspected [420] and provide an important example where GM-CSF is *not* necessary for survival in vitro for up to 3 weeks but *is* necessary for cell proliferation [421]. While studies on the nature of these cells have so far indicated that they are macrophages [103, 421], it may be that some of the colonies of macrophage-like cells grown from hemopoietic tissues are actually capable of elaborating regulatory factors.

The final studies worthy of comment are those indicating that fibroblast feeder layers derived from mouse embryos are able to stimulate GM-colony formation in which significant numbers of CFUs may be present [71]. In an extension of this study, it was shown that the embryo-derived fibroblasts or media conditioned by them were able to activate CFUs into cell cycle and to stimulate reasonably good self-maintenance of CFUs by proliferation [422, 127]. These studies did not employ cloned populations of fibroblasts, nor for that matter were the fibroblast-like cells proved to be fibroblasts. However, they do constitute encouraging evidence that factors can be derived from embryonic fibroblast-like cells that have an influence on CFUs. These studies are worthy of extension using fibroblast colonies derived from mouse embryo populations, with subsequent selection and testing of the progeny of individual colonies.

Comment

The whole subject of hemopoietic stromal colonies is barely in its early infancy. Little of concrete nature has been established, but there are encouraging leads that fibroblast-like cells not only can be cloned from hemopoietic populations but, by a number of tests, appear to be able to influence CFU and progenitor cell populations.

Because the morphology of these stromal cells is likely to be nondescript, their characterization will require a series of functional tests which presumably will depend heavily on semisolid cultures of various hemopoietic cells.

For the same reasons that make colonies of hemopoietic cells superior to liquid cultures of the same cells, it can be concluded that the proper analysis of stromal cells is going to require the use of stromal cell colonies where cloned populations derived from individual cells can be studied.

Possibly the most important achievement of the studies to date has been to break down a mental barrier which existed regarding the impossible complexity of local control systems operating on stem and progenitor cells. No doubt these will prove to be highly complex, but the above studies suggest that the processes may well be capable of analysis using relatively simple models.

Chapter 14

General Discussion

All the major subpopulations of hemopoietic cells can now be grown as cloned colonies in semisolid culture. With the intelligent use of these cloning systems, it should now be possible to analyze most of the biological processes occurring as progenitor cells proliferate and differentiate to eventually form the mature end cells in each hemopoietic subpopulation.

Not all the techniques have yet been adapted to permit the culture of human cells, and it is a matter of urgency to develop cloning systems for human megakaryocyte and B-lymphocyte colony-forming cells.

The present state of the in vitro cloning systems for mouse hemopoietic cells is summarized in Figure 54. In general, the colony-forming cells in each hemopoietic family appear to be specific progenitor cells. The cells forming clusters or smaller aggregates are slightly more mature cells occupying the intermediate area between progenitor cells and the morphologically recognizable cells, and in fact some are probably members of this latter group. Note that the location of cells forming B and T-lymphocyte colonies is uncertain, but most are likely to be relatively mature cells. Note also that the cells in the peritoneal cavity and other organs that form macrophage colonies appear to be relatively mature cells in the GM-series. The shaded areas showing the location of the different differentiation stages of hemopoietic cells overlap, indicating the occurrence of cells with intermediate properties. Note also that erythroid and GM-populations exhibit a special interrelationship somewhere in the stem cell compartment.

The scheme shown in Figure 54 represents the interpretation most workers in the field

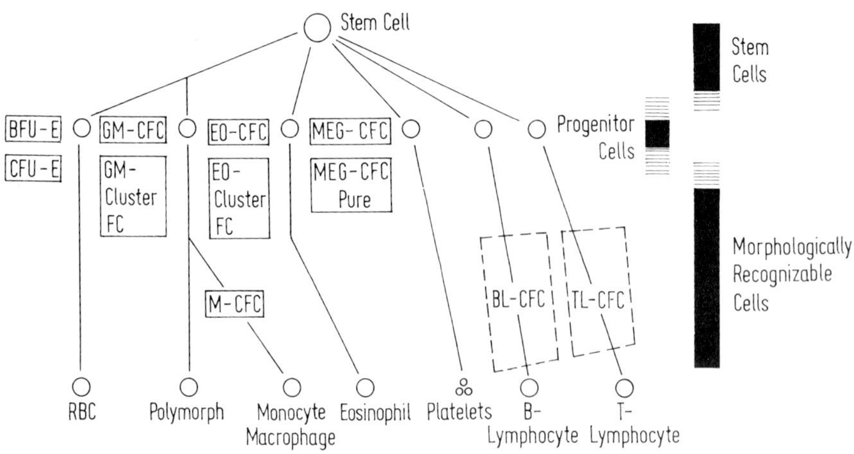

Fig. 54. Schematic representation of the various hemopoietic populations and the level of differentiation of the various colony-forming cells

currently place on the available data. It should be added, however, that opposing proposals have been advanced and have not been completely excluded. For example, under some circumstances progenitor cells may be able to move laterally, e.g., change from erythroid to GM-progenitor cells. The available in vitro data indicate strongly that lateral movement after the colony-forming cell stage does not occur but cannot exclude this possibility at the colony-forming cell or precolony-forming cell levels.

An extreme view held by a few workers is that there is only one type of progenitor cell and which pathway the cell enters is determined by random effective contact of the cell with one or other specific regulator molecule. This hypothesis would require that all progenitor cells exhibit specific receptors for all regulators, an improbable but perhaps not impossible situation. If the "one progenitor cell hypothesis" is correct, it should be possible, for example, to deplete a marrow population of erythroid colony-forming cells by preincubation of the marrow with very high concentrations of GM-CSF. Experiments of this type are now technically feasible using purified preparations of erythropoietin and GM-CSF.

The outstanding failure so far has been the inability to develop a cloning system for multipotential hemopoietic stem cells. It is not yet certain whether this is a genuine failure to grow such colonies or a failure to *recognize* colonies as being derived from or composed of stem cells. Bone marrow-derived colonies are extremely heterogeneous in size and composition, and for example, in cultures of mouse marrow cells stimulated by endotoxin serum, there are many colonies which have not been convincingly identified. If stem cell colonies were relatively small and failed to generate differentiating progeny, these colonies would be quite inconspicuous, and if they contained a population of nondescript mononuclear cells, they might well be mistakenly classified as a macrophage or early granulocytic colonies.

Perhaps the most promising starting population for attempts to grow stem cell colonies would be the hemopoietic cells of the mouse fetal liver. Preliminary observations on the culture of mouse fetal liver cells have revealed curious colonies which might well contain cells of more than one lineage, and these need further investigation. Properties of colonies which might indicate an origin from stem cells are: (1) formation by cells of relatively slow sedimentation velocity, (2) capacity of colonies for sustained proliferation to form populations of very large size, (3) presence in colonies of cells of more than one lineage, e.g., erythroid or megakaryocyte cells in addition to granulocytic and macrophage cells, and (4) presence of colony-forming cells in such colonies.

In this context, it is of interest that, in cultures of mouse marrow cells stimulated by crude preparations of mouse lung-conditioned medium, cells forming colonies that are capable of extensive growth to a large size during the 2nd week of incubation have been shown to have a slower sedimentation rate than typical GM-CFCs and more closely approximate the sedimentation profiles of CFUs (METCALF, D., unpublished data).

The above postulated properties of stem cell-derived colonies are of course predictions based on the behavior of CFU-derived spleen colonies in vivo. It may well be that in vitro a quite different growth pattern is observed, and it is wise to approach the search for a stem cell colony with a quite open mind. Because of the known capacity of fibroblast underlayers and fibroblast-conditioned medium to activate CFUs into cell cycle [127, 422], it seems wise to pay particular attention to these materials in attempts to grow CFU-derived colonies.

Few studies have yet made maximum use of the potential offered by semisolid cultures—the capacity to work with the progeny of *single* hemopoietic cells. As cell separation and micromanipulation methods are improved, it will become of increasing importance to work with single hemopoietic cells so that interactions between purified regulator molecules and specific target cells can be analyzed free of all possible interactions with adjacent cells.

One of the exciting possibilities clearly emerging from studies so far is the capacity to induce leukemia at will in vitro and to work immediately with the cloned progeny of such transformed cells. Depending on the cell population being used, it is now reasonable to claim that the development of leukemia can be documented by characteristic changes in in vitro growth patterns, and assay of the cells in vivo is no longer necessary. In view of the long latent period and multiple-step nature of leukemia development in vivo, it might be considered of doubtful value to work with an artificial in vitro system in which leukemogenesis or transformation of the infected hemopoietic cells is almost instantaneous. However, provided these systems are used with caution and common sense, they offer exciting possibilities not only for analyzing the direct effects of the leukemia virus on selected semipurified target cells but also for analyzing interactions between leukemia viruses and purified regulator molecules. So far, in vitro transformation has been described for erythroid cells using Friend virus [11], granulocytic cells using Friend virus (DEXTER, T. M., personal communication), lymphoid cells using Abelson virus (SCHER, C. D., personal communication), and human leukocytes by the Epstein-Barr virus [400], and this list must certainly be able to be extended. It may also be possible to develop a transformation system using various chemical carcinogens known to be active in provoking leukemia development in vivo.

The in vitro cloning systems have provided important new information on the nature of leukemia—particularly myeloid leukemia in humans. Two major discoveries have been: (1) the demonstration that previously suppressed normal granulopoietic populations rebound during remission, and (2) the demonstration that myeloid leukemic cells remain dependent on the normal regulator GM-CSF. Important questions yet to be resolved are whether abnormal forms of GM-CSF exist and are of importance in such patients and whether the leukemic cells in AML can be made to differentiate. This latter question is of great practical importance in devising methods to restrict the progressive proliferation of leukemic populations.

Despite the existence of at least one mouse model indicating that leukemic cells can be forced to differentiate to nonproliferating cells by culture with GM-CSF, the data from cultures of human AML cells appear contradictory. In the culture systems used so far, proliferating human AML cells have failed to differentiate normally, and it is not yet clear whether the restricted capacity for proliferation they exhibit is a phenomenon controlled by GM-CSF or results from the abnormal in vitro culture systems used. The present data suggest strongly that human AML cells do not simply exhibit a failure to differentiate but have such serious somatic genetic derangements that any differentiation attempted results in the formation of highly abnormal progeny. It is not impossible, however, that these apparently irreversible derangements could be correct by altering the environment of cells, i.e., supplying missing metabolites, cofactors, or regulatory factors.

These questions are certainly worth intensive study using modifications of existing semisolid culture systems. Even if AML cells cannot be induced to differentiate normally, it may at least prove possible to force them to differentiate to nondividing end cells.

Studies carried out so far on patients with myeloproliferative disorders that are potentially preleukemic have documented what appears to be the successive emergence and dominance of more and more abnormal granulopoietic populations as the diseases progress. These findings are compatible with current general concepts of carcinogenesis and warrant extension. It is a matter of some urgency to identify factors or circumstances favoring the expansion of such populations at the expense of the existing populations, and information on some aspects of this should be able to be gathered from a careful analysis of the cells in semisolid cultures.

Related to these problems is the role played by regulators in the development and progression in leukemia. From the fragmentary evidence available at present, it is clear enough that specific regulators are involved as cofactors in leukemia development, presumably in association with the interaction between leukemia viruses and hemopoietic target cells of an appropriately susceptible genotype (see review, 349).

However, work using semisolid cultures has raised more complex questions which future studies will need to resolve. Do abnormal forms of the regulator molecules exist in preleukemic or leukemic patients, and are preleukemic or leukemic cells peculiarly responsive to such factors? Does an abnormally high level of a regulatory factor like GM-CSF increase the probability of leukemia development in a virus-infected population? Which population becomes dominant under conditions of very high or very low GM-CSF levels — leukemic or normal granulopoietic populations?

Before any therapeutic manipulation of GM-CSF levels can be contemplated in patients, it is essential that extensive tests be carried out in semisolid cultures to determine the probable outcome of long-term manipulations of regulator levels. Allied to this question is the need to understand more clearly the function and role of the inhibitory lipoproteins in human and mouse serum. Is the observed inhibitory activity in a number of cloning systems simply an in vitro artifact, or do these lipoproteins represent specific inhibitions modulating the effects of other regulators?

Although experience has shown that the semisolid culture systems can be applied to clinical material to produce information of practical value in the diagnosis and management of hemopoietic diseases, it must be admitted that in few centers are these techniques being applied optimally. In general hospitals not associated with research institutes or university departments, insufficient support facilities exist to guarantee continuity in the staff to perform and analyze the cultures or to ensure adequate standards in media preparation and general culture techniques. Conversely, many research groups with a long-term involvement in hemopoietic cloning techniques are not able to get adequate access to clinical material because they do not have direct control of the patients under investigation.

While the culture techniques are relatively simple, they do require a minimum level of technology and experience, and the techniques can only be used effectively by full-time graduates with a genuine interest in hematology. The culture procedures cannot be performed and analyzed by technicians, and many of the incorrect reports confusing the literature at present have originated from data generated by unsupervised technicians.

The present frustrations preventing a proper application of available semisolid culture technology to today's patients with diseases of hemopoiesis are to a large degree a reflection of teething problems in organisational structure and originate in part from the developmental stage of the techniques, e.g., the unavailability at present of commercially prepared standard human GM-CSF. No doubt a number of these problems will be resolved as the techniques are used more routinely.

One of the major findings coming from the use of semisolid cloning cultures has been the demonstration that hemopoietic populations are highly heterogeneous, even within single hemopoietic families. This heterogeneity is unexpected but it must serve a purpose. The most likely reason for the heterogeneity is that it provides a method for producing subpopulations of end cells whose functions differ significantly one from the other. It becomes of importance therefore to develop functional assays for hemopoietic populations like macrophages and neutrophils that can be applied to individual cells and to all the cells from selected in vitro colonies. Such an approach has already been pioneered by STEWART and co-workers [421, 423, 424] and could clearly be extended.

An obvious comment that scarcely needs making is that, for a proper analysis of the regulatory factors controlling hemopoietic populations, each identified regulator needs to be purified, then checked for activity against other target cells or in other assay systems. The confusion surrounding products released by activated lymphocytes (lymphokines) stems mainly from a failure to purify any of these factors for cross-testing. While most would accept the validity of these statements, few people are aware that each purification is a major undertaking that can be expected to take at least 2–5 years.

Decisions to commit a sizeable fraction of a laboratory's resources to the purification of a particular factor with activity in one or other in vitro cloning system cannot be taken lightly. Two sets of questions have to be answered:

1. Is this factor likely to function in vivo as a significant regulator of hemopoiesis?
2. Does the starting material have a sufficiently high specific activity to warrant purification attempts?

In vitro culture systems are notoriously prone to detect artifacts of no conceivable in vivo significance. This is particularly true of apparent inhibitory factors where, at the very least, some evidence of selectivity or specificity is needed in a battery of in vitro assays before even contemplating purification work. Major considerations in reaching a decision on the value of characterizing and purifying a particular factor should be:

1. Is this factor demonstrable in vivo, either in the serum or the tissues?
2. Do levels of this factor fluctuate under conditions known to involve perturbations in the cell system involved?
3. Does the injection of crude material produce an effect in vivo similar to those seen in vitro?

Answers to at least two of these three questions need to be affirmative before any major purification study is warranted.

Since multiple-step purification procedures usually yield low recoveries of active material (1–10%) and factors of this type usually are present in starting material in extremely low concentrations (e.g. 1 ng/ml), purification studies often run into difficulties simply because of the unavailability of sufficient starting material or the presence of too high a level of contaminating proteins in the crude material. These considerations will not in themselves influence a decision to engage in a particular purification project but certainly should influence the choice of starting material.

Despite these cautionary remarks, it cannot be overemphasized that it is of critical importance to progress in this field to purify each regulator detected, despite the effort and frustration involved.

Similar comments are, of course, equally valid regarding improvement in methods for fractionating hemopoietic populations. The introduction of fluorescence-activated cell sorters can be expected to revolutionize these techniques since the use of many new parameters permitting selective separation can be envisaged and the cell yields will be more than sufficient to allow subsequent analysis in semisolid culture systems. Progress in determining whether various subpopulations are related to one another or can generate other populations now depends heavily on improvement in cell separation methods.

It has been said a number of times in this book that there is a need to develop matrix culture systems which might be able to mimic the cell contact or microenvironmental control systems influencing hemopoiesis, particularly from the stem cell to progenitor cell stages. This may be an overly pessimistic view, and it may well be that nothing more complex than a monolayer of microenvironmental cells is required to selectively activate the transition from CFU to progenitor cell. Since it is technically feasible to produce monolayers from cloned hemopoietic stromal cells, it is certainly worth extensive study to determine whether they can function as rudimentary control systems. Of course, the observed role of local factors in determining the localization and type of hemopoiesis in various tissues does not require that the inductive events committing stem cells necessarily involve cell contact processes. A similar pattern could also result from the focal production and diffusion of specific factors. Because of this, efforts should certainly be made to detect and characterize humoral factors released by stromal cells that can possibly influence these biological events.

Concluding Remarks

The introduction of selective semisolid culture systems for all major hemopoietic subpopulations has transformed cellular hematology.

The difficulties inherent in the use of intact animals and the strictures on investigations in human patients can largely be circumvented by use of such primary culture systems. The continued application of these techniques can be expected to produce a very rapid increase in knowledge in the next few years concerning the nature of the various proliferative disorders of hemopoiesis, particularly leukemia and allied disorders.

There has always been an acknowledged risk that information obtained from in vitro cultures might be misleading because of the inherent artificiality of the systems or the operation of artifacts. While some of the data derived from semisolid cultures have been novel and unexpected, so far there has been no indication that the data are irrelevant or misleading for the in vivo processes.

It should be possible with the proper use of these cloning systems in the next decade to characterize all the major humoral regulators controlling hemopoiesis and to determine the details of the interaction between these regulators and the various target hemopoietic populations.

For any young graduate with an interest in hemopoiesis or a broader interest in cell biology these are exciting times that will probably never be repeated. Fascinating cell populations can now be analyzed in detail even at the single cell level, and differentiation processes can be monitored by a battery of sophisticated marker systems—regulators have been identified and are waiting to be characterized by purification methods already available. For hematologists, the golden days of endocrinology are upon us with the equivalent of a new insulin or growth hormone lying around every corner. *Andiamo!*

References

1. MACPHERSON, I.: The characteristics of animal cells transformed in vitro. Advanc. Cancer Res. *13*, 169–209 (1970).
2. HINUMA, Y., GRACE, G. T.: Cloning of Burkitt lymphoma cells cultured in vitro. Cancer (Philad.) *22*, 1089–1095 (1968).
3. PUCK, T. T., MARCUS, P. I.: A rapid method for viable cell titration and clone production with Hela cells in tissue culture: The use of X-irradiated cells to supply conditioning factors. Proc. nat. Acad. Sci. (Wash.) *41*, 432–437 (1955).
4. BRADLEY, T. R., METCALF, D.: The growth of mouse bone marrow cells in vitro. Aust. J. exp. Biol. med. Sci. *44*, 287–300 (1966).
5. ICHIKAWA, Y., PLUZNIK, D. H., SACHS, L.: In vitro control of the development of macrophage and granulocyte colonies. Proc. nat. Acad. Sci. (Wash.) *56*, 488–495 (1966).
6. PLUZNIK, D. H., SACHS, L.: The cloning of normal "mast" cells in tissue culture. J. cell. comp. Physiol. *66*, 319–324 (1965).
7. PLUZNIK, D. H., SACHS, L.: The induction of clones of normal mast cells by a substance from conditioned medium. Exp. Cell Res. *43*, 553–563 (1966).
8. STEPHENSON, J. R., AXELRAD, A. A., MCLEOD, D. L., SHREEVE, M. M.: Induction of colonies of hemoglobin-synthesising cells by erythropoietin in vitro. Proc. nat. Acad. Sci. (Wash.) *68*, 1542–1546 (1971).
9. MCLEOD, D. L., SHREEVE, M. M., AXELRAD, A. A.: Improved plasma culture system for production of erythrocytic colonies in vitro: quantitative assay method for CFU-E. Blood *44*, 517–534 (1974).
10. LIAO, S-K, AXELRAD, A. A.: Erythropoietin-independent erythroid colony formation in vitro by hemopoietic cells of mice infected with Friend virus. Int. J. Cancer *15*, 467–482 (1975).
11. CLARKE, B. J., AXELRAD, A. A., SHREEVE, M. M., MCLEOD, D. L.: Erythroid colony induction without erythropoietin by Friend leukemia virus in vitro. Proc. nat. Acad. Sci. (Wash.) *72*, 3556–3560 (1975).
12. PIKE, B. L., ROBINSON, W. A.: Human bone marrow colony growth in agar gel. J. cell. Physiol. *76*, 77–84 (1970).
13. CHERVENICK, P. A., BOGGS, D. R.: In vitro growth of granulocytic and mononuclear cell colonies from blood of normal individuals. Blood *37*, 131–135 (1971).
14. ICHIKAWA, Y.: Differentiation of a cell line of myeloid leukemia. J. cell. Physiol. *74*, 223–234 (1969).
15. ICHIKAWA, Y.: Further studies on the differentiation of a cell line of myeloid leukemia. J. cell. Physiol. *76*, 175–184 (1970).
16. METCALF, D., MOORE, M. A. S., WARNER, N. L.: Colony formation in vitro by myelomonocytic leukemic cells. J. nat. Cancer Inst. *43*, 983–1001 (1969).
17. MCNEILL, T. A.: Release of bone marrow colony stimulating activity during immunological reactions in vitro. Nature (New Biol.) *244*, 175–176 (1973).
18. PARKER, J. W., METCALF, D.: Production of colony-stimulating factors in mitogen-stimulated lymphocyte cultures. J. Immunol. *112*, 502–510 (1974).
19. METCALF, D., PARKER, J., CHESTER, H. M., KINCADE, P. W.: Formation of eosinophilic-like granulocytic colonies by mouse bone marrow cells in vitro. J. cell. Physiol. *84*, 275–290 (1974).
20. METCALF, D., MACDONALD, H. R., ODARTCHENKO, N., SORDAT, B.: Growth of mouse megakaryocyte colonies in vitro. Proc. nat. Acad. Sci. (Wash.) *72*, 1744–1748 (1975).
21. METCALF, D.: Formation in agar of fibroblast-like colonies by cells from the mouse pleural cavity and other sources. J. cell. Physiol. *80*, 409–420 (1972).
22. FRIEDENSTEIN, A. J., DERIGLASOVA, U. F., KULAGINA, N. N., PANASUK, A. F., RUDAKOWA, S. F., LURIA, E. A., RUDAKOW, I. A.: Precursors for fibroblasts detected in different populations of hematopoietic cells as detected by the in vitro colony assay method. Exp. Hemat. *2*, 83–92 (1974).
23. METCALF, D.: Colony formation in agar by murine plasmacytoma cells: potentiation by hemopoietic cells and serum. J. cell. Physiol. *81*, 397–410 (1973).

24. CLICK, R. E., BENCK, L., ALTER, B. J.: Enhancement of antibody synthesis in vitro by mercaptoethanol. Cell Immunol. *3*, 156–160 (1972).
25. BROOME, J. D., JENG, M. M.: Promotion of replication in lymphoid cells by specific thiols and disulfides in vitro. Effects on mouse lymphoma cells in comparison with splenic lymphocytes. J. exp. Med. *138*, 574–592 (1973).
26. METCALF, D.: The serum factor stimulating colony formation in vitro by murine plasmacytoma cells: response to antigens and mineral oil. J. Immunol. *113*, 235–243 (1974).
27. METCALF, D., WARNER, N. L., NOSSAL, G. J. V., MILLER, J. F. A. P., SHORTMAN, K., RABELLINO, E.: Growth of B-lymphocyte colonies in vitro from mouse lymphoid organs. Nature (Lond.) *255*, 630–632 (1975).
28. METCALF, D., NOSSAL, G. J. V., WARNER, N. L., MILLER, J. F. A. P., MANDEL, T. E., LAYTON, J. E., GUTMAN, G. A.: Growth of B-lymphocyte colonies in vitro. J. exp. Med. *142*, 1534–1549 (1975).
29. ROZENSZAJN, L. A., SHOHAM, D., KALECHMAN, I.: Clonal proliferation of PHA-stimulated human lymphocytes in soft agar culture. Immunology *29*, 1041–1055 (1975).
30. METCALF, D., MOORE, M. A. S.: Haemopoietic Cells. Amsterdam: North-Holland (1971).
31. PARMLEY, R. T., OGAWA, M., SPICER, S. G., WRIGHT, N. J.: Ultrastructure and cytochemistry of bone marrow granulocytes in culture. Exp. Hemat. *4*, 75–89 (1976).
32. METCALF, D., MOORE, M. A. S., SHORTMAN, K.: Adherence column and buoyant density separation of bone marrow stem cells and more differentiated cells. J. cell. Physiol. *78*, 441–450 (1971).
33. SHORTMAN, K.: The separation of different cell classes from lymphoid organs. II. The purification and analysis of lymphocyte populations by equilibrium density gradient centrifugation. Aust. J. exp. Biol. med. Sci. *46*, 375–396 (1968).
34. MILLER, R. G., PHILLIPS, R. A.: Separation of cells by velocity sedimentation. J. cell. Physiol. *73*, 191–201 (1969).
35. MACDONALD, H. R., MILLER, R. G.: Synchronisation of mouse L-cells by a velocity sedimentation technique. Biophysics *10*, 834–842 (1970).
36. METCALF, D., MACDONALD, H. R.: Heterogeneity of in vitro colony -and cluster-forming cells in the mouse marrow. Segregation by velocity sedimentation. J. cell. Physiol. *85*, 643–654 (1975).
37. HANNIG, K.: Separation of cells and particles by continuous free-flow electrophoresis. In: Techniques of Biochemical and Biophysical Morphology. Glick, D., Rosenbaum, R. (eds.). New York: Wiley 1972, Vol. I, pp. 191–232.
38. VAN DEN ENGH, G. J., GOLUB, E. S.: Antigenic differences between hemopoietic stem cells and myeloid progenitors. J. exp. Med. *139*, 1621–1627 (1974).
39. KIM, H. C., MARKS, P. A., RIFKIND, R. A., MANIATIS, G. M., BANK, A.: Isolation and in vitro differentiation of human erythroid precursor cells. Blood *47*, 767–776 (1976).
40. PARISH, C. R., HAYWARD, J. A.: The lymphocyte surface. I. Relation between F_c receptors, C'3 receptors and surface immunoglobulin. Proc. roy. Soc. B. *187*, 47–63 (1974).
41. PARISH, C. R., KIROV, S. M., BOWERN, N., BLANDEN, R. V.: A one-step procedure for separating mouse T and B-lymphocytes. Europ. J. Immunol. *4*, 808–815 (1974).
42. MOORE, M. A. S., WILLIAMS, N.: Physical separation of colony stimulating cells from in vitro colony-forming cells in hemopoietic tissue. J. cell. Physiol. *80*, 195–206 (1972).
43. MOORE, M. A. S., WILLIAMS, N., METCALF, D.: Purification and characterisation of the in vitro colony forming cell in monkey hemopoietic tissue. J. cell. Physiol. *79*, 283–292 (1972).
44. MOORE, M. A. S., WILLIAMS, N., METCALF, D.: In vitro colony formation by normal and leukemic human hematopoietic cells. Interaction between colony-forming and colony-stimulating cells. J. nat. Cancer Inst. *50*, 591–602 (1973).
45. MESSNER, H. A., TILL, J. E., MCCULLOCH, E. A.: Interacting cell populations affecting granulopoietic colony formation by normal and leukemic human marrow cells. Blood *42*, 701–710 (1973).
46. BROXMEYER, H. E., BAKER, F. L., GALBRAITH, P. R.: In vitro regulation of granulopoiesis in human leukemia: application of an assay for colony-inhibiting cells. Blood *47*, 389–402 (1976).
47. HARRIS, J. E.: Effect of l-asparagine on the ability of normal mouse bone marrow to form soft agar colonies. Nature (Lond.) *223*, 850–851 (1969).
48. METCALF, D., MACDONALD, H. R., CHESTER, H. M.: Serum potentiation of granulocytic and macrophage colony formation in vitro. Exp. Hemat. *3*, 261–273 (1975).
49. METCALF, D.: Acute antigen-induced elevation of serum colony stimulating factor (CSF) levels. Immunology *21*, 427–436 (1971).
50. SHERIDAN, J. W., METCALF, D.: A low molecular weight factor in lung conditioned medium stimulating granulocyte and monocyte colony formation in vitro. J. cell. Physiol. *81*, 11–24 (1973).
51. STANLEY, E. R., BRADLEY, T. R., SUMNER, M. A.: Properties of mouse embryo conditioned medium

factor(s) stimulating colony formation by mouse bone marrow cells grown in vitro. J. cell. Physiol. *78*, 301–318 (1971).
52. Stanley, E. R., Metcalf, D., Maritz, J. S., Yeo, G. F.: Standardised bioassay for bone marrow colony stimulating factor in human urine: levels in normal man. J. Lab. clin. Med. *79*, 657–668 (1972).
53. Iscove, N. N., Senn, J. S., Till, J. E., McCulloch, E. A.: Colony formation by normal and leukemic human marrow cells in culture: effect of conditioned medium from human leukocytes. Blood *37*, 1–5 (1971).
54. Paran, M., Sachs, L., Barak, Y., Resnitsky, P.: In vitro induction of granulocyte differentiation in hematopoietic cells from leukemic and non-leukemic patients. Proc. nat. Acad. Sci. (Wash.) *67*, 1542–1549 (1970).
55. Aye, M. T., Niko, Y., Till, J. E., McCulloch, E. A.: Studies of leukemic cell populations in culture. Blood *44*, 205–219 (1974).
56. Prival, J. T., Paran, M., Gallo, R. C., Wu, A. M.: Colony-stimulating factors in cultures of human peripheral blood cells. J. nat. Cancer Inst. *53*, 1583–1588 (1974).
57. Burgess, A. W., Wilson, E. C., Metcalf, D.: Stimulation by human placental conditioned medium of hemopoietic colony formation by human marrow cells. Blood *49*, 573–583 (1977).
58. Dodge, W. H., Moscovici, C.: Colony formation by chicken hematopoietic cells and virus-induced myeloblasts. J. cell. Physiol. *81*, 371–386 (1973).
59. Bradley, T. R., Siemienowicz, R.: Colony growth of rat bone marrow cells in vitro. Aust. J. exp. Biol. med. Sci. *46*, 595–605 (1968).
60. Marsh, J. C., Levitt, M., Katzenstein, A.: The growth of leukocyte colonies in vitro from dog bone marrow. J. Lab. clin. Med. *79*, 1041–1050 (1972).
61. Metcalf, D.: Role of mercaptoethanol and endotoxin in stimulating B-lymphocyte colony formation in vitro. J. Immunol. *116*, 635–638 (1976).
62. Iscove, N. N., Sieber, F.: Erythroid progenitors in mouse bone marrow detected by macroscopic colony formation in culture. Exp. Hemat. *3*, 32–43 (1975).
63. Iscove, N. N., Sieber, F., Winterhalter, K. H.: Erythroid colony formation in cultures of mouse and human bone marrow. Analysis of the requirement for erythropoietin by gel filtration and affinity chromatography on agarose-concanavalin A. J. cell. Physiol. *83*, 309–320 (1974).
64. Van den Engh, G. J., Bol, S.: The presence of a CSF enhancing activity in the serum of endotoxin-treated mice. Cell Tiss. Kinet. *8*, 579–587 (1975).
65. Bradley, T. R., Telfer, P. A., Fry, P. A.: The effect of erythrocytes on mouse bone marrow colony development in vitro. Blood *38*, 353–359 (1971).
66. Metcalf, D.: Potentiation of bone marrow colony growth in vitro by the addition of lymphoid or bone marrow cells. J. cell. Physiol. *72*, 9–20 (1968).
67. Dicke, K. A., Spitzer, G., Ahearn, M. J.: Colony formation in vitro by leukaemic cells in acute myelogenous leukaemia with phytohaemagglutinin as stimulating factor. Nature (Lond.) *259*, 129–130 (1976).
68. Stanners, C. P., Eliceiri, G. L., Green, H.: Two types of ribosome in mouse-hamster hybrid cells. Nature (New Biol.) *230*, 52–54 (1971).
69. Gordon, M. Y.: Quantitation of haemopoietic cells from normal and leukaemic RFM mice using an in vivo colony assay. Brit. J. Cancer *30*, 421–428 (1974).
70. Gordon, M. Y., Blackett, N. M., Douglas, I. D. C.: Colony formation by human haemopoietic precursor cells cultured in semi-solid agar in diffusion chambers. Brit. J. Haemat. *31*, 103–110 (1975).
71. Dicke, K. A., Platenburg, M. G. C., Van Bekkum, D. W.: Colony formation in agar: in vitro assay for hemopoietic stem cells. Cell Tiss. Kinet. *4*, 463–477 (1971).
72. Metcalf, D., Bradley, T. R., Robinson, W.: Analysis of colonies developing in vitro from mouse bone marrow cells stimulated by kidney feeder layers or leukemic serum. J. cell. Physiol. *69*, 93–108 (1967).
73. Testa, N. G., Lord, B. I.: A technique for the morphological examination of hemopoietic cells grown in agar. Blood *36*, 586–589 (1970).
74. Rabellino, E. M., Metcalf, D.: Receptors for C3 and IgG on macrophage, neutrophil and eosinophil colony cells grown in vitro. J. Immunol. *115*, 688–692 (1975).
75. Shoham, D., Ben David, E., Rozenszajn, L. A.: Cytochemical and morphologic identification of macrophages and eosinophils in tissue cultures of normal human bone marrow. Blood *44*, 221–233 (1974).
76. Spurr, A. R.: A low viscosity epoxy resin embedding medium for electronmicroscopy. J. Ultrastruct. Res. *26*, 31–43 (1969).

77. VAN NOORD, M. J., BLANSJAAR, N., NAKEFF, A.: The processing of mammalian haemopoietic cells in thin layer agar cultures for electron microscopy. Stain Technol. *48*, 239–246 (1973).
78. METCALF, D., FOSTER, R.: Behavior on transfer of serum stimulated bone marrow colonies. Proc. Soc. exp. Biol. (N.Y.) *126*, 758–762 (1967).
79. PARAN, M., SACHS, L.: The continuous requirement for inducer for the development of macrophage and granulocyte colonies. J. cell. Physiol. *72*, 247–250 (1968).
80. METCALF, D.: Transformation of granulocytes to macrophages in bone marrow colonies. J. cell. Physiol. *77*, 277–280 (1971).
81. METCALF, D., MOORE, M. A. S.: Regulation of growth and differentiation in haemopoietic colonies growing in agar. In: Haemopoietic Stem Cells. CIBA Foundation Symposium 13. Wolstenholme, G. E. W. (ed.). Amsterdam: Associated Scientific Publishers 1973, pp. 157–182.
82. METCALF, D.: Studies on colony formation in vitro by mouse bone marrow cells. I. Continuous cluster formation and relation of clusters to colonies. J. cell. Physiol. *74*, 323–332 (1969).
83. METCALF, D.: Studies on colony formation in vitro by mouse bone marrow cells. II. Action of colony stimulating factor. J. cell. Physiol. *76*, 89–100 (1970).
84. METCALF, D.: Effect of thymidine suiciding on colony formation in vitro by mouse hematopoietic cells. Proc. Soc. exp. Biol. (N.Y.) *139*, 511–514 (1972).
85. MOORE, M. A. S., WILLIAMS, N., METCALF, D.: In vitro colony formation by normal and leukemic human hematopoietic cells: Characterisation of the colony-forming cells. J. nat. Cancer Inst. *50*, 603–623 (1973).
86. ZUCKER-FRANKLIN, D., GRUSKY, G.: Ultrastructural analysis of hematopoietic colonies derived from human peripheral blood. J. Cell Biol. *63*, 855–863 (1974).
87. CLINE, M. J., WARNER, N. L., METCALF, D.: Identification of the bone marrow colony mononuclear phagocyte as a macrophage. Blood *39*, 326–330 (1972).
88. MCLEOD, D. L., SHREEVE, M. M., AXELRAD, A. A.: Induction of megakaryocyte colonies with platelet formation in vitro. Nature (Lond.) *261*, 492 (1976).
89. SREDNI, B., KALECHMAN, Y., MICHLIN, H., ROZENSZAJN, L. A.: Development of colonies in vitro of mitogen-stimulated mouse T-lymphocytes. Nature (Lond.) *259*, 130–132 (1976).
90. LEVI-MONTALCINI, R., ANGELETTI, P. U.: Nerve growth factor: evaluation and perspectives. In: Nerve Growth Factor and Its Antiserum Zaimis, E., Knight, J. (eds.). London: Athlone Press 1972 pp. 46–58.
91. BURGESS, A. W., METCALF, D.: The effect of colony stimulating factor on the synthesis of ribonucleic acid by mouse bone marrow cells in vitro. J. cell. Physiol. *90*, 471–484 (1977).
92. GROSS, M. GOLDWASSER, E.: On the mechanism of action of erythropoietin-induced differentiation. V. Characterisation of the ribonucleic acid formed as a result of erythropoietin action. Biochemistry *8*, 1795–1805 (1969).
93. MOORE, M. A. S., WILLIAMS, N.: Functional, morphologic and kinetic analysis of the granulocytic-macrophage progenitor cell. In: Hemopoiesis in Culture. Robinson, W. A. (ed.). Washington: DHEW Publication No. 74–205, 1973, pp. 17–27.
94. BURGESS, A. W., CAMAKARIS, J., METCALF, D.: The purification and properties of colony stimulating factor from mouse lung conditioned medium. J. biol. Chem. *252*, 1998–2003 (1977).
95. ROBINSON, W., METCALF, D., BRADLEY, T. R.: Stimulation by normal and leukemic mouse sera of colony formation in vitro by mouse bone marrow cells. J. cell. Physiol. *69*, 83–92 (1967).
96. MOORE, M. A. S., METCALF, D.: Ontogeny of the haemopoietic system. Yolk sac origin of in vivo and in vitro colony forming cells in the developing mouse embryo. Brit. J. Haemat. *18*, 279–296 (1970).
97. SILINI, G., POZZI, L. V., PONS, S.: Studies on the haematopietic stem cells of mouse foetal liver. J. Embryol. exp. Morph. *17*, 303–318(1967).
98. HAYS, E. F., FIRKIN, F. C., KOGA, Y., HAYS, D. M.: Hemopoietic colony forming cells in regenerating liver. J. cell. Physiol. *86*, 213–220 (1975).
99. TESTA, N. G., HENDRY, J. H.: Radiation-induced haemopoiesis in adult mouse liver. Exp. Hemat. *5*, 136–140 (1977).
100. BRADLEY, T. R., FRY, P., SUMNER, M. A. MCINERNEY, E.: Factors determining colony forming efficiency in agar suspension cultures. Aust. J. exp. Biol. med. Sci. *50*, 813–818 (1972).
101. METCALF, D., STEVENS, S.: Influence of age and antigenic stimulation on granulocyte and macrophage progenitor cells in the mouse spleen. Cell Tiss. Kinet. *5*, 433–446 (1972).
102. METCALF, D., RUSSELL, S.: Inhibition by mouse serum of hemopoietic colony formation in vitro. Exp. Hemat. *4*, 339–353 (1976).

103. Lin, H. S., Stewart, C. C.: Peritoneal exudate cells. I. Growth requirement of cells capable of forming colonies in soft agar. J. cell. Physiol. *83*, 369–378 (1974).
104. Dodge, W. H. Silva, R. F. Moscovici, C.: The origin of chicken hematopoietic colonies as assayed in semisolid agar. J. cell. Physiol. *85*, 25–30 (1975).
105. Lajtha, L. G., Pozzi, L. V., Schofield, R., Fox, M.: Kinetic properties of haemopoietic stem cells. Cell Tiss. Kinet. *2*, 39–49 (1969).
106. Rickard, K. A., Shadduck, R. K. Howard, D. E., Stohlman, F: A differential effect of hydroxyurea on hemopoietic stem cell colonies in vitro and in vivo. Proc. Soc. exp. Biol. (N.Y.) *134*, 152–156 (1970).
107. Iscove, N. N., Till, J. E. McCulloch, E. A.: The proliferative states of mouse granulopoietic progenitor cells. Proc. Soc. exp. Biol. (N.Y.) *134*, 33–36 (1970). 108. Williams, N., Van den Engh, G. J. :Separation of subpopulations of in vitro colony forming cells from mouse marrow by equilibrium density centrifugation. J. cell. Physiol. *86*, 237–245 (1975).
109. Senn, J. S. McCulloch, E. A: Radiation sensitivity of human bone marrow cells measured by a cell culture method. Blood *35*, 56–60 (1970).
110. Metcalf, D.: Cortisone action on serum colony-stimulating factor and bone marrow in vitro colony forming cells. Proc. Soc. exp. Biol. (N.Y.) *132*, 391–394 (1969).
111. McNeill, T. A.: Effect of methisazone and other drugs on mouse hemopoietic colony formation in vitro. Antimicrob. Agents Chemother. *1*, 6–11 (1972).
112. Brown, C. H., Carbone, P. P.: Effects of chemotherapeutic agents on normal mouse bone marrow grown in vitro. Cancer Res. *31*, 185–190 (1970).
113. Haskill, J. S. McNeill, T. A., Moore, M. A. S.: Density distribution analysis of in vivo and in vitro colony-forming cells in bone marrow. J. cell. Physiol. *75*, 167–180 (1970).
114. McCulloch, E. A., Till, J. E.: Effects of short term culture on populations of hemopoietic progenitor cells from mouse marrow. Cell Tiss. Kinet. *4*, 11–20 (1971).
115. Sumner, M. A., Bradley, T. R., Hodgson, G. S., Cline, M. J., Fry, P. A., Sutherland, L.: The growth of bone marrow cells in liquid culture. Brit. J. Haemat. *23*, 221–234 (1972).
116. Testa, N. G., Lajtha, L. G.: Comparison of the kinetics of colony forming units in spleen (CFU_s) and culture (CFU_c). Brit. J. Haemat. *24*, 367–376 (1973).
117. Sutherland, D. J. A., Till, J. E., McCulloch, E. A.: Short term cultures of mouse marrow cells separated by velocity sedimentation. Cell Tiss. Kinet. *4*, 479–490 (1971).
118. Dicke, K. A., Van Noord, M. J., Maat, B., Schaefer, U. W., Van Bekkum, D. W.: Identification of cells in primate bone marrow resembling the hemopoietic stem cell in the mouse. Blood *42*, 195–208 (1973).
119. Johnson, G. R., Metcalf, D.: Characterization of mouse foetal liver granulocyte-macrophage colony-forming cells (GM-CFC) by velocity sedimentation at unit gravity. Exp. Hemat. (1977).
120. Metcalf, D., Wilson, J.: Endotoxin-induced size change in bone marrow progenitors of granulocytes and macrophages. J. cell. Physiol. *89*, 381–392 (1976).
121. Metcalf, D., Johnson, G. R., Wilson, J.: Radiation-induced enlargement of granulocytic and macrophage progenitor cells in the mouse bone marrow. Exp. Hemat. (1977).
122. Rickard, K., Brown, B., Kronenberg, H.: Radiation and the human agar colony forming cell. Pathology *6*, 169–181 (1974).
123. Niho, Y., Till, J. E., McCulloch, E. A.: Effect of arabinosyl cytosine on granulopoietic colony formation by marrow cells from leukemic and non-leukemic patients. Exp. Hemat. *4*, 63–69 (1976).
124. Rickard, K. A., Shadduck, R. K. Morley, A., Stohlman, F.: In vitro and in vivo colony technics in the study of granulopoiesis. In: Hemopoietic Cellular Proliferation. Stohlman, F. (ed.). New York: Grune and Stratton 1970, pp. 238–248.
125. Rickard, K. A., Morley, A., Howard, D., Stohlman, F.: The in vitro colony forming cell and the response to neutropenia. Blood *37*, 6–13 (1971).
126. Wu, A. M., Siminovitch, L., Till, J. E. McCulloch, E. A.: Evidence for a relationship between mouse hemopoietic stem cells and cells forming colonies in culture. Proc. nat. Acad. Sci. (Wash.) *59*, 1209–1215 (1968).
127. Lowenberg, B., Dicke, K. A.: Studies on the in vitro proliferation of pluripotent haemopoietic stem cells. In: Leukemia and, Aplastic Anemia. Metcalf, D., Condorelli, M., Peschle, C. (eds.). Rome: Il Pensiero Scientifico 1976, pp. 377–391.
128. Worton, R. G., McCulloch, E. A., Till, J. E.: Physical separation of hemopoietic stem cells from cells forming colonies in culture. J. cell. Physiol. *74*, 171–182 (1969).
129. Bennett, M., Cudkowicz, G., Foster, R. S., Metcalf, D.: Hemopoietic progenitor cells in W anemic mice studied in vivo and in vitro. J. cell. Physiol. *71* , 211–226 (1968).
130. Testa, N. G., Hendry, J. H., Lajtha, L. G.: The response of mouse haemopoietic colony formers

to acute or continuous gamma irradiation. Biomedicine *19*, 183–186 (1973).
131. LORD, B. I., TESTA, N. G., HENDRY, J. H.: The relative spatial distributions of the CFUs and CFUc in the normal mouse femur. Blood *46*, 65–72 (1975).
132. METCALF, D., STANLEY, E. R.: Haematological effects in mice of partially purified colony stimulating factor (CSF) prepared from human urine. Brit. J. Haemat. *21*, 481–492 (1971).
133. METCALF, D.: Regulation by colony-stimulating factor of granulocyte and macrophage colony formation in vitro by normal and leukemic cells. In: Control of Proliferation in Animal Cells. Baserga, R. (ed.). New York: Cold Spring Harbor Laboratory 1974, pp. 887–905.
134. MOORE, M. A. S., SPITZER, G., METCALF, D., PENINGTON, D. G.: Monocyte production of colony stimulating factor in familial cyclic neutropenia. Brit. J. Haemat. *27*, 47–55 (1974).
135. NELSON, D. S.: Macrophages and Immunity. Amsterdam: North-Holland 1969.
136. SHERIDAN, J. W., STANLEY, E. R. Tissue sources of bone marrow colony stimulating factor. J. cell. Physiol. *78*, 451–459 (1971).
137. BRADLEY, T. R., SUMNER, M. A.: Stimulation of mouse bone marrow colony growth in vitro by conditioned medium. Aust. J. exp. Biol. Med. Sci. *46*, 607–618 (1968).
138. BRADLEY, T. R., STANLEY, E. R., SUMNER, M. A.: Factors from mouse tissues stimulating colony growth of mouse bone marrow cells in vitro. Aust. J. exp. Biol. med. Sci. *49*, 595–603 (1971).
139. GUEZ, M., SACHS, L.: Purification of the protein that induces cell differentiation to macrophages and granulocytes. Febs Lett. *37*, 149–154 (1973).
140. AUSTIN, P. E., MCCULLOCH, E. A., TILL, J. E.: Characterisation of the factor in L-cell conditioned medium capable of stimulating colony formation by mouse marrow cells in culture. J. cell. Physiol. *77*, 121–133 (1971).
141. ROBINSON, W. A., STANLEY, E. R., METCALF, D.: Stimulation of bone marrow colony growth in vitro by human urine. Blood *33*, 396–399 (1969).
142. KNUDTZON, S., MORTENSEN, B. T.: Growth stimulation of human bone marrow cells in agar culture by vascular cells. Blood *46*, 937–943 (1975).
143. CHAN, S. H., METCALF, D.: Local production of colony-stimulating factor within the bone marrow. Role of non-hematopoietic cells. Blood *40*, 646–653 (1972).
144. GOLDE, D. W., CLINE, M. J.: Identification of the colony-stimulating cell in human peripheral blood. J. Clin. invest. *52*, 2981–2983 (1972).
145. CHERVENICK, P. A., LOBUGLIO, A. F.: Human blood monocytes: stimulators of granulocyte and mononuclear formation in vitro. Science *178*, 164–166 (1972).
146. LUTTON, J. D., OSBORN, D. C. ZANJANI, E. D., WASSERMAN, L. R.: Stimulation and inhibition of granulocyte and mononuclear colony formation in vitro by conditioned medium from mouse peritoneal cells. J. reticuloendoth. Soc. *18*, 186–195 (1975).
147. DALE, D. C., BROWN, C. H., CARBONE, P., WOLF, S. M.: Cyclic urinary leukopoietic activity in gray collie dogs. Science *173*, 152–153 (1971).
148. GATTI, R. A., ROBINSON, W. A., DEINARD, A. S., NESBIT, M., MCCULLOGH, J. J., BULLOW, M., GOOD, R. A.: Cyclic leucocytosis in chronic myelogenous leukemia: new perspectives on pathogenesis and therapy. Blood *41*, 771–782 (1973).
149. GUERRY, D., ADAMSON, J. W., DALE, D. C., WOLFF, S. M.: Human cyclic neutropenia: urinary colony-stimulating factor and erythropoietin levels. Blood *44*, 257–262 (1974).
150. EAVES, A. C., BRUCE, W. R.: In vitro production of colony-stimulating activity. I. Exposure of mouse peritoneal cells to endotoxin. Cell Tiss. Kinet. *7*, 19–30 (1974).
151. SHERIDAN, J. W., METCALF, D.: CSF production and release following endotoxin. In: Hemopoiesis In Culture. Robinson, W. A. (ed.). Washington: DHEW Publication No. (NIH) 74–205, 1973, pp. 135–143.
152. PARKER, J. W., METCALF, D.: Production of colony-stimulating factor in mixed leucocyte cultures. Immunology *26*, 1039–1049 (1974).
153. CLINE, M. J., GOLDE, D. W.: Production of colony-stimulating activity by human lymphocytes. Nature (Lond.) *248*, 703–704 (1974).
154. RUSCETTI, F. W., CHERVENICK, P. A.: Regulation of the release of colony-stimulating activity from mitogen-stimulated lymphocytes. J. Immunol. *114*, 1513–1517 (1975).
155. RUSCETTI, F. W., CHERVENICK, P. A.: Release of colony-stimulating activity from thymus-derived lymphocytes. J. clin. Invest. *55*, 520–527 (1975).
156. CHAN, S. H., METCALF, D.: Local and systemic control of granulocytic and macrophage progenitor cell regeneration after irradiation. Cell Tiss. Kinet. *6*, 185–197 (1973).
157. SHERIDAN, J. W. METCALF, D.: Studies on the bone marrow colony stimulating factor (CSF). Relation of tissue CSF to serum CSF. J. cell. Physiol. *80*, 129–140 (1972).
158. SHERIDAN, J. W., METCALF, D., STANLEY, E. R.: Further studies on the factor in lung-conditioned

medium stimulating granulocyte and monocyte colony formation in vitro. J. cell. Physiol. *84*, 147–158 (1974).
159. SHADDUCK, R. K. METCALF, D.: Preparation and neutralisation characteristics of an anti-CSF antibody. J. cell. Physiol. *86*, 247–252 (1975).
160. GRANSTROM, M.: Conditions influencing inhibitors to the colony stimulating factor (CSF). Exp. Cell. Res. *87*, 307–312 (1974).
161. STANLEY, E. R., METCALF, D.: Partial purification and some properties of the factor in normal and leukaemic human urine capable of stimulating mouse bone marrow colony growth in vitro. Aust. J. exp. Biol. Med. Sci. *47*, 467–483 (1969).
162. STANLEY, E. R., METCALF, D.: Purification and properties of human urinary colony stimulating factor (CSF). In: Cell Differentiation. Harris, R., Viza, D. (eds.). Copenhagen: Munksgaard 1972, pp. 272–276.
163. STANLEY, E. R., METCALF, D. The molecular weight of colony stimulating factor (CSF) Proc. Soc. exp. Biol. (N.Y.) *137*, 1029–1031 (1971).
164. STANLEY, E. R., METCALF, D.: Enzyme treatment of colony stimulating factor. Evidence for a peptide component. Aust. J. exp. Biol. (N.Y.) Sci. *49*, 281–290 (1971).
165. KELLAR, K. L. VOGLER, W. R., KINKADE, J. M.: Colony stimulating factor (CSF) from human leukemic urine. Affinity chromatography and isoelectric focusing. Proc. Soc. exp. Biol. (N.Y.) *150*, 766–772 (1975).
166. STANLEY, E. R., HANSEN, G., WOODCOCK, J., METCALF, D.: Colony stimulating factor and the regulation of granulopoiesis and macrophage production. Fed. Proc. *34*, 2272–2278 (1975).
167. SHERIDAN, J. W., METCALF, D.: Purification of mouse lung-conditioned medium colony stimulating factor (CSF). Proc. Soc. exp. Biol. (N.Y.) *146*, 218–221 (1974).
168. STANLEY, E. R., CIFONE, M., HEARD, P. M., DEFENDI, V.: Factors regulating macrophage production and growth. Identity of colony stimulating factor and macrophage growth factor. J. exp. Med. *143*, 631–647 (1976).
169. VIROLAINEN, M., DEFENDI, V.: Dependence of macrophage growth in vitro upon interaction with other cell types. Wistar Inst. Symp. Monogr. *7*, 67–86 (1967).
170. MAUEL, J. DEFENDI, V.: Regulation of DNA synthesis in mouse macrophages. I. Sources, action and purification of the macrophage growth factor (MGF). Exp. Cell Res. *65*, 33–42 (1971).
171. MAUEL, J., DEFENDI, V.: Regulation of DNA synthesis in mouse macrophages. II. Studies on mechanisms of action of the macrophage growth factor. Exp. Cell Res. *65*, 377–385 (1971).
172. LANDAU, T., SACHS, L.: Activation of a differentiation-inducing protein by adenine and adenine-containing nucleotides. FEBS Lett. *17*, 339–341 (1971).
173. METCALF, D., STANLEY, E. R.: Serum half-life in mice of colony stimulating factor prepared from human urine. Brit. J. Haemat. *20*, 549–556 (1971).
174. BURGESS, A. W., METCALF, D.: Serum half-life and organ distribution of radiolabeled colony stimulating factor in mice. Exp. Hemat. (1977).
175. SHERIDAN, J. W., METCALF, D.: The bone marrow colony stimulating factor (CSF): relation of serum CSF to urine CSF. Proc. Soc. exp. Biol. (N.Y.) *144*, 785–788 (1973).
176. STANLEY, E. R., MCNEILL, T. A., CHAN, S. H.: Antibody production to the factor in human urine stimulating colony formation in vitro by bone marrow cells. Brit. J. Haemat. *18*, 585–590 (1970).
177. PRICE, G. B., SENN, J. S., MCCULLOCH, E. A., TILL, J. E.: The isolation and properties of granulocyte colony-stimulating activities from medium conditioned by human peripheral leucocytes. Biochem. J. *148*, 209–217 (1975).
178. PRICE, G. B., MCCULLOCH, E. A., TILL, J. E.: Cell membranes as sources of granulocyte colony stimulating activities. Exp. Hemat. *3*, 227–233 (1975).
179. PRICE, G. B., MCCULLOCH, E. A., TILL, J. E.: A new low molecular weight granulocyte colony stimulating activity. Blood *42*, 341–348 (1973)
180. PRICE, G. B., SENN, J. S., MCCULLOCH, E. A., TILL, J. E.: Heterogeneity of molecules with low molecular weight isolated from media conditioned by human leukocytes and capable of stimulating colony formation by human granulopoietic progenitor cells. J. cell. Physiol. *84*, 383–396 (1974).
181. LIND, D. E., BRADLEY, M. L., GUNZ, F. W., VINCENT, P. C.: The non-equivalence of mouse and human marrow culture in assay of granulopoietic stimulatory factors. J. cell. Physiol. *83*, 35–42 (1974).
182. METCALF, D.: Stimulation by human urine or plasma of granulopoiesis by human marrow cells in agar. Exp. Hemat. *2*, 157–173 (1974).
183. MOORE, M. A. S., WILLIAMS, N.: Analysis of proliferation and differentiation of foetal granulocyte-macrophage progenitor cells in haemopoietic tissue. Cell Tiss. Kinet. *6*, 461–476 (1973).
184. MOORE, M. A. S., MCNEILL, T. A., HASKILL, J. S.: Density distribution analysis of in vivo and in

vitro colony forming cells in developing fetal liver. J. cell. Physiol. *75*, 181–192 (1970).
185. HASKILL, J. S., MOORE, M. A. S.: Two dimensional cell separation: comparison of embryonic and adult haemopoietic stem cells. Nature (Lond.) *226*, 853–854 (1970).
186. METCALF, D.: Antigen-induced proliferation in vitro of bone marrow precursors of granulocytes and macrophages. Immunology *20*, 727–738 (1971).
187. McNEILL, T. A.: Antigenic stimulation of bone marrow colony forming cells. III. Effect in vivo. Immunology *18*, 61–72 (1970).
188. METCALF, D.: Depressed responses of the granulocyte-macrophage system to bacterial antigens following preimmunization. Immunology *26*, 1115–1125 (1974).
189. PLUZNIK, D. H. ROTTER, V., SCHEINMAN, R.: Kinetics of proliferation of splenic macrophage precursor cells during the early primary immune response. J. reticuloendoth. Soc. *11*, 154–166 (1972).
190. HIBBERD, A. D., METCALF, D.: Proliferation of macrophage and granulocyte precursors in response to primary and transplanted tumors. Israel J. med. Sci. *7*, 202–210 (1971).
191. McNEILL, T. A., FLEMING, W. A., McCLURE, S. KILLEN, M.: Granulocyte-macrophage precursor cell responses in mice of different strain, age and sex. Immunology *25*, 91–101 (1973).
192. APTE, R. N. PLUZNIK, D. H.: Genetic control of lipopolysaccharide-induced generation of serum colony stimulating factor and proliferation of splenic granulocyte/macrophage precursor cells. J. cell. Physiol. *89*, 313–324 (1976).
193. APTE, R. N., PLUZNIK, D. H.: Control mechanisms of endotoxin and particulate material stimulation of hemopoietic colony forming cell differentiation. Exp. Hemat. *4*, 10–18 (1976).
194. TRUDGETT, A., McNEILL, T. A., KILLEN, M.: Granulocyte-macrophage precursor cell and colony stimulating factor responses of mice-infected with Salmonella typhymurium. Infect. Immun. *8*, 450–455 (1973).
195. ITURRIZA, R. G. SEIDEL, H. J.: Stem cell growth and production of colony stimulating factor in Rauscher virus-infected CBA/J mice. J. nat. Cancer Inst. *53*, 487–492 (1974).
196. KURNICK, J. E., ROBINSON, W. A.: Colony growth of human peripheral white blood cells in vitro. Blood *37*, 136–141 (1971).
197. PLUZNIK, D. H., FEIGIS, M.: Stimulation of macrophage precursor cell proliferation and its relation to phagocytic activity and immune suppression. J. reticuloendoth. Soc. *15*, 466–474 (1974).
198. PLUZNIK, D. H., ZILBER, D., FEIGIS, M.: Correlation between splenic phagocytic activity and increase in splenic granulocyte/macrophage progenitors. Exp. Hemat. *4*, 170–179 (1976).
199. ICHIKAWA, Y., PLUZNIK, D. H., SACHS, L.: Feedback inhibition of the development of macrophage and granulocyte colonies. I. Inhibition by macrophages. Proc. nat. Acad. Sci. (Wash.) *58*, 1480–1486 (1967).
200. PLUZNIK, D. H., ZILBER, D.: Increase in splenic macrophage precursor cells and its relation to a decrease in inhibitor activity. J. reticuloendoth. Soc. *18*, 160–166 (1975).
201. WALKER, W. S.: Functional heterogeneity of macrophages in the induction and expression of acquired immunity. J. reticuloendoth. Soc. *20*, 57–65 (1976).
202. BRADLEY, T. R., ROBINSON, W., METCALF, D.: Colony production in vitro by normal polycythemic and anaemic bone marrow. Nature (Lond.) *213*, 511 (1967).
203. METCALF, D.: The effect of bleeding on the number of in vitro colony forming cells in the bone marrow. Brit. J. Haemat. *16*, 397–407 (1969).
204. HODGSON, G. S., BRADLEY, T. R., TELFER, P. A.: Haemopoietic stem cells in experimental haemolytic anaemia. Cell Tiss. Kinet. *5*, 283–288 (1972).
205. QUESENBERRY, P. J., MORLEY, A., STOHLMAN, F., RICKARD, K., HOWARD, D., SMITH, M.: Effect of endotoxin on granulopoiesis and colony stimulating factor. New Engl. J. Med. *286*, 227–232 (1972).
206. GOLDE, D. W., CLINE, M. J.: Endotoxin-induced release of colony-stimulating activity in man. Proc. Soc. exp. Biol. (N.Y.) *149*, 845–848 (1975).
207. QUESENBERRY, P., HALPERIN, J., RYAN, M., STOHLMAN, F.: Tolerance to the granulocyte-releasing and colony-stimulating factor elevating effects of endotoxin. Blood *45*, 789–800 (1975).
208. APTE, R. N., GALANOS, C., PLUZNIK, D. H.: Lipid A, the active part of bacterial endotoxins in inducing serum colony stimulating activity and proliferation of splenic granulocyte/macrophage progenitor cells. J. cell. Physiol. *87*, 71–78 (1976).
209. McNEILL, T. A.: Antigenic stimulation of bone marrow colony forming cells. I. Effects of antigens on normal bone marrow cells in vitro. Immunology *18*, 39–47 (1970).
210. McNEILL, T. A.: The effect of synthetic double-stranded polyribonucleotides on haemopoietic colony-forming cells in vitro. Immunology *21*, 741–750 (1971).
211. RUSCETTI, F. W., CYPESS, R. H., CHERVENICK, P. A.: Specific release of neutrophilic -and eosinophilic-stimulating factors from sensitized lymphocytes. Blood *47*, 757–765 (1976).
212. HALL, B. M.: The effects of whole body irradiation on serum colony stimulating factor and in vitro

colony-forming cells in the bone marrow. Brit. J. Haemat. *17*, 553–561 (1969).
213. Morley, A. A., Rickard, K. A., Howard, D., Stohlman, F.: Studies on the regulation of granulopoiesis. IV. Possible humoral regulation. Blood *37*, 14–22 (1971).
214. Metcalf, D., Foster, R., Pollard, M.: Colony stimulating activity of serum from germfree normal and leukemic mice. J. cell. Physiol. *70*, 131–132 (1967).
215. Morley, A. A., Quesenberry, P. J., Bealmear, P., Stohlman, F., Wilson, R.: Serum colony stimulating factor levels in irradiated germfree and conventional CFW mice. Proc. Soc. exp. Biol. (N.Y.) *140*, 478–480 (1972).
216. Chang, C. F., Pollard, M.: Effects of microbial flora on levels of colony stimulating factor in serum of irradiated CFW mice. Proc. Soc. exp. Biol. (N.Y.) *144*, 177–180 (1973).
217. Gordon, M. Y., Blackett, W. M.: Stimulation of granulocytic colony formation in agar diffusion chambers implanted in cyclophosphamide pretreated mice. Brit. J. Cancer *32*, 51–59 (1975).
218. Foster, R., Metcalf, D., Kirchmyer, R.: Induction of bone marrow colony-stimulating activity by a filtrable agent in leukemic and normal mouse serum. J. exp. Med. *127*, 853–866 (1968).
219. Foster, R., Metcalf, D., Robinson, W. A., Bradley, T. R.: Bone marrow colony stimulating activity in human sera. Results of two independent surveys in Buffalo and Melbourne. Brit. J. Haemat. *15*, 147–159 (1968).
220. Metcalf, D., Wahren, B.: Bone marrow colony-stimulating activity of sera in infectious mononucleosis. Brit. med. J. *3*, 99–101 (1968).
221. Metcalf, D., Bradley, T. R.: Factors regulating in vitro colony formation by hematopoietic cells. In: Regulation of Hematopoiesis. Gordon, A. S. (ed.). New York: Appleton-Century-Crofts 1970, pp. 187–215.
222. Granstrom, M.: Studies on inhibitors of bone marrow colony formation in normal human sera and during a viral infection. Exp. Cell Res. *82*, 426–432 (1972).
223. Metcalf, D., Chan, S. H., Gunz, F. W., Vincent, P., Ravich, R. B. M.: Colony stimulating factor and inhibitor levels in acute granulocytic leukemia. Blood *38*, 143–152 (1971).
224. Robinson, W. A.: Granulocytosis in neoplasia. Ann. N.Y. Acad. Sci. *230*, 212–218 (1974).
225. Myers, A. M., Robinson, W. A.: Colony stimulating factor levels in human serum and urine following chemotherapy. Proc. Soc. exp. Biol. (N.Y.) *148*, 694–700 (1975).
226. Chan, S. H.: Studies on colony-stimulating factor (CSF): role of the kidney in clearing serum CSF. Proc. Soc. exp. Biol. (N.Y.) *134*, 733–737 (1970).
227. Foster, R. S., Mirand, E. A.: Bone marrow colony stimulating factor following ureteral ligation in germfree mice. Proc. Soc. exp. Biol. (N.Y.) *133*, 1223–1227 (1970).
228. Tisman, G., Herbert, V., Rosenblatt, S.: Evidence that lithium induces human granulocyte proliferation. Elevated serum B_{12} binding capacity in vivo and granulocyte colony proliferation in vitro. Brit. J. Haemat. *24*, 767–771 (1973).
229. Gupta, R. C., Robinson, W. A., Kurnick, J. E.: Felty's syndrome. Effect of lithium on granulopoiesis. Amer. J. Med. *61*, 29–32 (1976).
230. Mangalik, A., Robinson, W. A.: Cyclic neutropenia. The relationship between urine granulocyte colony stimulating activity and neutrophil count. Blood *41*, 79–84 (1973).
231. Shadduck, R. K. Nagabhushananm, N. G.: Granulocyte colony stimulating factor. I. Response to acute granulocytopenia. Blood *38*, 559–568 (1971).
232. Wewerka, J. R., Dale, D. C.: Colony-stimulating factor in patients with chronic neutropenia. Blood *47*, 861–867 (1976).
233. Amato, D., Freedman, M. H., Saunders, E. F.: Granulopoiesis in severe congenital neutropenia. Blood *47*, 531–538 (1976).
234. Mabry, J., Carbone, P. P., Bull, J. M.: Amplification of colony stimulating activity in human serum by interaction with CSA from other sources. Exp. Hemat. *3*, 354–361 (1975).
235. Vogler, W. R., Winton, E. F.: Humoral granulopoietic inhibitors. A review. Exp. Hemat. *3*, 337–353 (1975).
236. Stanley, E. R., Robinson, W. A., Ada, G. L.: Properties of the colony stimulating factor in leukaemic and normal mouse serum. Aust. J. exp. Biol. med. Sci. *46*, 715–726 (1068).
237. Metcalf, D., Foster, R.: Bone marrow colony-stimulating activity of serum from mice with viral-induced leukemia. J. nat. Cancer Inst. *39*, 1235–1245 (1967).
238. Chan, S. H.: Influence of serum inhibitors on colony development in vitro by bone marrow cells. Aust. J. exp. Biol. med. Sci. *47*, 553–564 (1971).
239. Chan, S. H., Metcalf, D., Stanley, E. R.: Stimulation and inhibition by normal human serum of colony formation in vitro by bone marrow cells. Brit. J. Haemat. *20*, 329–341 (1971).
240. McNeill, T. A., Fleming, W. A.: Cellular responsiveness to stimulation in vitro. Strain differences in hemopoietic colony forming cell responsiveness to stimulating factor and suppresson of

responsiveness by glucocorticoids. J. cell. Physiol. *82*, 49–58 (1973).
241. BERAN, M.: The influence of mouse sera on colony formation and on the production of colony stimulating factor in vitro. Exp. Hemat. *3*, 309–318 (1975).
242. CHAN, S. H., METCALF, D.: Inhibition of bone marrow colony formation by normal and leukaemic human serum. Nature (Lond.) *227*, 845–846 (1970).
243. GRANSTROM, M., WAHREN, B., GAHRTON, G., KILLANDER, D., FOLEY, G. E.: Inhibitors of the bone marrow colony formation in sera of patients with leukemia. Int. J. Cancer *10*, 482–488 (1972).
244. RYTOMAA, T., KIVINIEMI, K.: Regulator system of blood cell production. In: Control of Cellular Growth in Adult Organisms. London: Academic Press 1967, pp. 106–138.
245. RYTOMAA, T., KIVINIEMI, K.: Control of granulocyte production. I. Chalone and anti-chalone, two specific humoral regulators. Cell Tiss. Kinet. *1*, 329–340 (1968).
246. SHADDUCK, R. K.: Granulocyte stimulating activity from neutrophils (PMN's): Possible dual feedback control of granulopoiesis. Blood *38*, 820 (1971).
247. MACVITTIE, T. J., MCCARTHY, K. F.: Inhibition of granulopoiesis in diffusion chambers by a granulocyte chalone. Exp. Hemat. *2*, 182–194 (1974).
248. PARAN, M., ICHIKAWA, Y., SACHS, L.: Feedback inhibition of the development of macrophage and granulocyte colonies. II. Inhibition of granulocytes. Proc. nat. Acad. Sci. (Wash.) *62*, 81–87 (1969).
249. HASKILL, J. S., MCKNIGHT, R. D., GALBRAITH, P. R.: Cell-cell stimulating and inhibiting cells from human bone marrow. Blood *40*, 391–399 (1972).
250. LORD, B. I. CERCEK, L., CERCEK, B., SHAH, G. P., DEXTER, T. M., LAJTHA, L. G.: Inhibitors of haemopoietic cell proliferation? Specificity of action within the haemopoietic system. Brit. J. Cancer *29*, 168–175 (1974).
251. LORD, B. I., CERCEK, L., CERCEK, B., SHAH, G. P. LAJTHA, L. G.: Inhibitors of haemopoietic cell proliferation: reversibility of action. Brit. J. Cancer *29*, 407–409 (1974).
252. PAUKOVITS, W. R.: Control of granulocyte production: separation and chemical identification of a specific inhibitor (chalone). Cell Tiss. Kinet. *4*, 539–547 (1971).
253. PAUKOVITS, W. R.: Granulopoiesis-inhibiting factor. Demonstration and preliminary chemical and biological characterisation of a specific polypeptide (chalone). Nat. Cancer Inst. Monog. *38*, 147–155 (1973).
254. METCALF, D.: Inhibition of bone marrow colony formation in vitro by dialysable products of normal and neoplastic haemopoietic cells. Aust. J. exp. Biol. med. Sci. *49*, 351–363 (1971).
255. KURLAND, J., MOORE, M. A. S.: Inhibition of normal and neoplastic hemopoietic proliferation by a diffusible factor from activated macrophages. In: Experimental Hematology Today. Ed. S. J. Baum, S. J. (ed.). New York: Springer-Verlag 1976.
256. LOZZIO, C. B., LOZZIO, B. B.: Cytotoxicity of a factor isolated from human spleen. J. nat. Cancer Inst. *50*, 535–538 (1973).
257. FLEMING, W. A., MCNEILL, T. A., KILLEN, M.: The effects of an inhibiting factor (interferon) on the in vitro growth of granulocyte and macrophage colonies. Immunology *23*, 429–437 (1972).
258. MCNEILL, T. A., GRESSER, I.: Inhibition of haemopoietic colony growth by interferon preparations from different sources. Nature (New Biol.) *244*, 173–174 (1973).
259. ROTHSTEIN, G., HUGL, E. H., CHERVENICK, P. A., ATHENS, J. W., MACFARLANE, J.: Humoral stimulators of granulocyte production. Blood *41*, 73–78 (1973).
260. BRADLEY, T. R., METCALF, D., SUMNER, M., STANLEY, R.: Characteristics of in vitro colony formation by cells from haemopoietic tissues. In: Hemic Cells in vitro. Farnes, P. (ed.) Baltimore: Williams and Wilkins 1969, pp. 22–35.
261. ATHENS, J. W.: Granulocyte kinetics in health and disease. Nat. Cancer. Inst. Monog. *30*, 135–155 (1969).
262. BROWN, R. D., RICKARD, K. A., KRONENBERG, H.: Granulopoietic activity and the human bone marrow colony forming cell. Aust. J. Med. Technol. *4*, 183–190 (1973).
263. KURNICK, J. E., ROBINSON, W. A., DICKEY, C. A.: In vitro granulocytic colony-forming potential of bone marrow from patients with granulocytopenia and aplastic anemia. Proc. Soc. exp. Biol. (N.Y.) *137*, 917–920 (1971).
264. MINTZ, U., SACHS, L.: Normal granulocyte colony-forming cells in the bone marrow of Yemenite Jews with genetic neutropenia. Blood *41*, 745–751 (1973).
265. ICHIKAWA, Y.: Differentiation of a cell line of myeloid leukemia. In: The Nature of Leukaemia. Vincent, P. C. (ed.). Sydney: Australian Cancer Society 1972, p. 187.
266. STOCKDALE, F., OKAZAKI, K., NAMEROFF, M., HOLTZER, H.: 5-bromodeoxyuridine: effects on myogenesis in vitro. Science *146*, 533–535 (1964).
267. ABBOT, J., HOLTZER, H.: The loss of phenotypic traits by differentiated cells. V. The effect of 5-bromodeoxyaridine on cloned chondrocytes. Proc. nat. Acad. Sci. (Wash.) *59*, 1144–1151 (1968).

268. COLEMAN, A. W., COLEMAN, J. R., KANKEL, D., WERNER, I.: The reversible control of animal cell differentiation by the thymidine analog, 5-bromodeoxyuridine. Exp. Cell Res. *59*, 319–328 (1970).
269. FIBACH, E., LANDAU, T., SACHS, L.: Normal differentiation of myeloid leukaemic cells induced by a differentiation-inducing protein. Nature (Lond.) *237*, 276–278 (1972).
270. FIBACH, E., HAYASHI, M., SACHS, L.: Control of normal differentiation of myeloid leukemic cells to macrophages and granulocytes. Proc. nat. Acad. Sci. (Wash.) *70*, 343–346 (1973).
271. HAYASHI, M., FIBACH, E., SACHS, L.: Control of normal differentiation of myeloid leukemic cells. V. Normal differentiation in aneuplioid leukemic cells and the chromosome banding pattern of D+ and D− clones. Int. J. Cancer *14*, 40–48 (1974).
272. FIBACH, E., SACHS, L.: Control of normal differentiation of myeloid leukemic cells. IV. Induction of differentiation by serum from endotoxin treated mice. J. cell. Physiol. *83*, 177–186 (1974).
273. FIBACH, E., SACHS, L.: Control of normal differentiation of myeloid leukemic cells. VII. Induction of differentiation to mature granulocytes in mass culture. J. cell. Physiol. *86*, 221–230 (1975).
274., LOTEM, J., SACHS, L.: Control of normal differentiation of myeloid leukemic cells. VI. Inhibition of cell multiplication and the formation of macrophages. J. cell. Physiol. *85*, 587–594 (1975).
275. LOTEM, J., SACHS, L.: Different blocks in the differentiation of myeloid leukemic cells. Proc. nat. Acad. Sci. (Wash.) *71*, 3507–3511 (1974).
276. LOTEM, J., SACHS, L.: Induction of specific changes in surface membrane of myeloid leukemic cells by steroid hormones. Int. J. Cancer *15*, 731–740 (1975).
277. WARNER, N. L., MOORE, M. A. S., METCALF, D.: A transplantable myeomonocytic leukemia in BALB/c mice: cytology, karyotype and muramidase content. J. natl. Cancer Inst. *43*, 963–982 (1969).
278. METCALF, D., MOORE, M. A. S.: Factors modifying stem cell proliferation of myelomonocytic leukemic cells in vitro and in vivo. J. nat. Cancer Inst. *44*, 801–808 (1970).
279. CLINE, M. J., METCALF, D.: Cellular differentiation in a murine myelomonocytic leukemia. Blood *39*, 771–777 (1972).
280. NOOTER, K., BENTVELSEN, P.: In vitro growth characteristics of virally transformed murine myeloid cells. Cancer Res. *36*, 1246–1250 (1976).
281. GOLDMAN, J. M., TH'NG, K. H., LOWENTHAL, R. M.: In vitro colony-forming cells and colony stimulating factor in chronic granulocytic leukaemia. Brit. J. Cancer *30*, 1–12 (1974).
282. MOBERG, C., OLOFSSON, T., OLSSON, I.: Granulopoiesis in chronic myeloid leukaemia. I. In vitro cloning of blood and bone marrow cells in agar culture. Scand. J. Haemat. *12*, 381–390 (1974).
283. SHADDUCK, R. K., NANKIN, H. R.: Cellular origin of granulocytic colonies in chronic myeloid leukaemia. Lancet (1971) II, 1097–1098.
284. MOORE, M. A. S., METCALF, D.: Cytogenetic analysis of human acute and chronic myeloid leukemic cells cloned in agar culture. Int. J. Cancer *11*, 143–152 (1973).
285. CHERVENICK, P. A., ELLIS, C. D., PAN, S. F., LAWSON, A. L.: Human leukemic cells: in vitro growth of colonies containing the Philadelphia (Ph^1) chromosome. Science *174*, 1134–1136 (1971).
286. METCALF, D., MOORE, M. A. S., SHERIDAN, J. W., SPITZER, G.: Responsiveness of human granulocytic leukemic cells to colony-stimulating factor. Blood *43*, 847–859 (1974).
287. HURDLE, A. D. F., GARSON, O. M., BUIST, D. G.: Clinical and cytogenetic studies in chronic myelomonocytic leukemia. Brit. J. Haemat. *32*, 733–782 (1972).
288. MOORE, M. A. S., WILLIAMS, N., METCALF, D., GARSON, O. M., HURDLE, A. D. F.: Control of human leukemic cell proliferation and differentiation in agar culture. In: Cell Differentiation. Harris, R., Viza, D. (eds.). Munksgaard 1972, pp. 144–150.
289. MOORE, M. A. S.: Marrow culture — a new approach to classification of leukemias. In: Unclassifiable Leukemias. Bessis, M., Brecher, G. (eds.). Berlin: Springer-Verlag, 1975, pp. 149–158.
290. BROWN, C. H., CARBONE, P. P.: In vitro growth of normal and leukemic human bone marrow. J. nat. Cancer Instit. *46*, 989–1000 (1971).
291. BOGGS, D. R.: Hematopoietic stem cell theory in relation to possible lymphoblastic conversion of chronic myeloid leukemia. Blood *44*, 449–453 (1974).
292. SENN, J. S., MCCULLOCH, E. A., TILL, J. E.: Comparison of colony-forming ability of normal and leukaemic human marrow in cell culture. Lancet (1967) II, 597–598.
293. ROBINSON, W. A., PIKE, B. L.: Colony growth of human bone marrow cells in vitro. In: Hemopoietic Cellular Proliferation. Stohlman, F. (ed.). New York: Grune and Stratton, 1970, pp. 249–259.
294. GREENBERG, P. L., NICHOLS, W., SCHRIER, S. L.: Granulopoiesis in acute myeloid leukemia and preleukemia. New Eng. J. Med. *284*, 1225–1232 (1971).
295. ROBINSON, W. A., ENTRINGER, M. A.: Correlation of clinical disease and colony growth of human leukemic cells in vitro. In: Hemopoiesis in Culture. Robinson, W. A. (ed.). Washington: DHEW Publication No. (NIH) 74-205, 1973, pp. 288–300.

296. Bull, J. M., Duttera, M. J., Stashick, E. D., Northrup, J., Henderson, E., Carbone, P. P.: Serial in vitro marrow culture in acute myelocytic leukemia. Blood *42*, 679–686 (1973).
297. Sultan, C., Marquet, M., Joffroy, Y.: Etude des leucemies aiques myeloblastiques en pousse et en remission par culture de moelle in vitro. Nouv. Rev. franc, Hématol. *13*, 641–648 (1973).
298. Moore, M. A. S., Spitzer, G., Williams, N., Metcalf, D., Buckley, J.: Agar culture studies in 127 cases of untreated acute leukemia: the prognostic value of reclassification of leukemia according to in vitro growth characteristics. Blood *44*, 1–18 (1974).
299. Robinson, W. A., Entringer, M. A., Otsuka, A. L.: In vitro studies in acute granulocytic leukemia. In: The Nature of Leukemia. Vincent, P. C. (ed.). Sydney: Australian Cancer Society, 1972, pp. 151–161.
300. Killmann, S. A.: Acute leukemia: the kinetics of leukemic blast cells in man. An analytical review. Ser. Haemat. *1*, 38–102 (1968).
301. Whang, J., Frei, E., Tjio, J. H., Carbone, P. P., Brecher, G.: The distribution of the Philadelphia chromosome in patients with chronic myelogenous leukemia. Blood *22*, 664–673 (1963).
302. Clein, G. P., Flemans, R. J.: Involvement of the erythroid series in blastic crisis of chronic myeloid leukemia. Further evidence for the presence of Philadelphia chromosome in erythroblasts. Brit. J. Haemat. *12*, 754–758 (1966).
303. Tough, I. M., Jacobs, P. A., Court-Brown, W. M., Baikie, A. G., Williamson, E. R. D.: Cytogentic studies on bone marrow in chronic myeloid leukemia. Lancet (1963) II, 844–846.
304. Fialkow, P. J., Gartler, S. M., Yoshida, A.: Clonal origin of chronic myelocytic leukemia in man. Proc. nat. Acad. Sci. (Wash.) *58*, 1468–1471 (1967).
305. Moore, M. A. S., Ekert, H., Fitzgerald, M. G., Carmichael, A.: Evidence for the clonal origin of chronic myeloid leukemia from a sex chromosome mosaic: clinical cytogenetic and marrow culture studies. Blood *43*, 15–22 (1974).
306. Krogh Jenson, M., Killmann, S. A.: Additional evidence for chromosome abnormalities in the erythroid precursors in acute leukaemia. Acta med. scand. *189*, 97–100 (1971).
307. Duttera, M. J., Whang-Peng, J., Bull, J. M. C., Carbone, P. P.: Cytogenetically abnormal cells in vitro in acute leukemia. Lancet, (1972) I, 715–718.
308. Spitzer, G., Dicke, K. A., Gehan, E. A., Smith, T., McCredie, K. B.: The use of the Robinson in vitro agar culture assay in adult acute leukemia. Blood Cells *2*, 139–148 (1976).
309. Chervenick, P. A.: In vitro colony formation and clinical response in acute leukemia. In: Workshop on Prognostic Factors in Human Acute Leukemia. Fliedner, T. M., Perry, S. (eds.). Vieweg: Permagon Press 1975, pp. 229–236.
310. Robinson, W. A., Entringer, M. A.: Correlation of clinical factors with colony growth of human leukemic cells in vitro. In: Workshop on Prognostic Factors in Human Acute Leukemia. Fliedner, T. M., Perry, S. (eds.). Vieweg: Permagon Press 1975, pp. 249–257.
311. Spitzer, G., Schwarz, M. A., Dicke, K. A., Trujillo, J. M., McCredie, K. B.: Significance of PHA-induced clonigenic cells in chronic myeloid leukemia and early acute myeloid leukemia. Blood Cells *2*, 149–159 (1976).
312. Mack, T., Robinson, W. A., Holton, C. P.: Colony growth of peripheral blood cells from patients with acute lymphocytic leukemia. Cancer Res. *32*, 2054–2057 (1972).
313. Duttera, M., Bull, J., Northup, J., Stashick, E., Henderson, E., Carbone, P. P.: Serial in vitro marrow culture in acute lymphocytic leukemia. Blood *42*, 687–699 (1973).
314. Ragab, A. H., Gilkerson, E., Myers, M., Choi, S. L.: The culture of colony forming units from the peripheral blood and bone marrow of children with acute lymphocytic leukemia. Cancer (Philad.), *34*, 663–669 (1974).
315. Harris, J., Freireich, E. J.: In vitro growth of myeloid colonies from bone marrow of patients with acute leukemia in remission. Blood *35*, 61–63 (1970).
316. Cowan, D. H., Clarysse, A., Abu-Zahra, H., Senn, J. S., McCulloch, E. A.: The effect of remission induction in acute myeloblastic leukemia on efficiency of colony formation in culture. Ser. Hemat, *5*, 179–188 (1972).
317. Moore, M. A. S.: In vitro studies in the myeloid leukemias. In: Advances in Acute Leukemia. Cleton, F. J., Crowther, D., Malpas, J. S. (eds.). Amsterdam: North-Holland 1975, pp. 161–227.
318. Mak, T. W., Aye, M. T., Messner, H. A., Sheinin, R., Till, J. E., McCulloch, E. A.: Reverse transcriptase activity: increase in marrow cultures from leukemic patients in relapse and remission. Brit. J. Cancer *29*, 433–437 (1974).
319. Gallagher, R. E., Salahuddin, S. Z., Hall, W. T., McCredie, K. B., Gallo, R. C.: Growth and differentiation in culture of leukemic leukocytes from a patient with acute myelogenous leukemia and reidentification of a Type C virus. Proc. nat. Acad. Sci. (Wash.) *72*, 4137–4141 (1975).
320. Finney, R., McDonald, G. A., Baikie, A. G., Douglas, A. S.: Chronic granulocytic leukaemia

with Ph[1] negative cells in bone marrow and a ten year remission after busulphan hypoplasia. Brit. J. Haemat. *23*, 283–288 (1972).
321. Hays, E. F., Craddock, C. G., Haskett, D., Newell, M.: In vitro colony-forming cells in the marrow of leukemic and preleukemic mice. Blood *47*, 603–610 (1976).
322. Metcalf, D., Furth, J., Buffett, R. F.: Pathogenesis of mouse leukemia caused by Friend virus. Cancer Res. *19*, 52–58 (1959).
323. Metcalf, D., Chan, S. H.: Abnormal regulation of granulopoiesis in human acute granulocytic leukemia. In: Unifying Concepts of Leukemia. Dutcher, R. M., Chieco-Bianchi, L. (eds.). Basel: Karger 1973, pp. 878–884.
324. Mintz, U., Sachs, L.: Differences in inducing activity for human bone marrow colonies in normal serum and serum from patients with leukemia. Blood *42*, 331–339 (1973).
325. Mangalik, A., Robinson, W. A.: The effect of serum from patients with acute granulocytic leukemia or granulocyte colony formation in vitro. A search for inhibitors. Proc. Soc. exp. Biol. (N.Y.) *141*, 515–518 (1972).
326. Paran, M., Ichikawa, Y., Sachs, L.: Production of the inducer for macrophage and granulocyte colonies by leukemic cells. J. cell. Physiol. *72*, 251–254 (1968).
327. Goldman, J. M., Th'ng, K. H., Catovsky, D., Galton, D. A. G.: Production of colony-stimulating factor by leukemic leukocytes. Blood *47*, 381–388 (1976).
328. Golde, D. W., Rothman, B., Cline, M. J.: Production of colony-stimulating factor by malignant leukocytes. Blood *43*, 749–756 (1974).
329. Aye, M. T., Till, J. E., McCulloch, E. A.: Interacting populations affecting proliferation of leukemic cells in culture. Blood *45*, 485–493 (1975).
330. Tanaka, T., Testa, N., Lajtha, L. G.: Leukemic stem cell kinetics in experimental animals. Bibl. haemat. (Basel) *39*, 984–991 (1973).
331. Hoelzer, D., Harriss, E. B., Haas, R. J.: The behaviour of resting bone marrow cells in rats with acute leukemia. Bibl. haemat. (Basel) *39*, 1008–1013 (1973).
332. Van Bekkum, D. W., Van Oosterom, P., Dicke, K. A.: In vitro colony formation of transplantable rat leukemias in comparison with human acute myeloid leukemia. Cancer Res. *36*, 941–946 (1976).
333. Chiyoda, S., Mizoguchi, H., Kosaka, K., Takaku, F., Miura, Y.: Influence of leukaemic cells on the colony formation of human bone marrow cells in vitro. Brit. J. Cancer *31*, 355–358 (1975).
334. Chiyoda, S., Mizoguchi, H., Asano, S., Takaku, F., Miura, Y.: Influence of leukaemic cells on the colony formation of human bone marrow cells in vitro. II. Suppressive effects of leukaemic cell extracts. Brit. J. Cancer *33*, 379–384 (1976).
335. Morris, T. C. M., McNeill, T. A., Bridges, J. M.: Inhibition of normal human in vitro colony forming cells by cells from leukaemic patients. Brit. J. Cancer *31*, 641–648 (1975).
336. Bull, J. M., Rosenblum, A., Carbone, P. P.: In vitro culture studies in patients with acute myelocytic leukemia. In: Hemopoiesis in Culture. Robinson, W. A. (ed.). Washington DHEW Publication No. (NIH) 74–205, 1973, pp. 335–341.
337. Gray, J. L., Robinson, W. A.: In vitro colony formation by human bone marrow cells after freezing. J. Lab. clin. Med. *81*, 317–322 (1973).
338. Moore, M. A. S., Spitzer, G.: In vitro studies in the myeloproliferative disorders. In: Lympohcyte Recognition and Effector Mechanisms. Proceedings of Eighth Leucocyte Culture Conference. Lindahl-Kiessling, K., Osoba, D. (eds.). New York: Academic Press 1974, pp. 431–437.
339. Dicke, K. A., Lowenberg, B.: In vitro analysis of pancytopenia: its relevance to the clinic. In: Prognostic Factors in Human Acute Leukemia. Advances in the Biosciences 14. Fliedner, T. M., Perry, S. (eds.). Vieweg: Permagon Press 1975, pp. 259–270.
340. Vilter, R. W., Will, J. J., Jarrold, T.: Refractory anemia with hyperplastic bone marrow (Aregenerative anemia) Semin. Hemat. *4*, 175–193 (1967).
341. Greenberg, P., Mara, B., Bax, I., Brossel, R. Schrier, S.: The myeloproliferative disorders: correlation between clinical evolution and alterations of granulopoiesis. Amer. J. Med. *61*, 878–891 (1976).
342. Senn, J. S., Pinkerton, P. H.: Defective in vitro colony formation by human bone marrow preceding overt leukemia. Brit. J. Haemat. *23*, 277–281 (1972).
343. Killman, S. A.: Chronic myelogenous leukemia: preleukemia or leukemia. Haematologica *57*, 641–649 (1972).
344. Pederson, B.: Annotation. The blastic crisis of chronic myeloid leukaemia: acute transformation of a preleukaemic condition? Brit. J. Haemat. *25*, 141–145 (1973).
345. Prchal, J. F. (personal communication).
346. Upton, A. C., Furth, J.: Transmissable disease of mice characterised by anemia, leukopenia,

splenomegaly and myelosclerosis. Acta haemat. (Basel) *13*, 65–76 (1955).
347. KAPLAN, H. S.: On the natural history of the murine leukemias. Cancer Res. *27*, 1325–1340 (1967).
348. HARDY, W. D., OLD, L. J., HESS, P. W., ESSEX, M., COTTER, S.: Horizontal transmission of feline leukemia virus. Nature (Lond.) *244*, 266–269 (1973).
349. METCALF, D.: Humoral regulators in the development and progression of leukemia. Advanc. Cancer Res. *14*, 181–230 (1971).
350. BASTEN, A., BEESON, P. B.: Mechanism of eosinophilia. II. Role of the lymphocyte. J. exp. Med. *131*, 1288–1305 (1970).
351. PORTER, R. P., GENGOZIAN, N.: In vitro proliferation and differentiation of hemic precursor cells from marrow and blood of naturally chimeric marmosets. J. cell. Physiol. *79*, 27–41 (1972).
352. NAKEFF, A., DICKE, K. A., VAN NOORD, M. J.: Megakaryocytes in agar cultures of mouse bone marrow. Ser. Haemat. *8*, 4–21 (1975).
353. NAKEFF, A., DANIELS-MCQUEEN, S.: In vitro colony assay for a new class of megakaryocyte precursor: colony-forming unit megakaryocyte (CFU-M). Proc. Soc. exp. Biol. (N.Y.) *151*, 587–590 (1976).
354. NAKEFF, A., VAN NOORD, M. J., BLANSJAAR, N.: Electron microscopy of megakaryocytes in thin-layer agar cultures of mouse bone marrow. J. Ultrastruct. Res. *49*, 1–10 (1974).
355. NAKEFF, A.: Colony forming unit megakaryocyte (CFU-M). Its use in elucidating the kinetics and humoral control of the megakaryocytic committed progenitor cell compartment. In: Experimental Hematology Today. Baum, S. J. (ed.). New York: Springer-Verlag 1977.
356. EBBE, S.: Megakaryocytopoiesis. In: Regulation of Hematopoiesis. Gordon, A. S. (Ed.). New York: Appleton-Century-Crofts 1970, pp. 1587–1610.
357. COOPER, G. W.: The regulation of thrombopoiesis. In: Regulation of Hematopoiesis. Gordon, A. S. (ed.). New York: Appleton-Century-Crofts 1970, pp. 1611–1629.
358. DE GABRIELE, G., PENINGTON, D. G.: Regulation of platelet production: Thrombopoietin. Brit. J. Haemat. *13*, 210–215 (1967).
359. CEROTTINI, J. C., ENGERS, H. D., MACDONALD, H. R., BRUNNER, K. T.: Generation of cytotoxic T-lymphocytes in vitro. I. Response of normal and immune mouse spleen cells in mixed leucocyte cultures. J. exp. Med. *140*, 703–717 (1974).
360. HEATH, D. S., AXELRAD, A. A., MCLEOD, D.L., SHREEVE, M. M.: Separation of the erythropoietin-responsive progenitors BFU-E and CFU-E in mouse bone marrow by unit gravity sedimentation. Blood *47*, 777–792 (1976).
361. COOPER, M. C., LEVY, J., CANTOR, L. N., MARKS, P. A., RIFKIND, R. A.: The effect of erythropoietin on colonial growth of erythroid precursor cells in vitro. Proc. nat. Acad. Sci. (Wash.) *71*, 1677–1680 (1974).
362. GREGORY, C. J., MCCULLOCH, E. A., TILL, J. E.: Erythropoietic progenitors capable of colony formation in culture. State of differentiation. J. cell. Physiol. *81*, 411–420 (1973).
363. AXELRAD, A. A., MCLEOD, D. L., SHREEVE, M. M., HEATH, D. S.: Properties of cells that produce erythrocytic colonies in vitro. In: Hemopoiesis in Culture. Robinson, W. A. (ed.). Washington: DHEW Publication No. (NIH) 74-205, 1973, pp. 226–234.
364. ZUCALI, J. R., STEVENS, V., MIRAND, E. A.: In vitro production of erythropoietin by mouse fetal liver. Blood *46*, 85–90 (1975).
365. SINGER, J. W., SAMUELS, A. I., ADAMSON, J. W.: Steroids and hematopoiesis. I. The effect of steroids on in vitro erythroid colony growth: structure/activity relationships. J. cell. Physiol. *88*, 127–134 (1976).
366. SINGER, J. W., ADAMSON, J. W.: Steroids and hematopoiesis. II. The effect of steroids on in vitro erythroid colony growth: evidence for different target cells for different classes of steroids. J. cell. Physiol. *88*, 135–144 (1976).
367. PLUZNIK, D. H., SACHS, L., RESNITZKY, P.: The mechanisms of leukemogenesis by the Rauscher leukemia virus. In: Conference on Murine Leukemia. Nat. Cancer Inst. Monogr. *22*, pp. 3–12 (1966).
368. ZAJDELA, F.: Contribution a l'etude de la cellule de Friend. Bull. Cancer *49*, 351–373 (1962).
369. STEVENS, R. A., MIRAND, E. A., THOMSON, S., AVILA, L.: Enhancement of spleen focus formation and virus reputation in Friend virus infected mice. Cancer Res. *29*, 1111–1116 (1969).
370. SASSA, S., TAKAKU, F., NAKAO, K.: Regulation of erythropoiesis in the Friend leukemia mouse. Blood *31*, 758–765 (1968).
371. MIRAND, E. A., STEEVES, R. A., LANGE, R. D., GRACE, J. T.: Virus-induced polycythemia in mice: erythropoiesis without erythropoietin. Proc. Soc. exp. Biol. (N.Y.) *128*, 844–849 (1968).
372. NOOTER, K., GHIO, R.: Hormone-independent in vitro erythroid colony formation by bone marrow cells from Rauscher virus-infected mice. J. nat. Cancer Inst. *55*, 56–64 (1975).
373. EBERT, B., MAESTRI, N. E., CHIRIGOS, M. A.: Erythropoietic responses of mice to infection with

Rauscher leukemia virus. Cancer Res. *32*, 41–47 (1972).
374. TEPPERMAN, A. D., CURTIS, J. E., MCCULLOCH, E. A.: Erythropoietic colonies in cultures of human marrow. Blood *44*, 659–669 (1974).
375. FRIEND, C., SCHER, W., HOLLAND, J., SATO, T.: Hemoglobin synthesis in murine virus-induced leukemic cells in vitro. Stimulation of erythroid differentiation by dimethylsulfoxide. Proc. nat. Acad. Sci. (Wash.) *68*, 378–382 (1971).
376. PATULEIA, M. C., FRIEND, C.: Tissue culture studies on murine virus-induced leukemia cells: isolation of single cells in agar-liquid medium. Cancer Res. *27*, 726–730 (1967).
377. GOLDSTEIN, K., PREISLER, H. D., LUTTON, J. D., ZANJANI, E. D.: Erythroid colony formation in vitro by dimethylsulfoxide-treated erythroleukemic cells. Blood *44*, 831–836 (1974).
378. PRCHAL, J. F., AXELRAD, A. A.: Bone marrow responses in polycythemia vera. New Engl. J. Med. *290*, 1382 (1974).
379. ROBINSON, W. A., MARBROOK, J., DIENER, E.: Primary stimulation and measurement of antibody production to sheep red blood cells in vitro. J. exp. Med. *126*, 347–356 (1967).
380. KINCADE, P. W., RALPH, P., MOORE, M. A. S.: Growth of B-lymphocyte clones in semisolid culture is mitogen dependent. J. exp. Med. *143*, 1265–1270 (1976).
381. METCALF, D., WILSON, J. W., SHORTMAN, K., MILLER, J. F. A. P., STOCKER, J.: The nature of the cells generating B-lymphocyte colonies in vitro. J. cell. Physiol. *88*, 107–116 (1976).
382. METCALF, D., KOLBER, S.: Stimulation of B-lymphocyte colony formation in vitro by sera from patients with leukaemia or lymphoma. Brit. J. Cancer *34*, 465–475 (1976).
383. DUTTON, R. W., FALKOFF, R., HIRST, J. A., HOFFMAN, M., KAPPLER, J. K., KETTERMAN, J. R., LESLEY, J. F., VANN, D.: Is there evidence for a non-antigen specific diffusible chemical mediator from the thymus-derived cell in the initiation of the immune response? In: Progress in Immunology. Amos, B. (ed.). New York: Academic Press, Vol. I (1971) p. 355.
384. KASAKURA, S., LOWENSTEIN, L.: A factor stimulating DNA synthesis derived from medium of leucocyte cultures. Nature (Lond.) *208*, 794–795 (1965).
385. BEN-YAAKOV, M., HARAN-GHERA, N.: T and B lymphocytes in thymus of SJL/J mice. Nature (Lond.) *255*, 64–66 (1975).
386. CLAESSON, M. H., METCALF, D.: B-lymphocyte colony-forming cells in the SJL/J mouse thymus. J. Immunol. *118*, 1208–1212 (1977).
387. JOHNSON, G. R., METCALF, D., WILSON, J. W.: Development of B-lymphocyte colony-forming cells in foetal mouse tissues. Immunology *30*, 907–914 (1976).
388. ROZENSZAJN, L. A., SREDNI, B., MICHILIN, H., KALECHMAN, Y.: Colony growth in vitro of B-lymphocytes. J. Immunol. (1976).
389. FIBACH, E., GERASSI, E., SACHS, L.: Induction of colony formation in vitro by human lymphocytes. Nature (Lond.) *259*, 127–129 (1976).
390. MOLLER, G., COUTINHO, A.: Factors influencing activation of B cells in immunity. Ann. N.Y. Acad. Sci. *249*, 68–88 (1975).
391. BUJADOUX, M., SABOLOVIC, D., BURG, C.: Proliferation des colonies a partir du thymus in vitro. Exp. Cell Res. *74*, 175–178 (1972).
392. RABINOWITZ, W.: Separation of lymphocytes on glass columns including tissue culture observations. Blood *23*, 811–828 (1964).
393. WILSON, J. D., DALTON, G.: Human T lymphocyte colonies in agar. A comparison with other T cell assays in healthy subjects and cancer patients. Aust. J. exp. Biol. med. Sci. *54*, 27–34 (1976).
394. CLAESSON, M. H., RODGER, L., JOHNSON, G. R., WITTINGHAM, S., METCALF, D.: Colony formation by human T-lymphocytes in agar medium. Clin. exp. Immunol. (1977). (in press).
395. METCALF, D., JOHNSON, G. R.: Clonal analysis of B-lymphocyte development in the spleen. In: Immunoaspects of the Spleen. Batisto, J. R., Streilein, J. W. (eds.). Amsterdam: Elsevier/North-Holland 1976 pp. 27–34.
396. ZOLLA, S.: The effect of plasmacytomas on the immune response of mice. J. Immunol. *108*, 1039–1048 (1972).
397. HENLE, W., DIEHL, V., KOHN, G., ZUR HAUSEN, H., HENLE, G.: Herpes-type virus and chromosome marker in normal leukocytes after growth with irradiated Burkitt cells. Science *157*, 1064–1065 (1967).
398. POPE, J. H., HORNE, M. K., SCOTT, W.: Transformation of foetal human leukocytes in vitro by filtrates of a human leukaemic cell line containing herpes-like virus. Int. J. Cancer *3*, 857–866 (1968).
399. HINUMA, Y., GRACE, J. T.: Cloning of immunoglobulin-producing human leukemic and lymphoma cells in long-term cultures. Proc. Soc. exp. Biol. (N.Y.) *124*, 107–111 (1967).
400. YAMAMOTO, N., HINUMA, Y.: Clonal transformation of human leukocytes by Epstein-Barr virus in soft agar. Int. J. Cancer *17*, 191–196 (1976).

401. SCHARFF, M. D., BARGELLESI, A., BAUMAL, R., BUXBAUM, J., COFFINO, P., LASKOV, R.: Variations in the synthesis and assembly of immunoglobulins by mouse myeloma cells: a genetic and biochemical analysis. J. cell. Physiol. *76*, 331–348 (1970).
402. PARK, C. H., BERGSAGEL, D. E., MCCULLOCH, E. A.: Ascorbic acid: a culture requirement for colony formation by mouse plasmacytoma cells. Science *174*, 720–722 (1971).
403. PARK, C. H., BERGSAGEL, D. E., MCCULLOCH, E. A.: Mouse myeloma tumor stem cells: a primary culture assay. J. nat. Cancer Inst. *46*, 411–422 (1971).
404. COFFINO, P., BAUMAL, R., LASKOV, R., SCHARFF, M. D.: Cloning of mouse myeloma cells and detection of rare variants. J. cell. Physiol. *79*, 429–440 (1972).
405. POTTER, M., PUMPHREY, J. C., WALTERS, J. L.: Growth of primary plasmacytomas in mineral oil-conditioned peritoneal environment. J. nat. Cancer Inst. *49*, 305–308 (1972).
406. NAMBA, Y., HANAOKA, M.: Immunocytology of cultured IgM-forming cells of mouse. I. Requirement of phagocytic cell factor for the growth of IgM-forming tumor cells in tissue culture. J. Immunol. *109*, 1193–1200 (1972).
407. POTTER, M.: Immunoglobulin-producing tumors and myeloma proteins of mice. Physiol. Rev. *52*, 631–719 (1972).
408. MCINTYRE, K. R., PRINCLER, G. L.: Prolonged adjuvant stimulation in germfree BALB/c mice. Development of plasma cell neoplasia. Immunology *17*, 481–487 (1969).
409. SCHER, C. D., SIEGLER, R.: Direct transformation of 3T3 cells by Abelson murine leukaemia virus. Nature (Lond.) *253*, 729–731 (1975).
410. RASCHKE, W. C., RALPH, P. WATSON, J., SKLAR, M., COON, H.: Oncogenic transformation of murine lymphoid cells by in vitro infection with Abelson leukemia virus. J. nat. Cancer Inst. *54*, 1249–1253 (1975).
411. ROSENBERG, N., BALTIMORE, D., SCHER, C. D.: In vitro transformation of lymphoid cells by Abelson murine leukemia virus. Proc. nat. Acad. Sci., (Wash.) *72*, 1932–1936 (1975).
412. HAAS, W., LAYTON, J. E.: Separation of antigen-specific lymphocytes. I. Enrichment of antigen-binding cells. J. exp. Med. *141*, 1004–1014 (1975).
413. DEXTER, T. M., ALLEN, T. D., LAJTHA, L. G., SCHOFIELD, R., LORD, B. I.: Stimulation of differentiation and proliferation of haemopoietic cells in vitro. J. cell. Physiol. *82*, 461–473 (1973).
414. DEXTER, T. M., LAJTHA, L. G.: Proliferation of haemopoietic stem cells in vitro. Brit. J. Haemat. *28*, 525–530 (1974).
415. DEXTER, T. M., TESTA, N. G.: Differentiation and proliferation of haemopoietic cells in culture. In: Methods in Cell Biology 14. Prescott, D. M. (ed.). New York: Academic Press (in press).
416. FRIEDENSTEIN, A. J., CHAILAKHYAN, R. K. Lalykina, K. S.: The development of fibroblast colonies in monolayer cultures of guinea pig bone marrow and spleen cells. Cell Tiss. Kinet. *3*, 393–403 (1970).
417. FRIEDENSTEIN, A. J., CHAILAKHYAN, R. K., LATSINIK, N. V., PANASYUK, A. F., KEILISS-BOROK, I. V.: Stromal cells responsible for transferring the microenvironment of the hemopoietic tissues. Transplantation *17*, 331–340 (1974).
418. WILSON, F. D., O'GRADY, L., MCNEILL, C. J., MUNN, S. L.: The formation of bone marrow derived fibroblastic plaques in vitro: preliminary results contrasting these populations to CFU-C. Exp. Hemat. *2*, 343–354 (1974).
419. LIN, H-S, FREEMAN, P. G.: Peritoneal exudate cells. IV. Characterisation of colony forming cells. J. cell. Physiol. *90*, 407–413 (1977).
420. LIN, H-S.: Peritoneal exudate cells. II. Kinetics of appearance of colony-forming cells. J. cell. Physiol. *84*, 159–164 (1974).
421. STEWART, C. C., LIN, H-S, ADLES, C.: Proliferation and colony-forming ability of peritoneal exudate cells in liquid culture. J. exp. Med. *141*, 1114–1132 (1975).
422. LOWENBERG, B.: Fetal liver cell transplantation. M.D. Thesis, University of Rotterdam. Radiobiological Institute TNO Rijswijk (1975).
423. LAGWINSKA, E., STEWART, C. C., ADLES, C., SCHLESINGER, S.: Replication of lactic dehydrogenase virus and sindbis virus in mouse peritoneal macrophages. Induction of interferon and phenotypic mixing. Virology *65*, 204–214 (1975).
424. STEWART, C. C., ADLES, C., HIBBS, J. B.: Interaction of macrophages with tumor cells. In: The Reticuloendothelial System in Health and Disease. 1976, Vol. 73B.
425. HEIT, W., KERN, P., KUBANEK, B., HEIMPEL, H.: Some factors influencing granulocyte colony formation in vitro by human white blood cells. Blood *44*, 511–515 (1974).
426. GRANSTROM, M., GHARTON, G.: Colony-forming and colony-stimulating cells in normal human peripheral blood. Exp. Cell Res. *80*, 372–376 (1973).
427. AYE, M. T., TILL, J. E., MCCULLOCH, E. A.: Cytological studies of granulopoietic colonies from

two patients with chronic myelogenous leukemia. Exp. Hemat. *1*, 115–118 (1973).

428. Aye, M. T., Till, J. E., McCulloch, E. A.: Cytological studies of colonies in culture derived from the peripheral blood cells of two patients with acute leukemia. Exp. Hemat. *2*, 362–371 (1974).

Subject Index

Recent Results in Cancer Research

Sponsored by the Swiss League against Cancer. Editor in Chief: P. Rentchnick, Genève

For information about Vols. 1—9, please contact your bookseller or Springer-Verlag.

10 NELSON, R. S.: Radioactive Phosphorus in the Diagnosis of Gastrointestinal Cancer.
11 FREEMAN, R. G. and J. M. KNOX: Treatment of Skin Cancer.
12 LYNCH, H. T.: Hereditary Factors in Carcinoma.
13 Tumours in Children, 2nd Edition. Edited by H. B. MARSDEN and J. K. STEWARD.
14 ODARTCHENKO, N.: Production Cellulaire Erythropoïétique.
15 SOKOLOFF, B.: Carcinoid and Serotonin.
16 JACOBS, M. L.: Malignant Lymphomas and Their Management.
17 Normal and Malignant Cell Growth. Edited by R. J. M. FRY, M. L. GRIEM, and W. H. KIRSTEN (Symposium).
18 ANGLESIO, E.: The Treatment of Hodgkin's Disease.
19 BANNASCH, P.: The Cytoplasm of Hepatocytes during Carcinogenesis. Electron- and Lightmicroscopical Investigations of the Nitrosomorpholine-intoxicated Rat Liver.
20 Rubidomycin. A new Agent against Cancer. Edited by J. BERNARD, R. PAUL, M. BOIRON, C. JACQUILLAT, and R. MARAL.
21 Scientific Basis of Cancer Chemotherapy. Edited by G. MATHÉ (Symposium).
22 KOLDOVSKÝ, P.: Tumor Specific Transplantation Antigen.
23 FUCHS, W. A., J. W. DAVIDSON, and H. W. FISCHER: Lymphography in Cancer. With contributions by G. JANTET and H. RÖSLER.
24 HAYWARD, J.: Hormones und Human Breast Cancer. An Account of 15 Years Study.
25 ROY-BURMAN, P.: Analogues of Nucleic Acid Components. Mechanisms of Action.
26 Tumors of the Liver. Edited by G. T. PACK and A. H. ISLAMI.
27 SZYMENDERA, J.: Bone Mineral Metabolism in Cancer.
28 MEEK, E. S.: Antitumour and Antiviral Substances of Natural Origin.
29 Aseptic Environments and Cancer Treatment. Edited by G. MATHÉ (Symposium).
30 Advances in the Treatment of Acute (Blastic) Leukemias. Edited by G. MATHÉ (Symposium).
31 DENOIX, P.: Treatment of Malignant Breast Tumors. Indications and Results.
32 NELSON, R. S.: Endoscopy in Gastric Cancer.
33 Experimental and Clinical Effects of L-Asparaginase. Edited by E. GRUNDMANN and H. F. OETTGEN (Symposium).
34 Chemistry and Biological Actions of 4-Nitroquinolin 1-Oxide. Edited by H. ENDO, T. ONO, and T. SUGIMURA.
35 PENN, I.: Malignant Tumors in Organ Transplant Recipients.
36 Current Concepts in the Management of Lymphoma and Leukemia. Edited by J. E. ULTMANN, M. L. GRIEM, W. H. KIRSTEN, and R. W. WISSLER (Symposium).
37 CHIAPPA, S., R. MUSUMECI, and C. USLENGHI: Endolymphatic Radiotherapy in Malignant Lymphomas. With contributions by G. BONADONNA, B. DAMASCELLI, G. FAVA, F. PIZZETTI, U. VERONESI.
38 KOLLER, P. C.: The Role of Chromosomes in Cancer Biology.
39 Current Problems in the Epidemiology of Cancer and Lymphomas. Edited by E. GRUNDMANN and H. TULINIUS (Symposium).
40 LANGLEY, F. A. and A. C. CROMPTON: Epithelial Abnormalities of the Cervix Uteri.
41 Tumours in a Tropical Country. A Survey of Uganda (1964—1968). Edited by A. C. TEMPLETON.
42 Breast Cancer: A Challenging Problem. Edited by M. L. GRIEM, E. V. JENSEN, J. E. ULTMANN, and R. W. WISSLER (Symposium).
43 Nomenclature, Methodology and Results of Clinical Trials in Acute Leukemias. Edited by G. MATHÉ, P. POUILLART, L. SCHWARZENBERG (Symposium).

44 Special Topics in Carcinogenesis. Edited by E. GRUNDMANN (Symposium).
45 KOLDOVSKÝ, P.: Carcinoembryonic Antigens.
46 Diagnosis and Therapy of Malignant Lymphoma. Edited by K. MUSSHOFF (Symposium).
47 Investigation and Stimulation of Immunity in Cancer Patients. Edited by G. MATHÉ and R. WEINER (Symposium).
48 Platinum Coordination Complexes in Cancer Chemotherapy. Edited by T. A. CONNORS and J. J. ROBERTS (Symposium).
49 Complications of Cancer Chemotherapy. Edited by G. MATHÉ and R. K. OLDHAM (Symposium).
50 Cancer Registry. Edited by E. GRUNDMANN and E. PEDERSEN (Symposium).
51 Gliomas. Current Concepts in Biology, Diagnosis and Therapy. Edited by J. HEKMATPANAH (Symposium).
52 The Ambivalence of Cytostatic Therapy. Edited by E. GRUNDMANN and R. GROSS (Symposium).
53 A. CLARYSSE, Y. KENIS, and G. MATHÉ: Cancer Chemotherapy.
54 Malignant Bone Tumors. Edited by E. GRUNDMANN.
55 MATHÉ, G.: Cancer Active Immunotherapy, Immunoprophylaxis, and Immunorestoration.
56 Lymphocytes, Macrophages, and Cancer. Edited by G. MATHÉ, I. FLORENTIN, and M.-C. SIMMLER (Symposium).
57 Breast Cancer: A Multidisciplinary Approach. Edited by G. ST. ARNEAULT, P. BAND, and L. ISRAËL (Symposium).
58 B. S. SCHOENBERG: Multiple Primary Malignant Neoplasms.
59 Selective Heat Sensitivity of Cancer Cells. Edited by A. ROSSI-FANELLI, R. CAVALIERE, B. MONDOVI, and G. MORICCA.
60 Tumors of the Male Genital System. Edited by E. GRUNDMANN and W. VAHLENSIECK (Symposium).
61 D. METCALF: Hemopoietic Colonies.

Special Supplement: Biology of Amphibian Tumors. Edited by M. MIZELL.